METHODS IN PHARMACOLOGY AND TOXICOLOGY

Series Editor
Y. James Kang
University of Louisville
School of Medicine
Prospect, Kentucky, USA

For further volumes:
http://www.springer.com/series/7653

G Protein-Coupled Receptor Kinases

Edited by

Vsevolod V. Gurevich

Department of Pharmacology, Vanderbilt University, Nashville, TN, USA

Eugenia V. Gurevich

Department of Pharmacology, Vanderbilt University, Nashville, TN, USA

John J.G. Tesmer

Life Sciences Institute, University of Michigan, Ann Arbor, MI, USA

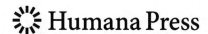 Humana Press

Editors
Vsevolod V. Gurevich
Department of Pharmacology
Vanderbilt University
Nashville, TN, USA

Eugenia V. Gurevich
Department of Pharmacology
Vanderbilt University
Nashville, TN, USA

John J.G. Tesmer
Life Sciences Institute
University of Michigan
Ann Arbor, MI, USA

ISSN 1557-2153   ISSN 1940-6053   (electronic)
Methods in Pharmacology and Toxicology
ISBN 978-1-4939-8142-7   ISBN 978-1-4939-3798-1   (eBook)
DOI 10.1007/978-1-4939-3798-1

Printed on acid-free paper

This Humana Press imprint is published by Springer Nature
The registered company is Springer Science+Business Media LLC New York

Preface

The signaling by most G protein-coupled receptors (GPCRs) is regulated by a conserved two-step mechanism: phosphorylation of active receptor by G protein-coupled receptor kinases (GRKs) followed by specific binding of an arrestin protein to the active phosphoreceptor. Arrestin binding blocks further coupling of the receptor to G proteins, promotes the recruitment of the complex to coated pits for internalization, and initiates a second, G protein-independent round of signaling. Whereas GPCRs, G proteins, and arrestins are getting a lot of attention, GRKs remain underestimated and under-investigated players in the regulation of GPCR signaling. For example, in recent years, biased GPCR signaling, i.e., differential signaling via G protein- and arrestin-dependent pathways, has been extensively investigated in the hope of designing GPCR-targeting drugs with fewer side effects. However, for a ligand to be biased toward arrestins, it must be biased toward GRKs first due to the fact that GRK phosphorylation in most cases is necessary for high-affinity arrestin binding. GRKs have numerous other functions in addition to phosphorylating GPCRs, some of which do and some do not require kinase activity. In this book, we include up-to-date descriptions of known GRK-dependent mechanisms, both associated with GPCR functions and receptor-independent. The chapters cover a wide range of studies from invertebrates to humans. Comprehensive mechanistic elucidation of GRK functions and their regulation in cells is necessary for a better understanding of cell biology, as well as for devising novel research approaches and therapeutic strategies.

Nashville, TN, USA   *Vsevolod V. Gurevich*
Nashville, TN, USA   *Eugenia V. Gurevich*
Ann Arbor, MI, USA   *John J.G. Tesmer*

Contents

Contributors

FAIZA BAAMEUR • *Division of Internal Medicine, Department of Symptom Research, The University of Texas M.D. Anderson Cancer Center, Houston, TX, USA*

SUMIT J. BANDEKAR • *Departments of Pharmacology and Biological Chemistry, University of Michigan, Ann Arbor, MI, USA; Department of Medicinal Chemistry, University of Michigan, Ann Arbor, MI, USA; Life Sciences Institute, University of Michigan, Ann Arbor, MI, USA*

TYLER S. BEYETT • *Program in Chemical Biology, University of Michigan, Ann Arbor, MI, USA; Departments of Pharmacology and Biological Chemistry, University of Michigan, Ann Arbor, MI, USA; Life Sciences Institute, University of Michigan, Ann Arbor, MI, USA*

ALESSANDRO CANNAVO • *Department of Pharmacology, Center for Translational Medicine, School of Medicine, Temple University, Philadelphia, PA, USA*

CHING-KANG JASON CHEN • *Department of Neuroscience, Baylor College of Medicine, Houston, TX, USA; Department of Ophthalmology, Baylor College of Medicine, Houston, TX, USA; Department of Biochemistry and Molecular Biology, Baylor College of Medicine, Houston, TX, USA*

MARTA CRUCES-SANDE • *Departamento de Biología Molecular and Centro de Biología Molecular Severo Ochoa (CSIC-UAM), Universidad Autónoma de Madrid, Madrid, Spain; Instituto de Investigación Sanitaria La Princesa, Madrid, Spain*

CAITRIN CRUDDEN • *Department of Oncology and Pathology, Cancer Center Karolinska, Karolinska Institutet, Karolinska University Hospital, Stockholm, Sweden*

DENISE M. FERKEY • *Department of Biological Sciences, University at Buffalo, Buffalo, NY, USA*

RAUL R. GAINETDINOV • *Institute of Translational Biomedicine, St. Petersburg State University, St. Petersburg, Russia; Skolkovo Institute of Science and Technology, Skolkovo, Moscow, Russia*

ADA GIRNITA • *Department of Oncology and Pathology, Cancer Center Karolinska, Karolinska Institutet, Karolinska University Hospital, Stockholm, Sweden*

LEONARD GIRNITA • *Department of Oncology and Pathology, Cancer Center Karolinska, Karolinska Institutet, Karolinska University Hospital, Stockholm, Sweden*

EUGENIA V. GUREVICH • *Department of Pharmacology, Vanderbilt University, Nashville, TN, USA*

VSEVOLOD V. GUREVICH • *Department of Pharmacology, Vanderbilt University, Nashville, TN, USA*

LIORA GUY-DAVID • *Department of Biomolecular Sciences, Weizmann Institute of Science, Rehovot, Israel*

COBI J. HEIJNEN • *Division of Internal Medicine, Department of Symptom Research, The University of Texas M.D. Anderson Cancer Center, Houston, TX, USA*

DAVID R. HIPFNER • *Epithelial Cell Biology Laboratory, Institut de Recherches Cliniques de Montréal (IRCM), Montréal, QC, Canada; Département de Médecine, Université de Montréal, Montréal, QC, Canada; Department of Anatomy & Cell Biology,*

McGill University, Montréal, QC, Canada; Department of Biology, McGill University, Montréal, QC, Canada

CHIH-CHUN HSU • Department of Neuroscience, Baylor College of Medicine, Houston, TX, USA

ANNEMIEKE KAVELAARS • Division of Internal Medicine, Department of Symptom Research, The University of Texas M.D. Anderson Cancer Center, Houston, TX, USA

WALTER J. KOCH • Department of Pharmacology, Center for Translational Medicine, School of Medicine, Temple University, Philadelphia, PA, USA

HONGDA LIU • Department of Pharmacology and Chemical Biology, University of Pittsburgh, Pittsburgh, PA, USA

ELISA LUCAS • Departamento de Biología Molecular and Centro de Biología Molecular Severo Ochoa (CSIC-UAM), Universidad Autónoma de Madrid, Madrid, Spain; Instituto de Investigación Sanitaria La Princesa, Madrid, Spain

CLAUDIO DE LUCIA • Department of Pharmacology, Center for Translational Medicine, School of Medicine, Temple University, Philadelphia, PA, USA

DOMINIC MAIER • Epithelial Cell Biology Laboratory, Institut de Recherches Cliniques de Montréal (IRCM), Montréal, QC, Canada

FEDERICO MAYOR JR. • Departamento de Biología Molecular and Centro de Biología Molecular Severo Ochoa (CSIC-UAM), Universidad Autónoma de Madrid, Madrid, Spain; Instituto de Investigación Sanitaria La Princesa, Madrid, Spain

CRISTINA MURGA • Departamento de Biología Molecular and Centro de Biología Molecular Severo Ochoa (CSIC-UAM), Universidad Autónoma de Madrid, Madrid, Spain; Instituto de Investigación Sanitaria La Princesa, Madrid, Spain

LAURA NOGUÉS • Departamento de Biología Molecular and Centro de Biología Molecular Severo Ochoa (CSIC-UAM), Universidad Autónoma de Madrid, Madrid, Spain; Instituto de Investigación Sanitaria La Princesa, Madrid, Spain

TIVADAR ORBAN • Department of Pharmacology, Cleveland Center for Membrane and Structural Biology, School of Medicine, Case Western Reserve University, Cleveland, OH, USA

KRZYSZTOF PALCZEWSKI • Department of Pharmacology, Cleveland Center for Membrane and Structural Biology, School of Medicine, Case Western Reserve University, Cleveland, OH, USA

PETRONILA PENELA • Departamento de Biología Molecular and Centro de Biología Molecular Severo Ochoa (CSIC-UAM), Universidad Autónoma de Madrid, Madrid, Spain; Instituto de Investigación Sanitaria La Princesa, Madrid, Spain

ADI RAVEH • Department of Biomedicine, University of Basel, Basel, Switzerland

CLARA REGLERO • Departamento de Biología Molecular and Centro de Biología Molecular Severo Ochoa (CSIC-UAM), Universidad Autónoma de Madrid, Madrid, Spain; Instituto de Investigación Sanitaria La Princesa, Madrid, Spain

EITAN REUVENY • Department of Biomolecular Sciences, Weizmann Institute of Science, Rehovot, Israel

VERÓNICA RIVAS • Departamento de Biología Molecular and Centro de Biología Molecular Severo Ochoa (CSIC-UAM), Universidad Autónoma de Madrid, Madrid, Spain; Instituto de Investigación Sanitaria La Princesa, Madrid, Spain

POOJA SINGHMAR • *Division of Internal Medicine, Department of Symptom Research, The University of Texas M.D. Anderson Cancer Center, Houston, TX, USA*

WILLIAM Z. SUO • *Laboratory for Alzheimer's Disease & Aging Research, Veterans Affairs Medical Center, Kansas City, MO, USA; Department of Neurology, University of Kansas Medical Center, Kansas City, KS, USA; Department of Molecular & Integrative Physiology, University of Kansas Medical Center, Kansas City, KS, USA; The University of Kansas Alzheimer's Disease Center, Kansas City, KS, USA*

JOHN J.G. TESMER • *Program in Chemical Biology, University of Michigan, Ann Arbor, MI, USA; Departments of Pharmacology and Biological Chemistry, University of Michigan, Ann Arbor, MI, USA; Life Sciences Institute, University of Michigan, Ann Arbor, MI, USA*

ROCÍO VILA-BEDMAR • *Departamento de Biología Molecular and Centro de Biología Molecular Severo Ochoa (CSIC-UAM), Universidad Autónoma de Madrid, Madrid, Spain; Instituto de Investigación Sanitaria La Princesa, Madrid, Spain*

JORDAN F. WOOD • *Department of Biological Sciences, University at Buffalo, Buffalo, NY, USA*

KUNHONG XIAO • *Department of Pharmacology and Chemical Biology, University of Pittsburgh, Pittsburgh, PA, USA*

Part I

Introduction

Chapter 1

G Protein-Coupled Receptor Kinases (GRKs) History: Evolution and Discovery

Vsevolod V. Gurevich and Eugenia V. Gurevich

Abstract

The discovery of rhodopsin kinase (GRK1) was a major conceptual breakthrough in visual biochemistry that was later found to be relevant to the whole GPCR field. The existence of GRKs and arrestins revealed the primary mechanism for termination of GPCR signaling. GRKs appeared in evolution long before animals, and it remains to be elucidated whether their first substrates were GPCRs or other proteins. It is also unclear whether and how GRKs are activated to phosphorylate non-receptor substrates. All mammals have far fewer GRK subtypes than GPCRs. Despite this fact, GRKs are not totally promiscuous: impressive receptor-specific phenotypes of GRK knockouts along with lack of dramatic receptor preference in vitro suggest that receptor specificity in vivo is largely determined by differential expression in various cell types, as well as subcellular localization of particular GRKs to compartments where certain GPCRs reside. Biological role of GRKs is wider than just phosphorylation of GPCRs: these kinases modify a variety of non-receptor substrates and regulate cell signaling via mechanisms that do not depend on their enzymatic activity.

Key words GPCRs, GRKs, Arrestins, Evolution, Phosphorylation, Kinase activation

1 Introduction: The Discovery of GRKs

G protein-coupled receptors (GPCRs) are the largest family of signaling proteins in animals, with >800 distinct subtypes in humans, and mediate cellular response to hormones, neurotransmitters, odorants, light, extracellular calcium, and many other stimuli [1]. Most GPCRs, as the name implies, couple to heterotrimeric G proteins, which specifically engage the active form of the receptor. Active GPCRs serve as guanyl nucleotide exchange factors for G proteins, catalyzing the release of bound GDP and its replacement with GTP [2]. GTP-liganded heterotrimeric G proteins leave the receptor and dissociate into Gα-GTP and Gβγ subunits. Active GPCRs can sequentially activate many G protein molecules [2]. G protein-mediated signaling by most GPCRs is terminated by a conserved two-step mechanism: receptor phosphorylation followed by arrestin binding [3]. The fact that this mechanism is designed

Vsevolod V. Gurevich et al. (eds.), *G Protein-Coupled Receptor Kinases*, Methods in Pharmacology and Toxicology,
DOI 10.1007/978-1-4939-3798-1_1, © Springer Science+Business Media New York 2016

for rapid regulation has led to a widely accepted belief that it must have been acquired by animals, which must be capable of quick responses [4].

1.1 GPCR Phosphorylation

GRKs as kinases that phosphorylate active GPCRs were essentially discovered twice. First, rhodopsin phosphorylation was described more than 40 years ago [5, 6]. Soon thereafter the "opsin kinase" responsible for this phenomenon (modern name GRK1) was identified [7], and the role of rhodopsin phosphorylation in rapid shut-off of its signaling was established [8]. It turned out that rhodopsin phosphorylation facilitates the binding of another protein, arrestin (called 48 kDa protein at the time) [9]. Later it was shown that arrestin binding to active phosphorylated rhodopsin, rather than phosphorylation per se, blocks further G protein activation [10].

The cloning of mammalian β2-adrenergic receptor (β2AR) [11] revealed its homology with rhodopsin, providing the first proof of the existence of a family of heptahelical rhodopsin-like receptors now called GPCRs [11]. The cloning of β2AR kinase (originally named β-adrenergic receptor kinase, or βARK; modern name GRK2) [12] showed that rhodopsin kinase also belongs to a family of related proteins. Interestingly, βARK was shown to selectively phosphorylate light-activated rhodopsin [13], similar to activation-dependent phosphorylation of β2AR [14], suggesting that GRKs have a common mechanism for recognizing the active state of different GPCRs [15]. Conserved structural rearrangement in GPCRs upon activation, including a large movement of the transmembrane helices that opens a cavity on the cytoplasmic side [16–18], is likely what GRKs use as a signal that the receptor is active.

1.2 The Discovery of Non-receptor GRK Substrates

Just when it seemed that the biological function of GRKs was clear, numerous reports documented phosphorylation by GRKs of a variety of other substrates. These include single transmembrane domain receptors, transcription factors, adapter proteins, and tubulin [19–21], the main component of the cytoskeleton, and synuclein, a protein with unclear function accumulated in Lewy bodies in the brain and implicated in neurodegeneration and dementia [22, 23]. Both α- and β-synuclein are phosphorylated by GRK2, whereas GRK5 prefers α-synuclein [22]. These paradigm-shifting discoveries suggested that the biological role of GRKs could be much wider than just enhancing the affinity of active GPCRs for arrestin (reviewed in ref. 24). Whereas the physiological role of GPCR phosphorylation by GRKs seems clear, many aspects of the biological functions of GRKs that are not associated with GPCR phosphorylation remain to be elucidated.

Another aspect of GRK activity towards non-GPCR substrates that remains obscure is the mechanism of GRK activation. So far, direct binding to active GPCRs, as established for rhodopsin kinase [25] and GRK2 [26], is the only documented mechanism of GRK activation. However, GRK activity towards tubulin [19, 20] and synuclein [22] greatly exceeds that towards peptide substrates, suggesting that physical interactions with other substrates might also activate GRKs. Lipids were shown to enhance GRK5 activity towards synuclein, and both lipids and Gβγ enhances GRK2 activity towards this substrate [22]. Thus, it is possible that membrane- or even GPCR-associated GRKs phosphorylate synuclein, but they are not activated by GPCRs, as their activity towards this substrate was detected in the absence of receptors in vitro [22]. Generally speaking, considering how diverse reported GRK substrates are, it is entirely possible that the mechanism of GRK activation might be substrate-dependent (reviewed in ref. 24).

Platelet-derived growth factor receptor-β (PDGFRβ) was the first non-GPCR cell membrane receptor reported to be phosphorylated by both GRK2 and 5 [27]. Interestingly, in this case the function of GRK phosphorylation was found to be the same as in case of GPCRs: it resulted in receptor desensitization [28, 29]. The picture is complicated by the fact that PDGFRβ phosphorylates and activates GRK2 [30], suggesting the existence of a feedback loop that has no precedent in GPCR field. Another related receptor tyrosine kinase, EGF receptor, was also shown to be GRK2 substrate, although no functional consequences of this phosphorylation could be detected [27].

Some GRK substrates reside and/or function in the nucleus. GRK5, which has an identifiable nuclear localization sequence [31], has been implicated in phosphorylation of class II histone deacetylases [32]. GRK2, which does not have a nuclear localization sequence, has been implicated in phosphorylation of transcription factors [33]. In this case, phosphorylation likely occurs in the cytoplasm, whereupon transcription factors translocate to the nucleus.

1.3 Nonenzymatic Functions of GRKs

Recent discoveries added yet another layer of complexity: GRKs regulate many branches of signaling via direct binding to other proteins, independently of their enzymatic activity. All GRKs have an RGS homology (RH) domain in their N-terminus, as first suggested by sequence analysis [34]. Only the RH domain of GRK2 and GRK3 have been shown to bind GTP-liganded Gα subunits of heterotrimeric G proteins [35]. Indeed, RH domain of GRK2 was shown to bind activated $G\alpha_q$ and inhibit G_q-mediated signaling [35, 36]. Subsequently a crystal structure of $G\alpha_q$ bound to GRK2 was solved, revealing fine molecular details of this interaction [37]. In contrast to classical RGS proteins that facilitate the GTPase activity of bound Gα, the GRK2 RH domain seems not to have significant GTPase-enhancing activity, but instead suppresses G_q-mediated signaling by sequestering active G_q [35]. The GRK2 RH domain was shown to be fairly selective for G_q, with fine discrimination even within the G_q subfamily of G protein α-subunits: it binds $G\alpha_q$, $G\alpha_{11}$, and $G\alpha_{14}$, but not $G\alpha_{16}$ [35, 38]. Mutagenesis studies identified eight residues in the GRK2 RH domain critical for $G\alpha_q$ binding, six of which are conserved in the GRK3 RH domain, but not in other members of GRK family [39]. RH-mediated inhibition of G_q-mediated signaling has been demonstrated in established cell lines [40] and in primary cells [41]. A recent study extended these findings in vivo: expression of GRK3, kinase-dead GRK3, as well as the isolated RH domain of GRK3 in the striatum of hemiparkinsonian rodents was shown to suppress the development of l-DOPA-induced dyskinesia [42], which is the most common side effect of l-DOPA therapy in Parkinson's disease. Interestingly, a GRK3 mutant defective in $G\alpha_q$ binding was ineffective [42].

GRK2 and GRK3 also have a pleckstrin homology domain in their C-termini, which binds Gβγ subunits of heterotrimeric G proteins [43, 44]. The crystal structure of GRK2 in complex with Gβγ revealed the molecular details of this interaction [45]. Originally, binding to Gβγ was believed to serve as a mechanism of the recruitment of GRK2 and GRK3 to the membrane where their substrate GPCRs reside [46–48]. Recently a different function of Gβγ binding by GRK2 was discovered: suppression of GPCR signaling by sequestration of Gβγ, similar to the effect of sequestration of $G\alpha_q$ [49]. It was shown that GRK2 binds Gβγ with high enough affinity to prevent its interaction with inwardly rectifying potassium channels, and that GRK2 reduces channel activation by GPCRs via this mechanism [49].

GRK interacting proteins (GITs) were identified during a search for GRK effectors [50]. GITs are complex multi-domain scaffolding proteins that also bind ARFs, other small GTPases, and several kinases [51]. GITs also interact with paxillin and other components of focal adhesions [51], suggesting that GRKs are recruited to these structures via GITs, and might play a role in cell adhesion and cytoskeleton remodeling. The recent finding that GRK2 promotes integrin-dependent migration of epithelial cells [52] supports this idea. Interestingly, members of the arrestin family of proteins, which were also originally discovered for their involvement in homologous GPCR desensitization, were found to play a role in cell adhesion and migration, directly regulating focal adhesion dynamics [53].

GRKs seem to play a role in many other biological processes via direct interactions with other proteins that are not their substrates (reviewed in ref. 24). Thus, GRKs cannot be viewed simply as specialized GPCR kinases that prepare these receptors for arrestin binding. Their versatility might explain why GRKs appeared fairly early in evolution, even before the emergence of multicellular organisms that evolved into Metazoa (Fig. 1).

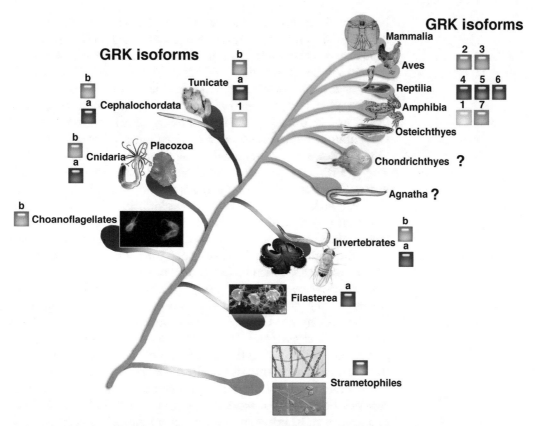

Fig. 1 Evolution of the GRK family. GRKs emerged by insertion of a kinase domain (KD), most closely related to the catalytic domain of the S6 kinase, into the loop of an ancestral RGS domain [56]. This apparently happened before the emergence of multicellularity in the branch of life that eventually gave rise to metazoans. This gene was likely duplicated early on, giving rise to the two main clades of GRKs: GRKb/2/3 and GRKa/1/4/5/6/7 (the latter is split into two lineages in vertebrates: visual GRK1/7 and non-visual GRK4/5/6). All known Metazoa retain both clades, and in vertebrates the number of GRK subtypes increased to seven. The presence of GRK isoforms in different clades is shown by respective squares. Unmistakable GRK proteins containing this RGS-KD arrangement found in the genomes of Stramenopiles (*Phytophthora infestans*, *Albugo laibachii*, *Ectocarpus siliculosus*), Filasterea (*Capsaspora owczarzaki*), Choanoflagellates (*Monosiga brevicollis*), Placozoa (*Trichoplax adhaerens*), several genomes of Cnidaria (jellyfish and sea anemones), various types of invertebrates, Cephalochordata (lancelet *Branchiostoma floridae*), Tunicate (*Ciona intestinalis*), and indicated groups of vertebrates. GRKs are likely present, although they have not yet been sequenced, in Agnatha (jawless fish) and Chondrichthyes (cartilage fish)

2 Evolution of GRKs

2.1 Evolution of the Kinase Domain (KD)

Based on sequence similarity, vertebrate GRKs are classified into three subfamilies: GRK1, comprising GRK1 (rhodopsin kinase) and GRK7 (cone opsin kinase); GRK2, comprising GRK2 and 3; and GRK4 comprising GRK4, 5, and 6. All GRKs are ~530-700 amino acid long multi-domain proteins consisting of a ~30-residue

N-terminal region specific for this family, followed by the RH domain [34], and a Ser-Thr protein kinase domain (KD) with high similarity to other AGC protein kinases, such as protein kinase A, protein kinase C, and Akt [54]. The C-termini of GRKs contain additional structural elements responsible for their membrane targeting: GRK1 and 7 carry C-terminal prenylation sequences; GRK2 and 3 contain pleckstrin homology (PH) domains that bind Gβγ subunits [44]; GRK4 and 6 carry palmitoylation sites, whereas GRK5 has positively charged lipid-binding amphipathic helix [54]. The C-terminal regions as well as the RH domains of some GRK isoforms contain regulatory phosphorylation sites [54].

Very little is known about the evolutional origin of GRKs. It has been observed that the kinase domain is the most conserved among the GRK families, whereas the RH and C-terminal domains show the highest degree of divergence [55]. The first evolutionary analysis of GRKs, which included only two nonmammalian species, *Caenorhabditis elegans* (*C. elegans*) and *Drosophila melanogaster* (*D. melanogaster*), demonstrated the split into two GRK subgroups, first comprising the GRK1/4/5/6 isoforms and second GRK2/3 isoforms. *C. elegans* and *D. melanogaster* each possessed two isoforms, one positioned in the foundation of the GRK2/3 clade and the other isoform at the root of the GRK1/4/5/6 clade [55].

A more extensive analysis that included a wider range of species was based on the sequence alignment of the KD [56]. The presence of an RH domain was obligatory for inclusion in the analysis but the RH domain itself was not used in the analysis because it was incomplete in several of the predicted proteins. The resulting Maximum-Likelihood analysis yielded two early splits that produced three statistically well-supported groups. The first split partitioned the ancestor of the GRK2/GRK3 group from the rest of the GRKs, whereas the second split separated GRK1/7 from GRK4/5/6 in vertebrates. Whenever a complete genome encodes two full-length GRKs, one of the two protein products belongs to the GRK2/3 clade and the other to the GRK(1/7)4/5/6 clade, in agreement with the earlier analysis [55]. However, in addition to vertebrates and most invertebrate species, such as cephalopod mollusks, insects, nematode *C. elegans*, chordates *Branchiostoma floridae* and *Ciona intestinalis*, Cnidaria sea anemone *Nematostella vectensis* as well as primitive metazoan Placozoa *Trichoplax adherens*, GRK-like RH+KD fusions were identified in non-metazoan species, including the opisthokont *Monosiga brevicollis*, thought to be the unicellular eukaryote closest to Metazoa [57] and another opisthokont *Capsaspora owczarzaki* (ATCC 30864), a unicellular amoeboid parasite of tropical snails, that has recently emerged as another candidate sister clade of Metazoa [58].

All sequenced genomes of invertebrates, of a cephalochordate, and of early Metazoan species (Cnidaria and Placozoa) have two GRK-like genes [55, 56], whereas the unicellular non-Metazoan organisms have only one [56]. A duplication of the ancestral GRK must have occurred before the emergence of Metazoa, to give rise to the lineage that includes GRK1/7/4/5/6 and the other to the GRK2/3 lineage. Because two unicellular opisthokont genomes appear to encode one GRK each, and these GRKs seem to belong to two different clades, it is possible that pre-GRK2/3 and pre-GRK1/7/4/5/6 emerged in the opisthokont lineage and preceded the advent of multicellularity. Following this duplication, *Monosiga brevicollis* may have lost one GRK clade and *Capsaspora owczarzaki* the other. In *C. elegans*, there are two GRK genes, one of which, called *grk-2*, encodes a product with 66% identity with human GRK3 and plays a role in chemosensation, apparently, via its RH domain [59]. In *Drosophila*, one of the two GRK isoforms, photoreceptor-enriched GRK1 (but present in all tissues), is highly similar to the mammalian GRK2 and GRK3 and has the same domain structure [60]. In the same clade are GRKs from cephalopod mollusks, which express exclusively in photoreceptors [61] and consequently have been annotated as invertebrate rhodopsin kinases, even though they belong to the GRK2/3 clade [56]. Thus, the GRK1/7 sub-clade seem to have evolved at the same time as vertebrate rhodopsins, which couple to transducin, with GRK2 clade members playing the role of rhodopsin kinase for invertebrate rhodopsins, which couple to $G\alpha_q$. But even in mammals, GRK2/3 as well as GRK5 effectively phosphorylate rhodopsin in vitro [62–64]. Interestingly, the sole known GRK-like protein in unicellular *Monosiga* is placed into the GRK2 clade on the basis of similarity in KD and the presence of a C-terminal PH domain [56].

The other clade is split into two subgroups, vertebrate-specific clade consisting of rhodopsin (GRK1) and cone opsin (GRK7) kinases, and the other clade comprising mammalian GRK4, 5, and 6 and their single-copy orthologs in lancelet and invertebrates [55, 56]. These proteins are more diverse than the members of the GRK2/3 clade. In C. elegans, this clade is represented by the grk-1 gene product and in *D. melanogaster* by a ubiquitously expressed GRK2 (referred to as Gprk2). The sole known GRK homolog from opisthokont *C. owczarzaki* is also placed into this clade [56]. The hemichordate *C. intestinalis* appears to represent an intermediate step in the evolution of the two clades. It has three GRKs, one of which is a basal member of GRK4/5/6 clade, another (GRK1) is a basal member of the "visual" branch in the same clade, and the third is the member of the GRK2/3 clade, where it mingles with the invertebrate GRK2/3 homologs. Thus, it appears that the duplication of the common GRK(1/7)/4/5/6 clade into two occurred in early chordate, since an apparently ancestral "visual" GRK is present in the urochordate *C. intestinalis* and no GRK1/7 genes are found in invertebrates. It has been proposed that vertebrates evolved through two rounds of whole-genome duplications (the "2R" hypothesis), the first occurring at the root of the vertebrate lineage and the second when jawless vertebrates brunched off [65–67]. The duplication in the GRK(1/7)/4/5/6 clade, splitting it into the GRK1/7 and GRK4/5/6 lineages, coincides with the first duplication. Further increase in the number of GRK isoforms is likely a part of the second duplication at the root of jawed vertebrates, since teleost fishes possess a full complement of GRK isoforms [56]. The analysis had been performed before fully sequenced genomes of *Leucoraja erinacea* (little skate) became available, and the genome of elephant shark (*Callorhinchus milii*) [68] was not yet fully annotated. The genome of sea lamprey (*Petromyzon marinus*) [69] is also relatively recent and has not yet been mined for GRK sequences. Cartilaginous fishes represent an oldest living group of jawed vertebrates and lampreys are representatives of an ancient vertebrate lineage, so these groups are important for understanding vertebrate evolution. Analyzing GRK sequences in these genomes will shed further light on the evolution of GRKs and GPCR signaling.

2.2 Evolution of the N-terminal Receptor-Binding Elements

The fact that GRKs have a highly conserved N-terminal extension preceding the RH domain, which was shown to be critical for the kinase phosphorylation of active GPCRs [70–72], suggests that GRKs evolved specifically as GPCR-binding kinases. In the GRK2/3 clade, multiple residues in the N-terminal sequence are highly conserved across species, including sea anemone *N. vectensis*, placozoan *T. adherens*, and non-metazoan *M. brevicollis* [56]. Furthermore, there is a significant conservation in this region across clades further stressing its key role in the receptor binding [73]. Importantly, many residues in this N-terminal region are also conserved in primitive GRKs from monocellular oomycetes *Phytophthora*, *Albugo*, and brown alga *Ectocarpus* further confirming that these are true GRKs likely to be ancestral to metazoan GRKs and to bind and phosphorylate GPCRs. Thus, it seems that this GRK-specific N-terminal extension was acquired soon after the emergence of the characteristic RH-KD arrangement, before the first gene duplication and separation of GRKs into two clades, or even was inherited from an ancestral RH domain that gave rise to it.

2.3 Evolution of the C-terminal Elements Mediating the Membrane Recruitment

GRK2/3 clade members have a C-terminal PH domain, which mediates their recruitment to the membrane via interaction with Gβγ [54]. This feature is well conserved in GRK evolution, because all proteins in the GRK2/3 clade, from opisthokont *Monosiga brevicollis* to primitive metazoans to vertebrates have a homologous PH domain [56]. The members of the GRK1/7 and GRK4/5/6 clades are characterized by specific C-terminal sequences that also ensure their localization to the plasma membrane: GRK1/7 have either farnesylation or geranylgeranylation

CAAX motifs [74, 75], whereas GRK4/5/6 possess either palmitoylation sites or lipid-binding motive such as amphipathic helix [55, 76–78]. These clade-specific membrane-targeting motives are well conserved in vertebrates and most invertebrate species and agree well with the placement by the KD sequences with the appropriate GRK clades [56]. In most invertebrates, including the early Metazoan *Trichoplax adherens* and opisthokont *Capsaspora owczarzaki*, the C-terminal motif is similar to that of GRK4 and includes palmitoylation sites as well as an easily recognizable amphipathic helix [56]. The only exception is the insect species that in the GRK4/5/6 clade evolved their own unique strictly conserved C-terminal arrangement, similar to that in the cnidarian *Nematostella vectensis* [56]. It is unclear whether such structural elements are able to mediate the attachment of these insect GRKs to the plasma membrane in a manner similar to that of the vertebrate GRK4/5/6 and other invertebrate species. Thus, the split of the ancient eukaryotic GRK into opisthokont-specific GRK2/3-like and GRK(1/7)/4/5/6-like seems to have been followed very closely by acquisition of two distinct C-terminal extensions, a PH domain in GRK in the first clade and alternative membrane-targeting sequences in the second.

2.4 The Origins of GRKs

The unusual structure of GRKs suggests that they emerged in evolution only once: in most multi-domain proteins, distinct domains are fused one after another, like beads in a necklace, whereas in case of GRKs, KD (homologous to those of AGC kinases, the group named after the protein kinase A, G, and C families (PKA, PKC, PKG)) is inserted into a loop in the RH domain [24, 34]. The KD sequence analysis demonstrated that the GRK kinase domain is most closely related to the kinases of the AGC kinase family ([79] and www.kinase.com), which are ubiquitous in unicellular eukaryotes. Thus, it is most likely that the KD region of GRKs has been produced by duplication of an AGC kinase. The provenance of the RH domain is much harder to establish because of the fast evolution of this relatively short region and the uncertain placement of the RH domain of GRKs in the phylogenetic tree of RGS proteins [80, 81], but it is notable that the RH domains are widespread in protists and were thus available for "domain tinkering".

The identification of GRK-like proteins in blight oomycete *Phytophthora infestans* and white rust oomycete *Albugo laibachii* Nc14, and brown alga *Ectocarpus siliculosus* suggested that the insertion of a kinase domain into the RH domain preceded the origin of *Metazoa* [56]. These pre-GRKs are quite similar to S6 kinase but display a recognizable N-terminal receptor-binding motif [56]. These earliest GRKs form their own clade loosely associated with the GRK2/3 subfamily on the basis of aligned KD domains. They lack recognizable lipid-binding motifs found in the GRK4/5/6 subfamily, nor do they possess a *bona fide* PH domain.

However, a C-terminal α-helix of the PH domain is discernible in GRKs from *Phytophthora infestans* and *Albugo laibachii*. Interestingly, both these GRKs also possess C-terminal geranyl-geranylation motives (CSIL and CILL, respectively) normally found in cone kinases (GRK7) that would allow for a semi-permanent association with the plasma membrane. Apparently, the single-copy GRKs of two oomycetes and brown alga represent the pre-duplication stage of GRK evolution before the split of the GRK2/3 and GRK(1/7)/4/5/6 clades. Although the genomic information that would permit connection of these early forms with pre-Metazoan and Metazoan GRKs is missing, it seems unlikely that GRKs appeared in evolution more than once. Most likely, these GRKs represent the earliest versions of GRKs with their key features already present.

2.5 Evolution of the GPCR Signaling Module and GRKs

GRKs have many substrates, but appear to be primarily specialized in phosphorylation of active seven transmembrane domain receptors [24]. Thus, it is interesting to compare the appearance of GRKs and GPCRs in evolution. Although comprehensive analysis of this issue still needs to be performed, existing evidence indicates that GRKs are a more recent and more restricted addition to the GPCR signaling pathways. Virtually every eukaryotic species has GPCRs responding an amazing variety of stimuli [1, 82–84]. As population studies show, the evolution of GPCR family continues [85]. The origin of some of the GRAFS (*G*lutamate, *R*hodopsin, *A*dhesion, *F*rizzled, *S*ecretin) GPCR families could be traced to common ancestor of Uniconts and Alveolates at the very root of eukaryote evolution [84, 86]. Whereas the relationship of prokaryotic seven transmembrane domain proteins, such as ion-pumping or sensory rhodopsins, with eukaryotic GPCRs is still debated, recent studies suggest that all these proteins might have evolved from a common ancestor [87, 88]. Thus, GPCR-like proteins seem to have emerged very early in the evolution of life.

Gα- and βγ-subunits also appeared at the root of the origin of eukaryotes [84, 89], and they are already diversified in unicellular opisthokonts [84]. RGS proteins were also found to be present in many eukaryotes in parallel with the appearance of subunits of heterotrimeric G proteins [84]. In contrast, no GRK-like kinases were found in prokaryotes and most branches of eukaryotes. GRKs were identified only in a few non-Metazoan species, such as brown algae *Ectocarpus siliculosus* and two oomycetes [56]. Thus, although GRKs apparently emerged before animals, this class was a relatively late addition to GPCR regulation machinery. The second element of the GPCR desensitization machinery acting in concert with GRKs, i.e., arrestin proteins, also seems to have appeared relatively late in evolution, and the arrestin family, similar to the GRK family, is represented by a small number of isoforms. "True" arrestins were found in unicellular opisthokonts [84, 90], whereas in earlier organisms arrestin domain-containing proteins, which share the arrestin domain fold [91], are abundant [84, 90]. Arrestin-like proteins have been identified in fungi [92, 93], but it remains unclear whether and how they relate functionally to animal arrestins.

The development of the complete GPCR desensitization system that includes both GRK-dependent receptor phosphorylation and arrestin binding to phosphorylated GPCRs may be linked with the expansion of the Rhodopsin GPCR family that also evolved from the common ancestor of Opisthokonts and enjoyed huge evolutionary success in the Metazoan lineage [83, 86, 94].

3   GRK Activation

Considering that the other two protein families that preferentially bind active GPCRs, heterotrimeric G proteins [17] and arrestins [18], both engage the inter-helical cavity that opens on the cytoplasmic side of GPCRs upon activation [16], it is likely that GRKs engage the same cavity to discriminate between active and inactive GPCRs [95, 96]. In receptor-bound G protein [17] and arrestin [18] the element interacting with this cavity is fully or partially disordered or has a different secondary structure in the inactive, unbound state, but likely forms an α-helix upon receptor binding [18, 97, 98]. The extreme N-terminal twenty amino acids of GRKs are not usually visible in crystal structures, but in the most active-like structure of GRK6 [72] this element becomes helical and interacts with both lobes of the kinase domain. This suggests that GPCR binding promotes GRK activity by helping to align catalytic residues contributed by the two lobes [71, 72] — a model consistent with the observation that binding to activated GPCRs directly activates GRKs, such that receptors serve as both substrates and allosteric activators [25, 26].

The role of GRKs in GPCR signaling is closely linked to the role of arrestins, which selectively bind active phosphorylated receptors [99], although the contribution to high-affinity arrestin binding of active conformation and receptor-attached phosphates varies in different GPCR subtypes [100]. It is arrestin bound to the phosphorylated receptor, rather than GRK-attached phosphates, that blocks further receptor coupling to cognate G proteins [101, 102]. Interestingly, arrestins apparently use the same cavity on the cytoplasmic side of GPCRs that opens upon receptor activation to identify active receptor molecules [18]. A loosely structured loop in the central crest of the receptor-binding side of all arrestin subtypes [103–106], called the "finger loop" [107], inserts itself into this cavity [18], likely also assuming helical conformation [18, 97, 98]. Both the formation of the helix in the finger loop, along with the flexibility of the long "legs" connecting this helix with the rest of the arrestin molecule, appear to be critical for receptor binding [108].

This mechanism differentiates GRKs from kinases that phosphorylate accessible residues (Ser, Thr, Tyr) in a particular sequence context and are not sensitive to the functional state of their substrate. Phosphorylation by GRKs of Ser and Thr residues is not strongly sequence context-specific, which matches the context-independent recognition of receptor-attached phosphates by arrestins [109]. Context-independence of the function of GRKs and arrestins helps to explain how few members of these two protein families can "serve" hundreds of GPCR subtypes. GRK activation by binding to an active GPCR ensures that GRKs phosphorylate nearby proteins with accessible loops, i.e., with highest probability the intracellular loops and tails of the receptor molecules they bind to. However, receptor-activated GRKs can more efficiently phosphorylate other substrates, such as exogenous peptides [25] and nearby inactive receptors [110]. The latter phenomenon is best observed in the visual system, where rhodopsin molecules are closely packed in the rod disk membrane, covering about half of its surface. In this case, activation of a single rhodopsin can result in phosphorylation of hundreds of inactive rhodopsin molecules ("high-gain phosphorylation") [110, 111], which is likely the consequence of rapidly diffusing GRK1-rhodopsin complexes [54, 112, 113].

For some time, selective phosphorylation of active GPCRs was believed to be the only function of GRKs. However, the identification of non-receptor substrates, such as tubulin [19, 20] or synuclein [22], as well as many non-GPCR receptors (reviewed in ref. 24), all of which are phosphorylated more efficiently than peptides derived from cognate GPCRs, suggested that there might be alternative mechanisms of GRK activation, which remain to be elucidated. It could be that any physicochemical environment that resembles that of the pockets found on activated GPCRs can favor GRK activation. One precedent for this is arrestin-3: its IP_6-induced trimerization induces its transition into an active (similar to receptor-bound) conformation, where the three finger loops of sister protomers create for each other an environment favoring α-helix formation [108]. In their inactive states, the two lobes of an AGC kinase domain are not perfectly aligned for phosphotransfer [114]. In most cases, phosphorylation of their so-called activation loops and the binding of ATP improve the alignment of the two lobes and enhances activity. In contrast, ATP or its analogs are not sufficient to force the GRK kinase domain into active conformation, nor is its activation loop subject to transphosphorylation [115, 116]. Interestingly, GRK5 [117, 118] and GRK6 [72, 73], both belonging to the GRK4 clade [56], crystallize in the presence of ATP and its analogs in a more "closed" (active-like) conformation [72], in contrast to GRK2, which belongs to GRK2/3 subfamily. Thus far, GRK6 is the only member of the family that has been crystallized in a conformation that approaches what is expected to be an active configuration, but this may be due to a unique crystal packing environment [72].

Importantly, the structural differences between the two GRK sub-families correlate with function. Significant activation-independent phosphorylation of several GPCRs in vitro and in cells was reported for GRK4 [119, 120], GRK5 [62, 121], and GRK6 [62], whereas GRK2 and GRK3 phosphorylate GPCRs in strictly activation-dependent manner [13, 14, 26, 62]. However, in some cases, such as the D_1 dopamine receptor, GRKs of both clades phosphorylate only the active form [62]. Considering that primates and bats have only ~800 GPCR subtypes, whereas most mammals have a lot more (>3400 in elephants; http://sevens.cbrc.jp/) distinct GPCRs [112, 113], these studies, which have thus far been performed on a limited number of receptors, should be expanded before general conclusions can be made.

4 Subcellular Localization and Receptor Specificity of GRKs

Whereas the typical RGS-kinase domain arrangement is shared by the whole GRK family, their C-terminal elements are quite different, mediating distinct means of membrane localization [24]. GRK2/3 are recruited to the membrane via the interaction of the pleckstrin homology domain in the C-terminus with G$\beta\gamma$ dimers [46, 47]. This makes sense biologically: G$\beta\gamma$ dimers are released upon the activation of heterotrimeric G proteins by GPCRs, and that seems to establish perfect timing, with GRKs recruited from the cytoplasm after the activation of cognate G proteins. However, both visual kinases, GRK1 ("opsin kinase") [74] and GRK7 [75], which are primarily expressed in rods and cones, have prenylation signatures at their C-termini and tend to be membrane-localized due to lipid modifications (although there is an equilibrium between soluble and membrane forms in both cases). The remaining GRKs have various types of membrane anchors. The C-termini of GRK4 and GRK6 are palmitoylated [78, 122, 123], whereas both GRK5 and GRK6 have lipid-binding amphipathic helices in their C-termini [122, 124]. A PIP_2 specific binding site is also observed near the N-terminus of the GRK4/5/6 clade. Subcellular localization of GRKs has primarily been studied in cultured HEK293 cells, with very few reports in the context of neurons which express much higher levels of GRKs [125]. Available data suggest that neurons employ additional mechanisms of sub-cellular localization of GRK subtypes. For example, GRK2 and GRK3 behave similarly in HEK293 cells, in that they are mostly cytoplasmic, whereas in the brain GRK3 is much more membrane-localized than GRK2 [126, 127]. Interestingly, GRK5 and GRK6 in the brain mostly localize to synaptic membranes [126, 128, 129], suggesting that there must be neuron-specific protein partners in the synapses that recruit these kinases. It is possible that specific localization of different GRK isoforms to particular compartments determines their receptor specificity, which seems to be much more pronounced in living animals [130, 131] than in cultured cells [62], and is virtually undetectable in vitro [132, 133].

Thus, despite tremendous progress in the last 20 years, there are many critical questions regarding the biological functions of GRKs in vivo that still need to be answered.

References

1. Bockaert J, Pin JP (1999) Molecular tinkering of G protein-coupled receptors: an evolutionary success. EMBO J 18:1723–1729
2. Dessauer CW, Posner BA, Gilman AG (1996) Visualizing signal transduction: receptors, G-proteins, and adenylate cyclases. Clin Sci (Lond) 91(5):527–537
3. Carman CV, Benovic JL (1998) G-protein-coupled receptors: turn-ons and turn-offs. Curr Opin Neurobiol 8:335–344
4. Gurevich EV, Gurevich VV (2006) Arrestins: ubiquitous regulators of cellular signaling pathways. Genome Biol 7(9):236
5. Bownds D, Dawes J, Miller J, Stahlman M (1972) Phosphorylation of frog photoreceptor membranes induced by light. Nature 237:125–127
6. Kühn H, Dreyer WJ (1972) Light dependent phosphorylation of rhodopsin by ATP. FEBS Lett 20:1–6
7. Weller M, Virmaux N, Mandel P (1975) Light-stimulated phosphorylation of rhodopsin in the retina: the presence of a protein kinase that is specific for photobleached rhodopsin. Proc Natl Acad Sci U S A 72:381–385
8. Liebman PA, Pugh ENJ (1980) ATP mediates rapid reversal of cyclic GMP phosphodiesterase activation in visual receptor membranes. Nature 287:734–736
9. Kuhn H, Hall SW, Wilden U (1984) Light-induced binding of 48-kDa protein to photoreceptor membranes is highly enhanced by phosphorylation of rhodopsin. FEBS Lett 176:473–478
10. Wilden U, Hall SW, Kühn H (1986) Phosphodiesterase activation by photoexcited rhodopsin is quenched when rhodopsin is phosphorylated and binds the intrinsic 48-kDa protein of rod outer segments. Proc Natl Acad Sci U S A 83:1174–1178
11. Dixon RA, Kobilka BK, Strader DJ, Benovic JL, Dohlman HG, Frielle T, Bolanowski MA, Bennett CD, Rands E, Diehl RE, Mumford RA, Slater EE, Sigal IS, Caron MG, Lefkowitz RJ, Strader CD (1986) Cloning of the gene and cDNA for mammalian beta-adrenergic receptor and homology with rhodopsin. Nature 321:75–79
12. Benovic JL, DeBlasi A, Stone WC, Caron MG, Lefkowitz RJ (1989) Beta-adrenergic receptor kinase: primary structure delineates a multigene family. Science 246:235–240
13. Benovic JL, Mayor FJ, Somers RL, Caron MG, Lefkowitz RJ (1986) Light-dependent phosphorylation of rhodopsin by beta-adrenergic receptor kinase. Nature 321:869–872
14. Benovic JL, Strasser RH, Caron MG, Lefkowitz RJ (1986) Beta-adrenergic receptor kinase: identification of a novel protein kinase that phosphorylates the agonist-occupied form of the receptor. Proc Natl Acad Sci U S A 83:2797–2801
15. Palczewski K (1997) GTP-binding-protein-coupled receptor kinases – two mechanistic models. Eur J Biochem 248:261–269
16. Farrens DL, Altenbach C, Yang K, Hubbell WL, Khorana HG (1996) Requirement of rigid-body motion of transmembrane helices for light activation of rhodopsin. Science 274:768–770
17. Rasmussen SG, DeVree BT, Zou Y, Kruse AC, Chung KY, Kobilka TS, Thian FS, Chae PS, Pardon E, Calinski D, Mathiesen JM, Shah ST, Lyons JA, Caffrey M, Gellman SH, Steyaert J, Skiniotis G, Weis WI, Sunahara RK, Kobilka BK (2011) Crystal structure of the β2 adrenergic receptor-Gs protein complex. Nature 477:549–555
18. Kang Y, Zhou XE, Gao X, He Y, Liu W, Ishchenko A, Barty A, White TA, Yefanov O, Han GW, Xu Q, de Waal PW, Ke J, Tan MHE, Zhang C, Moeller A, West GM, Van Eps N, Caro LN, Vishnivetskiy SA, Lee RJ, Suino-Powell KM, Gu X, Pal K, Ma J, Zhi X, Boutet

S, Williams GJ, Messerschmidt M, Gati C, Zatsepin NA, Wang D, James D, Basu S, Roy-Chowdhuty S, Conrad S, Coe J, Liu H, Lisova S, Kupitz C, Grotjohann I, Fromme R, Jiang Y, Tan M, Yang H, Li J, Wang M, Zheng Z, Li D, Zhao Y, Standfuss J, Diederichs K, Dong Y, Potter CS, Carragher B, Caffrey M, Jiang H, Chapman HN, Spence JCH, Fromme P, Weierstall U, Ernst OP, Katritch V, Gurevich VV, Griffin PR, Hubbell WL, Stevens RC, Cherezov V, Melcher K, Xu HE (2015) Crystal structure of rhodopsin bound to arrestin determined by femtosecond X-ray laser. Nature 523:561–567.

19. Carman CV, Som T, Kim CM, Benovic JL (1998) Binding and phosphorylation of tubulin by G protein-coupled receptor kinases. J Biol Chem 273:20308–20316

20. Pitcher JA, Hall RA, Daaka Y, Zhang J, Ferguson SS, Hester S, Miller S, Caron MG, Lefkowitz RJ, Barak LS (1998) The G protein-coupled receptor kinase 2 is a microtubule-associated protein kinase that phosphorylates tubulin. J Biol Chem 273:12316–12324

21. Haga K, Ogawa H, Haga T, Murofushi H (1998) GTP-binding-protein-coupled receptor kinase 2 (GRK2) binds and phosphorylates tubulin. Eur J Biochem 255:363–368

22. Pronin AN, Morris AJ, Surguchov A, Benovic JL (2000) Synucleins are a novel class of substrates for G protein-coupled receptor kinases. J Biol Chem 275:26515–26522

23. Sakamoto M, Arawaka S, Hara S, Sato H, Cui C, Machiya Y, Koyama S, Wada M, Kawanami T, Kurita K, Kato T (2009) Contribution of endogenous G-protein-coupled receptor kinases to Ser129 phosphorylation of alpha-synuclein in HEK293 cells. Biochem Biophys Res Commun 384:378–382

24. Gurevich EV, Tesmer JJ, Mushegian A, Gurevich VV (2012) G protein-coupled receptor kinases: more than just kinases and not only for GPCRs. Pharmacol Ther 133:40–69

25. Palczewski K, Buczylko J, Kaplan MW, Polans AS, Crabb JW (1991) Mechanism of rhodopsin kinase activation. J Biol Chem 266:12949–12955

26. Chen CY, Dion SB, Kim CM, Benovic JL (1993) Beta-adrenergic receptor kinase. Agonist-dependent receptor binding promotes kinase activation. J Biol Chem 268:7825–7831

27. Freedman NJ, Kim LK, Murray JP, Exum ST, Brian L, Wu L-H, Peppel K (2002) Phosphorylation of the platelet-derived growth factor receptor-β and epidermal growth factor receptor by G protein-coupled receptor kinase-2: mechanisms for selectivity of desensitization. J Biol Chem 277:48261–48269

28. Wu J-H, Goswami R, Cai X, Exum ST, Huang X, Zhang L, Brian L, Premont RT, Peppel K, Freedman NJ (2006) Regulation of the platelet-derived growth factor receptor-β by G protein-coupled receptor kinase-5 in vascular smooth muscle cells involves the phosphatase Shp2*. J Biol Chem 281:37758–37772

29. Hildreth KL, Wu L-H, Barak LS, Exum ST, Kim LK, Peppel K, Freedman NJ (2004) Phosphorylation of the platelet-derived growth factor receptor-β by G protein-coupled receptor kinase-2 reduces receptor signaling and interaction with the Na+/H+ exchanger regulatory factor. J Biol Chem 279:41775–41782

30. Wu J-H, Goswami R, Kim LK, Miller WE, Peppel K, Freedman NJ (2005) The platelet-derived growth factor receptor-β phosphorylates and activates G protein-coupled receptor kinase-2: a mechanisms for feedback inhibition. J Biol Chem 280:31027–31035

31. Johnson LR, Scott MG, Pitcher JA (2004) G protein-coupled receptor kinase 5 contains a DNA-binding nuclear localization sequence. Mol Cell Biol 24:10169–10179

32. Martini JS, Raake P, Vinge LE, DeGeorge BRJ, Chuprun JK, Harris DM, Gao E, Eckhart AD, Pitcher JA, Koch WJ (2008) Uncovering G protein-coupled receptor kinase-5 as a histone deacetylase kinase in the nucleus of cardiomyocytes. Proc Natl Acad Sci U S A 105:12457–12462

33. Ho J, Cocolakis E, Dumas VM, Posner BI, Laporte SA, Lebrun J-J (2005) The G protein-coupled receptor kinase-2 is a TGFβ-inducible antagonist of TGFβ signal transduction. EMBO J 24:3247–3258

34. Siderovski DP, Hessel A, Chung S, Mak TW, Tyers M (1996) A new family of regulators of G-protein-coupled receptors? Curr Biol 6:211–212

35. Carman CV, Parent JL, Day PW, Pronin AN, Sternweis PM, Wedegaertner PB, Gilman AG, Benovic JL, Kozasa T (1999) Selective regulation of Galpha(q/11) by an RGS domain in the G protein-coupled receptor kinase, GRK2. J Biol Chem 274:34483–34492

36. Usui H, Nishiyama M, Moroi K, Shibasaki T, Zhou J, Ishida J, Fukamizu A, Haga T, Sekiya S, Kimura S (2000) RGS domain in the amino-terminus of G protein-coupled receptor kinase 2 inhibits Gq-mediated signaling. Int J Mol Med 5(4):335–340

37. Tesmer VM, Kawano T, Shankaranarayanan A, Kozasa T, Tesmer JJ (2005) Snapshot of activated G proteins at the membrane: the Galphaq-GRK2-Gbetagamma complex. Science 310:1686–1690

38. Day PW, Carman CV, Sterne-Marr R, Benovic JL, Wedegaertner PB (2003) Differential interaction of GRK2 with members of the G alpha q family. Biochemistry 42:9176–9184

39. Sterne-Marr R, Tesmer JJ, Day PW, Stracquatanio RP, Cilente JA, O'Connor KE, Pronin AN, Benovic JL, Wedegaertner PB (2003) G protein-coupled receptor Kinase 2/G alpha q/11 interaction. A novel surface on a regulator of G protein signaling homology domain for binding G alpha subunits. J Biol Chem 278:6050–6058

40. Luo J, Busillo JM, Benovic JL (2008) M3 muscarinic acetylcholine receptor-mediated signaling is regulated by distinct mechanisms. Mol Pharmacol 74:338–347

41. Willets JM, Nash MS, Challiss RA, Nahorski SR (2004) Imaging of muscarinic acetylcholine receptor signaling in hippocampal neurons: evidence for phosphorylation-dependent and -independent regulation by G-protein-coupled receptor kinases. J Neurosci 24:4157–4162

42. Ahmed MR, Bychkov E, Li L, Gurevich VV, Gurevich EV (2015) GRK3 suppresses l-DOPA-induced dyskinesia in the rat model of Parkinson's disease via its RGS homology domain. Sci Rep 5:10920

43. Koch WJ, Inglese J, Stone WC, Lefkowitz RJ (1993) The binding site for the beta gamma subunits of heterotrimeric G proteins on the beta-adrenergic receptor kinase. J Biol Chem 268:8256–8260

44. Touhara K, Inglese J, Pitcher JA, Shaw G, Lefkowitz RJ (1994) Binding of G protein beta gamma-subunits to pleckstrin homology domains. J Biol Chem 269:10217–10220

45. Lodowski DT, Pitcher JA, Capel WD, Lefkowitz RJ, Tesmer JJ (2003) Keeping G proteins at bay: a complex between G protein-coupled receptor kinase 2 and Gbetagamma. Science 300:1256–1262

46. Haga K, Haga T (1992) Activation by G protein beta gamma subunits of agonist- or light-dependent phosphorylation of muscarinic acetylcholine receptors and rhodopsin. J Biol Chem 267:2222–2227

47. Pitcher JA, Inglese J, Higgins JB, Arriza JL, Casey PJ, Kim C, Benovic JL, Kwatra MM, Caron MG, Lefkowitz RJ (1992) Role of beta gamma subunits of G proteins in targeting the beta-adrenergic receptor kinase to membrane-bound receptors. Science 257:1264–1267

48. Li J, Xiang B, Su W, Zhang X, Huang Y, Ma L (2003) Agonist-induced formation of opioid receptor-G protein-coupled receptor kinase (GRK)-G beta gamma complex on membrane is required for GRK2 function in vivo. J Biol Chem 278:30219–30226

49. Raveh A, Cooper A, Guy-David L, Reuveny E (2010) Nonenzymatic rapid control of GIRK channel function by a G protein-coupled receptor kinase. Cell 143:750–760

50. Premont RT, Claing A, Vitale N, Freeman JLR, Pitcher JA, Patton WA, Moss J, Vaughan M, Lefkowitz RJ (1998) β2-Adrenergic receptor regulation by GIT1, a G protein-coupled receptor kinase-associated ADP ribosylation factor GTPase-activating protein. Proc Natl Acad Sci U S A 95:14082–14087

51. Hoefen RJ, Berk BC (2006) The multifunctional GIT family of proteins. J Cell Sci 119:1469–1475

52. Penela P, Ribas C, Aymerich I, Eijkelkamp N, Barreiro O, Heijnen CJ, Kavelaars A, Sánchez-Madrid F, Mayor FJ (2008) G protein-coupled receptor kinase 2 positively regulates epithelial cell migration. EMBO J 27:1206–1218

53. Cleghorn WM, Branch KM, Kook S, Arnette C, Bulus N, Zent R, Kaverina I, Gurevich EV, Weaver AM, Gurevich VV (2015) Arrestins regulate cell spreading and motility via focal adhesion dynamics. Mol Biol Cell 26(4):622–635

54. Gurevich VV, Hanson SM, Song X, Vishnivetskiy SA, Gurevich EV (2011) The functional cycle of visual arrestins in photoreceptor cells. Prog Retin Eye Res 30:405–430

55. Premont RT, Macrae AD, Aparicio SA, Kendall HE, Welch JE, Lefkowitz RJ (1999) The GRK4 subfamily of G protein-coupled receptor kinases. Alternative splicing, gene organization, and sequence conservation. J Biol Chem 274(41):29381–29389

56. Mushegian A, Gurevich VV, Gurevich EV (2012) The origin and evolution of G protein-coupled receptor kinases. PLoS One 7(3):e33806

57. King N, Westbrook MJ, Young SL, Kuo A, Abedin M, Chapman J, Fairclough S, Hellsten U, Isogai Y, Letunic I, Marr M, Pincus D, Putnam N, Rokas A, Wright KJ, Zuzow R, Dirks W, Good M, Goodstein D, Lemons D, Li W, Lyons JB, Morris A, Nichols S, Richter DJ, Salamov A, Sequencing JG, Bork P, Lim WA, Manning G, Miller WT, McGinnis W, Shapiro H, Tjian R, Grigoriev IV, Rokhsar D (2008) The genome of the choanoflagellate Monosiga brevicollis and the origin of metazoans. Nature 451:783–788

58. Ruiz-Trillo I, Lane CE, Archibald JM, Roger AJ (2006) Insights into the evolutionary origin and genome architecture of the unicellular opisthokonts Capsaspora owczarzaki and Sphaeroforma arctica. J Eukaryot Microbiol 53(5):379–384

59. Fukuto HS, Ferkey DM, Apicella AJ, Lans H, Sharmeen T, Chen W, Lefkowitz RJ, Jansen

G, Schafer WR, Hart AC (2004) G protein-coupled receptor kinase function is essential for chemosensation in C. elegans. Neuron 42:581–593

60. Cassill JA, Whitney M, Joazeiro CAP, Becker A, Zuker CS (1991) Isolation of Drosophila genes encoding G protein-coupled receptor kinases. Proc Natl Acad Sci U S A 88:11067–11070

61. Kikkawa S, Yoshida N, Nakagawa M, Iwasa T, Tsuda M (1998) A novel rhodopsin kinase in octopus photoreceptor possesses a pleckstrin homology domain and is activated by G protein betagamma-subunits. J Biol Chem 273:7441–7447

62. Li L, Homan KT, Vishnivetskiy SA, Manglik A, Tesmer JJ, Gurevich VV, Gurevich EV (2015) G protein-coupled receptor kinases of the GRK4 protein subfamily phosphorylate inactive G Protein-coupled Receptors (GPCRs). J Biol Chem 290(17):10775–10790

63. Benovic JL, Onorato JJ, Arriza JL, Stone WC, Lohse M, Jenkins NA, Gilbert DJ, Copeland NG, Caron MG, Lefkowitz RJ (1991) Cloning, expression, and chromosomal localization of beta-adrenergic receptor kinase 2. A new member of the receptor kinase family. J Biol Chem 266:14939–14946

64. Kunapuli P, Benovic JL (1993) Cloning and expression of GRK5: a member of the G protein-coupled receptor kinase family. Proc Natl Acad Sci U S A 90:5588–5592

65. Holland PWH, Garcia-Fernandez J, Williams NA, Sidow A (1994) Gene duplications and the origins of vertebrate development. Development 120:125–133

66. Furlong RF, Holland PW (2004) Polyploidy in vertebrate ancestry: Ohno and beyond. Biol J Linnean Soc 82:425–430

67. Donoghue PCJ, Purnell MA (2005) Genome duplication, extinction and vertebrate evolution. Trends Ecol Evol 20:312–319

68. Venkatesh B, Kirkness EF, Loh Y-H, Halpern AL, Lee AP, Johnson J, Dandona N, Viswanathan LD, Tay A, Venter JC, Strausberg RL, Brenner S (2007) Survey sequencing and comparative analysis of the elephant shark (Callorhinchus milii) genome. PLoS Biol 5(4):e101

69. Smith JJ, Kuraku S, Holt C, Sauka-Spengler T, Jiang N, Campbell MS, Yandell MD, Manousaki T, Meyer A, Bloom OE, Morgan JR, Buxbaum JD, Sachidanandam R, Sims C, Garruss AS, Cook M, Krumlauf R, Wiedemann LM, Sower SA, Decatur WA, Hall JA, Amemiya CT, Saha NR, Buckley KM, Rast JP, Das S, Hirano M, McCurley N, Guo P, Rohner N, Tabin CJ, Piccinelli P, Elgar G, Ruffier M, Aken BL, Searle SMJ, Muffato M, Pignatelli M, Herrero J, Jones M, Brown CT, Chung-Davidson Y-W, Nanlohy KG, Libants SV, Yeh C-Y, McCauley DW, Langeland JA, Pancer Z, Fritzsch B, de Jong PJ, Zhu B, Fulton LL, Theising B, Flicek P, Bronner ME, Warren WC, Clifton SW, Wilson RK, Li W (2013) Sequencing of the sea lamprey (Petromyzon marinus) genome provides insights into vertebrate evolution. Nat Genet 45(4):415–421

70. Pao CS, Barker BL, Benovic JL (2009) Role of the amino terminus of G protein-coupled receptor kinase 2 in receptor phosphorylation. Biochemistry 48:7325–7333

71. Huang CC, Orban T, Jastrzebska B, Palczewski K, Tesmer JJ (2011) Activation of G protein-coupled receptor kinase 1 involves interactions between its N-terminal region and its kinase domain. Biochemistry 50(11):1940–1949

72. Boguth CA, Singh P, Huang CC, Tesmer JJ (2010) Molecular basis for activation of G protein-coupled receptor kinases. EMBO J 29:3249–3259

73. Lodowski DT, Tesmer VM, Benovic JL, Tesmer JJ (2006) The structure of G protein-coupled receptor kinase (GRK)-6 defines a second lineage of GRKs. J Biol Chem 281:16785–16793

74. Inglese J, Glickman JF, Lorenz W, Caron MG, Lefkowitz RJ (1992) Isoprenylation of a protein kinase. Requirement of farnesylation/alpha-carboxyl methylation for full enzymatic activity of rhodopsin kinase. J Biol Chem 267(3):1422–1425

75. Hisatomi O, Matsuda S, Satoh T, Kotaka S, Imanishi Y, Tokunaga F (1998) A novel subtype of G-protein-coupled receptor kinase, GRK7, in teleost cone photoreceptors. FEBS Lett 424:159–164

76. Jiang X, Benovic JL, Wedegaertner PB (2007) Plasma membrane and nuclear localization of G protein coupled receptor kinase 6A. Mol Biol Cell 18:2960–2969

77. Thiyagarajan MM, Stracquatanio RP, Pronin AN, Evanko DS, Benovic JL, Wedegaertner PB (2004) A predicted amphipathic helix mediates plasma membrane localization of GRK5. J Biol Chem 279:17989–17995

78. Premont RT, Macrae AD, Stoffel RH, Chung N, Pitcher JA, Ambrose C, Inglese J, MacDonald ME, Lefkowitz RJ (1996) Characterization of the G protein-coupled receptor kinase GRK4. Identification of four splice variants. J Biol Chem 271:6403–6410

79. Manning G, Plowman GD, Hunter T, Sudarsanam S (2002) Evolution of protein kinase signaling from yeast to man. Trends Biochem Sci 27:514–520

80. Wilkie TM, Kinch L (2005) New roles for Galpha and RGS proteins: communication

continues despite pulling sisters apart. Curr Biol 15:R843–R854

81. Kimple AJ, Bosch DE, Giguère PM, Siderovski DP (2011) Regulators of G-protein signaling and their Gα substrates: promises and challenges in their use as drug discovery targets. Pharmacol Rev 63(3):728–749

82. Rompler H, Staubert C, Thor D, Schulz A, Hofreiter M, Schoneberg T (2007) G protein-coupled time travel: evolutionary aspects of GPCR research. Mol Interv 7:17–25

83. Fredriksson R, Schiöth HB (2005) The repertoire of G-protein-coupled receptors in fully sequenced genomes. Mol Pharmacol 67:1414–1425

84. de Mendoza A, Sebé-Pedrós A, Ruiz-Trillo I (2014) The evolution of the GPCR signaling system in eukaryotes: modularity, conservation, and the transition to metazoan multicellularity. Genome Biol Evol 6(3):606–619

85. Strotmann R, Schröck K, Böselt I, Stäubert C, Russ A, Schöneberg T (2011) Evolution of GPCR: change and continuity. Mol Cell Endocrinol 331(2):170–178

86. Krishnan A, Almén MS, Fredriksson R, Schiöth HB (2012) The origin of GPCRs: identification of mammalian like rhodopsin, adhesion, glutamate and frizzled GPCRs in fungi. PLoS One 7(e29817)

87. Mackin KA, Roy RA, Theobald DL (2014) An empirical test of convergent evolution in rhodopsins. Mol Biol Evol 31(1):85–95

88. Shalaeva DN, Galperin MY, Mulkidjanian AY (2015) Eukaryotic G protein-coupled receptors as descendants of prokaryotic sodium-translocating rhodopsins. Biol Direct 10:63

89. Anantharaman V, Abhiman S, de Souza RF, Aravind L (2011) Comparative genomics uncovers novel structural and functional features of the heterotrimeric GTPase signaling system. Gene 475(2):63–78

90. Alvarez CE (2008) On the origins of arrestin and rhodopsin. BMC Evol Biol 8:222–222

91. Shi H, Rojas R, Bonifacino JS, Hurley JH (2006) The retromer subunit Vps26 has an arrestin fold and binds Vps35 through its C-terminal domain. Nat Struct Mol Biol 13(6):540–548

92. Boase NA, Kelly JM (2004) A role for creD, a carbon catabolite repression gene from Aspergillus nidulans, in ubiquitination. Mol Microbiol 53(3):929–940

93. Herranz S, Rodríguez JM, Bussink H-J, Sánchez-Ferrero JC, Arst HN, Peñalva MA, Vincent O (2005) Arrestin-related proteins mediate pH signaling in fungi. Proc Natl Acad Sci U S A 102(34):12141–12146

94. Nordström KJ, Sällman Almén M, Edstam MM, Fredriksson R, Schiöth HB (2011) Independent HHsearch, Needleman-Wunsch-based, and motif analyses reveal the overall hierarchy for most of the G protein-coupled receptor families. Mol Biol Evol 28:2471–2480

95. Homan KT, Tesmer JJ (2014) Structural insights into G protein-coupled receptor kinase function. Curr Opin Cell Biol 27:25–31

96. Huang CC, Tesmer JJ (2011) Recognition in the face of diversity: interactions of heterotrimeric G proteins and G protein-coupled receptor (GPCR) kinases with activated GPCRs. J Biol Chem 286:7715–7721

97. Feuerstein SE, Pulvermüller A, Hartmann R, Granzin J, Stoldt M, Henklein P, Ernst OP, Heck M, Willbold D, Koenig BW (2009) Helix formation in arrestin accompanies recognition of photoactivated rhodopsin. Biochemistry 48(45):10733–10742

98. Szczepek M, Beyriere F, Hofmann KP, Elgeti M, Kazmin R, Rose A, Bartl FJ, von Stetten D, Heck M, Sommer ME, Hildebrand PW, Scheerer P (2014) Crystal structure of a common GPCR-binding interface for G protein and arrestin. Nat Commun 5:4801

99. Gurevich VV, Gurevich EV (2004) The molecular acrobatics of arrestin activation. Trends Pharmacol Sci 25:105–111

100. Gimenez LE, Kook S, Vishnivetskiy SA, Ahmed MR, Gurevich EV, Gurevich VV (2012) Role of receptor-attached phosphates in binding of visual and non-visual arrestins to G protein-coupled receptors. J Biol Chem 287(12):9028–9040

101. Lohse MJ, Andexinger S, Pitcher J, Trukawinski S, Codina J, Faure JP, Caron MG, Lefkowitz RJ (1992) Receptor-specific desensitization with purified proteins. Kinase dependence and receptor specificity of beta-arrestin and arrestin in the beta 2-adrenergic receptor and rhodopsin systems. J Biol Chem 267:8558–8564

102. Lohse MJ, Benovic JL, Codina J, Caron MG, Lefkowitz RJ (1990) beta-Arrestin: a protein that regulates beta-adrenergic receptor function. Science 248:1547–1550

103. Hirsch JA, Schubert C, Gurevich VV, Sigler PB (1999) The 2.8 A crystal structure of visual arrestin: a model for arrestin's regulation. Cell 97(2):257–269

104. Han M, Gurevich VV, Vishnivetskiy SA, Sigler PB, Schubert C (2001) Crystal structure of beta-arrestin at 1.9 A: possible mechanism of receptor binding and membrane translocation. Structure 9(9):869–880

105. Sutton RB, Vishnivetskiy SA, Robert J, Hanson SM, Raman D, Knox BE, Kono M, Navarro J, Gurevich VV (2005) Crystal struc-

ture of cone arrestin at 2.3Å: evolution of receptor specificity. J Mol Biol 354:1069–1080

106. Zhan X, Gimenez LE, Gurevich VV, Spiller BW (2011) Crystal structure of arrestin-3 reveals the basis of the difference in receptor binding between two non-visual arrestins. J Mol Biol 406:467–478

107. Kim M, Vishnivetskiy SA, Van Eps N, Alexander NS, Cleghorn WM, Zhan X, Hanson SM, Morizumi T, Ernst OP, Meiler J, Gurevich VV, Hubbell WL (2012) Conformation of receptor-bound visual arrestin. Proc Natl Acad Sci U S A 109(45):18407–18412

108. Chen Q, Gilbert NC, Perry NA, Zhuo Y, Vishnivetskiy SA, Berndt S, Klug CS, Gurevich VV, Iverson TM (2016) Structural basis for arrestin-3 activation by inositol hexakisphosphate. Cell, In revision

109. Vishnivetskiy SA, Paz CL, Schubert C, Hirsch JA, Sigler PB, Gurevich VV (1999) How does arrestin respond to the phosphorylated state of rhodopsin? J Biol Chem 274:11451–11454

110. Binder BM, Biernbaum MS, Bownds MD (1990) Light activation of one rhodopsin molecule causes the phosphorylation of hundreds of others. A reaction observed in electropermeabilized frog rod outer segments exposed to dim illumination. J Biol Chem 265:15333–15340

111. Binder BM, O'Connor TM, Bownds MD, Arshavsky VY (1996) Phosphorylation of non-bleached rhodopsin in intact retinas and living frogs. J Biol Chem 271:19826–19830

112. Gurevich VV, Gurevich EV (2008) GPCR monomers and oligomers: it takes all kinds. Trends Neurosci 31:74–81

113. Gurevich VV, Gurevich EV (2008) How and why do GPCRs dimerize? Trends Pharmacol Sci 29:234–240

114. Pearce LR, Komander D, Alessi DR (2010) The nuts and bolts of AGC protein kinases. Nat Rev Mol Cell Biol 11(1):9–22

115. Tesmer JJ, Tesmer VM, Lodowski DT, Steinhagen H, Huber J (2010) Structure of human G protein-coupled receptor kinase 2 in complex with the kinase inhibitor balanol. J Med Chem 53(4):1867–1870

116. Singh P, Wang B, Maeda T, Palczewski K, Tesmer JJ (2008) Structures of rhodopsin kinase in different ligand states reveal key elements involved in G protein-coupled receptor kinase activation. J Biol Chem 283(20):14053–14062

117. Homan KT, Waldschmidt HV, Glukhova A, Cannavo A, Song J, Cheung JY, Koch WJ, Larsen SD, Tesmer JJ (2015) Crystal structure of G protein-coupled receptor kinase 5 in complex with a rationally designed inhibitor. J Biol Chem 290(34):20649–20659

118. Komolov KE, Bhardwaj A, Benovic JL (2015) Atomic structure of GRK5 reveals distinct structural features novel for G protein-coupled receptor kinases. J Biol Chem 290(34):20629–20647

119. Ménard L, Ferguson SS, Barak LS, Bertrand L, Premont RT, Colapietro AM, Lefkowitz RJ, Caron MG (1996) Members of the G protein-coupled receptor kinase family that phosphorylate the beta2-adrenergic receptor facilitate sequestration. Biochemistry 35(13):4155–4160

120. Rankin ML, Marinec PS, Cabrera DM, Wang Z, Jose PA, Sibley DR (2006) The D1 dopamine receptor is constitutively phosphorylated by G protein-coupled receptor kinase 4. Mol Pharmacol 69(3):759–769

121. Inagaki S, Ghirlando R, Vishnivetskiy SA, Homan KT, White JF, Tesmer JJ, Gurevich VV, Grisshammer R (2015) G protein-coupled receptor kinase 2 (GRK2) and 5 (GRK5) exhibit selective phosphorylation of the neurotensin receptor in vitro. Biochemistry 54(28):4320–4329

122. Loudon RP, Benovic JL (1997) Altered activity of palmitoylation-deficient and isoprenylated forms of the G protein-coupled receptor kinase GRK6. J Biol Chem 272(43):27422–27427

123. Stoffel RH, Randall RR, Premont RT, Lefkowitz RJ, Inglese J (1994) Palmitoylation of G protein-coupled receptor kinase, GRK6. Lipid modification diversity in the GRK family. J Biol Chem 269(45):27791–27794

124. Pitcher JA, Fredericks ZL, Stone WC, Premont RT, Stoffel RH, Koch WJ, Lefkowitz RJ (1996) Phosphatidylinositol 4,5-bisphosphate (PIP2)-enhanced G protein-coupled receptor kinase (GRK) activity. Location, structure, and regulation of the PIP2 binding site distinguishes the GRK subfamilies. J Biol Chem 271:24907–24913

125. Gurevich EV, Benovic JL, Gurevich VV (2004) Arrestin2 expression selectively increases during neural differentiation. J Neurochem 91(6):1404–1416

126. Ahmed MR, Bychkov E, Gurevich VV, Benovic JL, Gurevich EV (2007) Altered expression and subcellular distribution of GRK subtypes in the dopamine-depleted rat basal ganglia is not normalized by l-DOPA treatment. J Neurochem 104:1622–1636

127. Bychkov E, Gurevich VV, Joyce JN, Benovic JL, Gurevich EV (2008) Arrestins and two receptor kinases are upregulated in Parkinson's disease with dementia. Neurobiol Aging 29:379–396

128. Bychkov ER, Ahmed MR, Gurevich VV, Benovic JL, Gurevich EV (2011) Reduced expression of G protein-coupled receptor kinases in schizophrenia but not in schizoaffective disorder. Neurobiol Dis 44(2):248–258

129. Ahmed MR, Berthet A, Bychkov E, Porras G, Li Q, Bioulac BH, Carl YT, Bloch B, Kook S, Aubert I, Dovero S, Doudnikoff E, Gurevich VV, Gurevich EV, Bezard E (2010) Lentiviral overexpression of GRK6 alleviates l-dopa-induced dyskinesia in experimental Parkinson's disease. Sci Transl Med 2:28ra28

130. Gainetdinov RR, Bohn LM, Sotnikova TD, Cyr M, Laakso A, Macrae AD, Torres GE, Kim KM, Lefkowitz RJ, Caron MG, Premont RT (2003) Dopaminergic supersensitivity in G protein-coupled receptor kinase 6-deficient mice. Neuron 38:291–303

131. Gainetdinov RR, Bohn LM, Walker JK, Laporte SA, Macrae AD, Caron MG, Lefkowitz RJ, Premont RT (1999) Muscarinic supersensitivity and impaired receptor desensitization in G protein-coupled receptor kinase 5-deficient mice. Neuron 24(4):1029–1036

132. Kim CM, Dion SB, Benovic JL (1993) Mechanism of beta-adrenergic receptor kinase activation by G proteins. J Biol Chem 268:15412–15418

133. Vishnivetskiy SA, Ostermaier MK, Singhal A, Panneels V, Homan KT, Glukhova A, Sligar SG, Tesmer JJ, Schertler GF, Standfuss J, Gurevich VV (2013) Constitutively active rhodopsin mutants causing night blindness are effectively phosphorylated by GRKs but differ in arrestin-1 binding. Cell Signal 25(11):2155–2162

Part II

GRK Structure, Mechanisms of Activation, and Interactions with GPCRs

Chapter 2

Structure and Function of G-Protein-Coupled Receptor Kinases 1 and 7

Tivadar Orban and Krzysztof Palczewski

Abstract

The importance of G protein-coupled receptor (GPCR) kinases (GRKs) as regulators of GPCR signaling has been widely recognized. In humans, GRKs constitute a family of seven protein kinases involved in the phosphorylation and desensitization of agonist-activated GPCRs in many physiological processes. The GPCR desensitization process is initiated by GRKs, but involves several subsequent steps including arrestin capping of phosphorylated receptors. High-resolution crystal structures were determined for four members of the GRK family, i.e., GRK1, GRK2, GRK5, and GRK6. This allowed decoding of the molecular basis of GRK activation and interactions with GPCR substrates, as well as the GRK interactions with cellular membranes and inhibitors. Here, we focused on retinal GRKs, or photopigment kinases, rhodopsin kinase (GRK1), and GRK7, in the context of major general advances in the GRK field.

Key words G protein-coupled receptors (GPCRs), Retinal G protein-coupled receptor kinases (GRKs), Visual signal transduction cascade, OGUCHI disease, GRK1–rhodopsin interaction, Structures of retinal GRKs and inhibitors

Abbreviations

CaM	Calmodulin
GPCRs	G protein-coupled receptors
GRKs	G protein-coupled receptor kinases
PDE	Phosphodiesterase
PKA	Protein kinase A
Rho	Rhodopsin
Rho*	Photoactivated rhodopsin

1 Introduction

1.1 G Protein-Coupled Receptors (GPCRs) and Their Kinases

G protein-coupled receptors (GPCRs) are important receptors involved in cell signaling. External signals received by cells, including small molecules, proteins, or light in the case of rhodopsin (Rho), interact with and activate GPCRs and thereby are trans-

Vsevolod V. Gurevich et al. (eds.), *G Protein-Coupled Receptor Kinases*, Methods in Pharmacology and Toxicology,
DOI 10.1007/978-1-4939-3798-1_2, © Springer Science+Business Media New York 2016

duced intracellularly through a system of proteins composed of G proteins, phosphodiesterases (PDEs), cation channels, and Ca^{2+} sensors, among others. To react on a limited timescale, an activated GRCR needs to be desensitized and returned to its unstimulated state. The desensitization process is typically carried out by a special class of protein kinases called G protein-coupled receptor kinases (GRKs) that preferentially recognize the activated state of their cognate GPCR [1]. GRKs are members of the A, G, and C (AGC) protein kinase family. Although different activated GPCRs initiate different intracellular processes, signal transmission and its consequent termination appear to be similar among them [2]. Pharmacological interventions that regulate GPCR activity are of great interest because GPCRs are involved in virtually all physiological processes. Defects, inhibition, or excessive activity of GRKs are thought to contribute to diseases such as hypertension [3], cardiac [4], Oguchi disease [5], and heart failure [6]. Further attesting to the importance of this class of kinases, the first biannual meeting dedicated to the GRK field was recently held [7].

1.2 Visual Transduction

When light enters the eye, specialized photoreceptor cells in the retina initiate the visual signaling cascade and together with other cell types such as Müller, horizontal, amacrine, bipolar, and ganglion cells transduce this information to the brain (Fig. 1a) [8, 9]. Signal transduction is accomplished by the polarization of photoreceptor cells, which are composed of three major domains: (1) an outer segment which contains the membrane disks where the phototransduction machinery is localized, (2) an inner segment where the protein synthetic apparatus is found, and (3) a synaptic region that connects with other neurons (Fig. 1a). The outer segment is the primary cilium of photoreceptor cells with the soma connected to the synaptic terminal domain. Photoreceptor cells are further categorized as either rods or cones (Fig. 1b), which have notable differences in shape, synaptic connections, and the type of visual photopigments they express.

Rod cells function as the primary visual detector cells under light conditions. Responsible for dim light (scotopic) vision, they are capable of detecting a single photon [10]. Cones are responsible for color (photopic) vision and they are about 100 times less sensitive to light than rods [11]. This decreased sensitivity permits cones to be active and photosensitive throughout the day even under high-intensity light conditions. Another distinguishing feature between rods and cones (Fig. 1b) is the time they need to readapt after light exposure. Rods are quickly desensitized and take about 1 h to recover to their pre-illumination state, whereas the recovery rate for cones is on a minute timescale. This property enables cone cells to quickly adjust to rapidly changing lighting conditions encountered throughout the day [12].

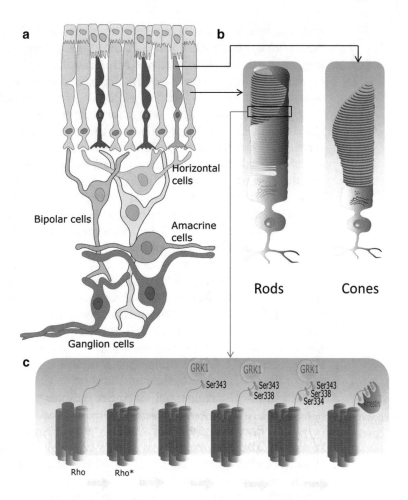

Fig. 1 Rod and cone photoreceptor cells. In the vertebrate system, rods specifically express GRK1 whereas cones express both GRK1 and GRK7. Panel **a** shows the layered organization of the retina with the major cell types involved in visual signal processing. Rods are shown in *grey*, and the three types of cones are colored in *red*, *blue*, and *green*, respectively. Following are the horizontal cells (*lime*), bipolar cells (*cyan* and *yellow*), amacrine cells (*green*), and ganglion cells (*orange*). Panel **b** shows a detailed view of the major components of the two types of photoreceptor cells: rods and cones. Rods possess a plasma membrane that covers the rod disks. Major differences between rods and cones include their shapes, and the cell specific set of gene products that affects responses under different light intensities. Panel **c** shows a simplified view of the Rho* activation and inactivation processes delineating the phosphorylation of residues catalyzed by GRK1 on Rho* and the subsequent binding and capping by arrestin

2   GRKs in Visual Transduction

2.1   The Role of GRKs in the Visual Signal Transduction Cascade   Vision is initiated when a photon of light interacts with the photosensitive chromophore of Rho and cone visual pigments [13]. The molecular mechanism of this event involves a series of sequential steps similar in both rod and cone photoreceptor cells that have been well characterized and reviewed elsewhere [14]. In addition, enzymes that contribute to signal transduction, Rho/cone pigment desensitization, and chromophore regeneration also have been extensively studied and summarized [15, 16]. Following activation of Rho (Rho*) and its interaction with its cognate G protein, G_t (transducin), visual cascade deactivation is achieved by multiple mechanisms. Rho* is inactivated by phosphorylation catalyzed by GRK1, and G_t is inactivated through its intrinsic GTPase activity. Phosphorylation of Rho* was found to be mainly located on its C-terminal domain with three added phosphates representing the optimal number [17] (Fig. 1c). The main effect of this phosphorylation is an increased interaction with arrestin that results in a diminished interaction of phosphorylated Rho* with G_t [18]. The interaction with G_t is further impaired by the subsequent binding of arrestin to phosphorylated Rho* [19, 20] resulting in inhibition of the signal transduction process [17].

Phosphorylation of Rho following light activation was first reported in the 1970s [21–24] and then reviewed in the late 1990s [25, 26]. Rho* phosphorylation correlated with the quenching of cGMP phosphodiesterase (PDE) activity [27], indicating that phosphorylation of Rho* was somehow related to the desensitization process [28]. GRK1 preferentially catalyzed the phosphorylation of Rho* with most of the phosphorylation sites at Ser residues located in the C-terminal tail. Such Ser residues were phosphorylated in the following order: Ser343, Ser338, and Ser334 [29–32] (Fig. 1c). Phosphorylation of Thr residues within the C-terminal region of Rho was recently shown to be involved in facilitating arrestin binding [33]. This phosphorylation desensitization mechanism is prototypical of that of other GPCRs [34]. Dephosphorylation of Rho*, catalyzed by phosphatase 2A (PP2A) [35], showed a similar order of phosphate removal in the Rho recycling pathway [29]. A Rho molecule lacking its C-terminal domain lost its ability to be phosphorylated [30]. The interaction of GRK1 with Rho* is needed for effective phosphorylation.

The mammalian family of GRKs is comprised of 7 members named GRK1 through 7 (Fig. 2). The family was divided into three groups based on their primary sequence homology. The first group contains Rho kinase (GRK1) and cone opsin kinase (GRK7), both expressed in vertebrate retina. GRK1 also was the first kinase characterized in the family [36] (Fig. 2a). The second group is composed of β-adrenergic receptor kinase 1 and 2 (GRK2 and GRK3) with a broad specific tissue expression profile (Fig. 2b). The third group consists of GRK4, GRK5, and GRK6 (Fig. 2c). Members of this group also have no specific tissue expression pattern except GRK4, which has the highest expression in testes.

GRK1 was the first member of the family shown to inhibit Rho's function through phosphorylation and the consequent binding of arrestin [19, 20] as well as the first to be purified and cloned [36]. GRK7 was discovered a decade later in retinas of cone-

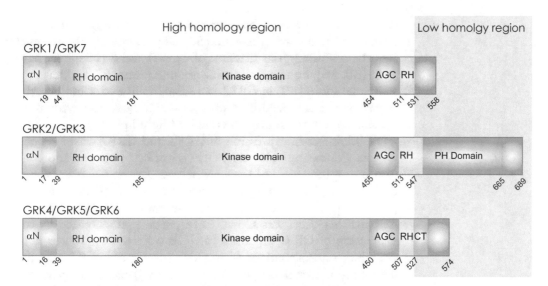

Fig. 2 Major domains and homology of GRK1 and 7 with other GRKs The principal domains of the seven GRK isoforms are shown as follows: α-domain (*blue*) and a connecting region (*red*) to the RH domain (*blue-green*). The AGC kinase domain is shown in magenta, the RH domain in *orange*, the PH domain (specific to GRK2/GRK3) in *dark blue*, and the C-terminal region in *violet*

dominant mammals [37, 38]. The expression pattern of GRK1 and GRK7 was found to be species-dependent [38–41]. All vertebrates express GRK1 in rods whereas in cones some vertebrates express either GRK7 alone or both GRK1 and GRK7 (reviewed in [42]). Mice and rats only express GRK1 in both rods and cones. In carp retina, there are four subtypes of GRK1 and GRK7, i.e., GRK1A-1a and 1A-1b, GRK1Ba and 1Bb, and two subtypes of GRK7-1a and 7-1b [43, 44]. GRK7 was designated as a cone-specific receptor kinase because its expression level was about ten times higher than that of rod-specific GRK1 [45] and its specific activity also was about ten times greater than that of GRK1. Knockdown of GRK7 in larval zebrafish demonstrated that this kinase is essential for cone-specific vision and that its absence resulted in a delayed cone response recovery and dark adaptation [46]. Co-expression of GRK7 in zebrafish rods with endogenously expressed GRK1 caused a considerable decrease in light sensitivity [47].

2.2 Deficiencies and Mutations in GRK1: Oguchi Disease

The gene for GRK1 is localized to chromosome 13, band q34, and encodes a protein composed of seven exons [48] (reviewed in [49]). Deficiencies in either GRK1 [50, 51] or arrestin [52, 53] were shown to cause prolonged insensitivity of rod-controlled vision after light exposure. The disease, termed Oguchi disease, is inherited as an autosomal recessive disorder. First described in Japanese patients, Oguchi disease was attributed to a homozygous deletion [52] with later reports of heterozygous nonsense mutations in the arrestin gene [53, 54]. Following these initial reports, a homozygous deletion of exon 5 and 3 [55], heterozygous [50, 56], homozygous missense mutations [57, 58], or nonsense mutations [59] in GRK1 were also implicated. Clinically, the disease is characterized by a progressive delayed dark adaptation accompanied by near normal vision in bright light [5].

Differences in expression of GRK1 and GRK7 exist between species. For example, in mice, *Grk1–/–* affects both rod and cone photoreceptors [60, 61], where it was shown to cause severe defects in rod and cone recovery and retinal degeneration [62] (similar to the *arrestin-1–/–* mouse model). In contrast, in humans this effect was shown to be partially ameliorated by the expression of GRK7 in cones [63]. Another mouse model with cone-like photoreceptors (double knockout of GRK1 and the neural retina leucine zipper, *Grk1–/–Nrl–/–*) also developed age-related retinal dystrophy in a light-independent manner, further supporting a role of GRK1 in the maintenance of proper cone health [64]. Though deletion of the *GRK1* gene negatively affected photoreceptor health, GRK1 overexpression failed to protect photoreceptors [65]. These findings in animal models indicate that excessive activity of the phototransduction cascade coupled with exposure to high-intensity light causes photoreceptor cell death [60]. A study that evaluated the effect of variable expression of GRK1 on the kinetics of recovery from dim light stimulation concluded that Rho* inactivation could indeed modulate such recovery [66].

3   GRK1 in Visual Transduction

3.1   Structure of GRK1

X-ray structures provide a fundamental basis for learning how enzymes work at the molecular level, and understanding such mechanisms in the field of vision was greatly enhanced by using this approach (reviewed in [67]). X-ray structures have been determined for several members of the GRK family including: GRK1, GRK2 [68], GRK5 [69, 70], and GRK6 [71–73]. Some of these structures were solved in the presence of inhibitors or ATP. Homologous domains in GRKs are categorized as: the RGS homology (RH) domain, the kinase domain, and the highly homologous N-terminal domain comprised of ~20 amino acids (Fig. 2). X-ray structures do not provide as much information on the N-terminal domain (reviewed in [74]) as the structure of this part is disordered in most of the crystallized GRK structures. The only two structures where the N-terminal region was detected (in one structure of GRK1 and one of GRK6) are distinct, an artifact that could result from differences in crystal packing. Because of this shortcoming, we still lack a definitive molecular view of this domain [75]. The function of GRK1 was suggested to be regulated by its N-terminal domain. The relevance of the N-terminal region was first described by following its interaction with specific antibodies, which inhibited the phosphorylation of Rho* but failed to prevent phosphorylation of synthetic peptides that had an identical sequence with Rho's C-terminal region [76]. A study that characterized the dynamics of GRK1 under a variety of conditions described a highly flexible molecule in the absence of ATP·Mg^{2+}. The dynamics of GRK1 in the presence of Rho, Rho*, ATP·Mg^{2+} reinforced the concept that conformational changes occur following interaction of GRK1 with either Rho* or ATP·Mg^{2+} [77]. Use of truncated GRK1 with the first 19 residues removed from the N-terminus provided further evidence about the importance of this sequence in the regulation of GRK1's function and interaction with Rho* [67, 76, 78, 79]. Because the interaction with a GPCR is expected to be similar for all GRKs, the same findings would pertain to other GRKs like GRK2 [80]. GRK1 is monomeric in solution, but crystallized in a dimeric form which was suggested to have a role in the function of GRKs. The dimer, also present in the GRK6 structure [72, 73], contained a hydrophobic patch conserved in all but GRK2 and GRK3. The GRK1-(L166K) mutant (a GRK1 with a mutation in the interface region of the dimer structure) crystallized in a novel space group as a monomer. This result is similar to that obtained with another GRK family member, GRK5 [69], which revealed a different conformation for the C-terminal region (amino acid residues 527–541). The structure of the C-terminal region contrasted with other structures reported for GRK1 and GRK6 but was similar to that of the GRK1-(L166K) mutant. In GRK5, however, the C-terminal structures were similar even though they were solved with a different crystal packing [69, 70].

One plausible working model by which GPCRs could activate GRKs is by inducing closure of the kinase domain. This would align the catalytic domain of the large lobe with the ATP-binding region of the small lobe. Conformational changes in GRK1 induced by binding of ATP could also favor closure in the kinase domain as evidenced by hydrogen-deuterium experiments [77] or as noted for other kinases such as protein kinase A (PKA) [81]. More experiments are needed to resolve the molecular details of GRK activation.

3.2 GRK1
Interactions
with Membranes

To fully exert their activity on activated GPCRs, GRKs require an interaction with negatively charged phospholipids. Specific details about the interactions of GRK1 and GRK7 with membranes are limited. The GRK interaction site with membranes is proposed to be a relatively flat surface that involves residues near the N-terminal domain, C-terminal tail, and a linker region between the N-terminal and RH domains [78]. Recent structures of GRK5 also provide evidence supporting an interaction with the membrane through its C-terminal region [69, 70]. With the current proposed arrangement, the N-terminal region would be inserted deeply into the membrane. This insertion is plausible for some GRK members because the N-terminal region contains several hydrophobic residues that would favorably interact with the hydrophobic membrane layer even though this region is not conserved and contains negatively charged residues in certain GRKs [78]. The C-terminal tails of GRKs are the least conserved regions among all GRKs and their involvement in the interaction with the phospholipid bilayer suggests the possibility of different recruiting mechanisms. Recent evidence suggests that in GRK5, interaction with the phospholipid membrane also involves a region from the RH domain (Leu135–Arg169), which appears to be conserved in GRK1 and GRK6 [82].

3.3 GRK1 Interaction with Rho

Because GRK1 competes with G_t to interact with Rho* (or constitutively active mutants of Rho [83]), some of the interaction regions on Rho* are expected to overlap [84]. Interaction of GRK1 with Rho* was described early as involving multiple sites [85]. Cytoplasmic loops I and II of Rho were shown to be needed for the interaction with GRK1 [86], in addition to cytoplasmic loop III previously found relevant for G_t binding [87, 88]. A 1:1 GRK1:Rho* stoichiometry sufficed for efficient phosphorylation of Rho* [89]. Likewise, a 1:1 ratio for the interaction of phosphorylated Rho* with arrestin was also reported [90]. Although a second Rho molecule does not seem strictly required for an interaction with arrestin or for GRKs to achieve full activity, a wealth of information indicates that Rho is dimeric in nature [91–94].

The first N-terminal 30 amino acids of GRK1 are involved in the interaction with Rho* (Fig. 3) [76, 77, 79, 95] together with a region of the C-terminal domain that encompasses residues 457 to 546 [96]. A recent study employing site-directed mutagenesis of the N-terminal region in GRK2 (Asp3-Glu18) evaluated the capability of mutated GRK2 to phosphorylate the β_2-adrenergic receptor. The interaction site with β_2-adrenergic receptor was found to involve the N-terminal domain together with an extension of the kinase domain including residues Gly475 to Ile485. This model of the GRK2-β_2-adrenergic receptor recapitulates that proposed for GRK1-Rho*-Rho [77] (Fig. 4).

3.4 High-Gain Phosphorylation of Rho

At low phosphorylation levels (<1%), as much as 50 mol of phosphate are incorporated per 1 mol of Rho* [97]. Similarly, when Rho was photoactivated at 0.04%, about 700 phosphates were incorporated per Rho* [98]. This effect is known as high-gain phosphorylation and one explanation could be that this "high-gain" reaction causes the phosphorylation of unbleached Rho molecules. High phosphorylation increases with elevated amounts of GRK1 and is quenched by the addition of recoverin and Ca^{2+} ions [65, 98]. High-gain phosphorylation, observed only under low illumination, exists because there are far less Rho* molecules than Rho molecules, and

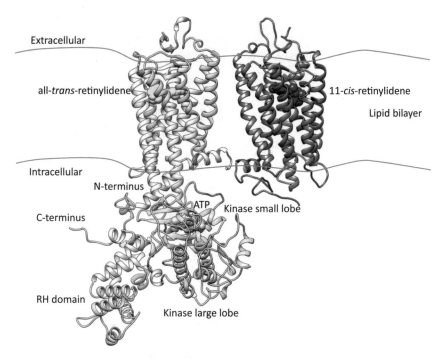

Fig. 3 Interaction of GRK1 with Rho*. The GRK1 molecule is modeled in a closed conformation. The position relative to Rho* was chosen based on the superposition of the N-terminal helix of GRK1 with the C-terminal helix of $G\alpha_s$ as described for the β_2-adrenergic receptor-G_s crystal structure [138]. Labeled GRK1 domains colored according to the code described in Fig. 1 are: the N-terminal region (Ser1-Arg19) in *light blue* and (Gly20-Leu44) in *pink*; the RH domain in *aquamarine* (Pro43 to Glu184 and Trp515 to Arg532); the kinase domain small lobe in *brown* (Asp185 to Asn268), and the large lobe in *green* (Gly269 to Pro514). The C-terminal region of GRK1 is depicted in *gray*. The homology model of the full GRK1 model was constructed using the GRK6·sangivamycin structure as a template [78]. The membrane wherein the Rho*-Rho heterodimer is inserted is depicted by wavy *grey lines*. A theoretical Rho*-Rho heterodimer is modeled in a helix 8-helix 8-dimer orientation. All-*trans*-retinylidene and 11-*cis*-retinylidene are depicted as *yellow* and *red spheres*, respectively. ATP bound to GRK1 is shown as light *grey spheres*. Dark state Rho is shown as a *dark grey cartoon*, whereas the light-activated monomer is in *light grey*

once activated by Rho*, GRK1 can also catalyze the phosphorylation of nearby Rho.

4   Regulation of GRK1

4.1   Post-translational Modifications

GRK1 from all species studied is post-translationally modified through farnesylation [99], except for chicken GRK1, which has a coding region that can be modified by geranylgeranylation in chicken liver extracts [100]. This modification of GRK1 could help direct the enzyme to the right locations in rods and cones because a non-farnesylated mutant had only a minimal effect on Rho* phosphorylation [101]. Consistent with the idea that lipid modification helps direct GRKs to appropriate compartments within photoreceptor

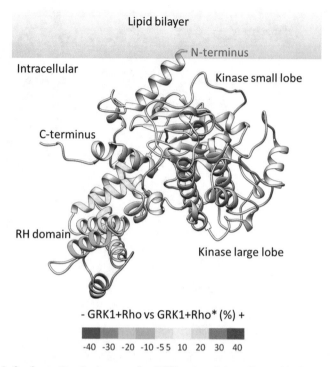

Fig. 4 Conformational changes in GRK1 upon interaction with Rho*. Low-resolution structural information obtained by hydrogen-deuterium exchange coupled to mass spectrometry provides the only information yet available that describes the conformational changes in GRK1 when complexed with Rho* [77]. The differences in normalized deuterium uptakes in the presence of either Rho or Rho* were mapped on the GRK1 molecule in an orientation similar to that described for the GRK1-Rho* model presented in Fig. 3. Color coding, defined as differences between the normalized deuterium uptakes, is shown for differences above the set threshold limit of 10 %. Positive differences (*yellow*, *orange*, and *red*) were assigned to the higher deuterium uptakes found in the case of GRK1 + Rho. Negative differences (*blue*, *cyan*, *light blue*, and *green*) denote higher uptakes in the GRK1 + Rho* sample

cells, GRK7 has a sequence predicted to be a geranylgeranyl modification site on its C-terminus. Post-translational modifications in GRK1 also involve C-terminal Cys residue α-carboxymethylation. Prenylation (addition of farnesyl or geranylgeranyl in the case of GRK1 and GRK7, respectively) followed by α-carboxymethylation thus could serve as hydrophobic anchors for GRK1 and GRK7 in membranes [102]. Increased GRK1 α-carboxymethylation in dark-adapted rods was found to be regulated by free nucleotides and high Ca^{2+} levels through their effects on recoverin, causing an increased association of GRK1 with recoverin and membranes [103]. As a consequence, increased GRK1 methylation in dark-adapted rods was attributed to increased Ca^{2+} levels. The increase of Ca^{2+} levels then additionally increases the association of GRK1 with both the membranes and recoverin, thereby providing a positive feedback decrease in the nonspecific phosphorylation of inactive Rho molecules.

This mechanism represents another option for increasing the light sensitivity of photoreceptors.

A third set of post-translational modifications of GRK1, other than prenylation and carboxymethylation, involves phosphorylation. Autophosphorylation of GRK1 [104] was found to affect GRK's affinity toward its substrates, both Rho* [105] and recoverin. Phosphorylated sites in GRK1 localized primarily on residues Ser488 and Thr489 [106]. The X-ray structure of GRK1 and further mass spectrometric analysis revealed two extra sites that also were phosphorylated, namely Ser5 and Thr8 [71]. However, GRK1 with mutations at these latter sites showed identical autophosphorylation rates with no obvious effects on ATP binding. This result suggests that these sites could be relevant for other functions of GRK1, such as membrane targeting and/or transport as evidenced by poor expression of some of the mutants [71]. In vitro phosphorylation of GRK1 by PKA at Ser21 and GRK7 at Ser23 and Ser36 in a cAMP-dependent fashion has also been reported [107]. These in vitro experiments were followed by in vivo studies which demonstrated that PKA-catalyzed phosphorylation of GRK1 was high in the dark-adapted state when cAMP levels also were elevated [108].

4.2 Protein Inhibitors

Recoverin is a Ca^{2+}-binding protein found to inhibit GRK1 function as part of the negative feedback of visual signal transduction [109–112] in both rods [113, 114] and cones [115]. Recoverin's interaction with GRK1 in the presence of Ca^{2+} was localized to the N-terminal region of both GRK1 (residues 1–25) [116, 117] and GRK7 [118], as reviewed in [119]. The interaction site on recoverin involved the C-terminal domain [120] together with a region of residues conserved among other Ca^{2+}-binding sensor proteins, suggesting that the binding site to GRKs would be partially conserved among Ca^{2+}-binding sensor proteins [121, 122]. The inhibitory efficacy of recoverin was also improved if this Ca^{2+}-binding protein was N-myristoylated [123]. These findings were mimicked by S-modulin, a recoverin ortholog in frogs, for both GRK1 and GRK7 [118, 124]. Another Ca^{2+}-binding protein, calmodulin (CaM), also can bind to GRK1 at residues between 150 and 175, although not with the same affinity as recoverin. In GRK5, CaM was shown to have a binding site localized between residues 20–39. In addition to the N-terminal region, the C-terminal region of GRK5 also was implicated in this interaction [125]. In the recently solved X-ray structure of GRK5, the positions of these two domains are in close proximity, suggesting that CaM might bind simultaneously to both [70]. This different binding pattern, as compared with GRK1, is due to the low homology in this region between these two GRKs, which explains the wide range of dissociation constants for CaM among various GRKs [126, 127]. Interactions of GRK1 with these two Ca^{2+}-binding proteins are synergistic, as evidenced by their different binding sites on GRK1 and the broader range of Ca^{2+}-sensing capabilities when compared to recoverin alone [125, 128]. In carp, visinin (an S-modulin analog in cones) was shown to inhibit GRK7 with a greater potency than GRK1 was inhibited by S-modulin [129]. In addition to the native recoverin/CaM inhibition, antibodies developed initially for purification purposes were also found to inhibit the function of GRK1. This inhibition resulted from interactions with the kinase C-terminal region [130]. Finally, caveolins were shown to inhibit GRK1 activity: peptides derived from caveolin-1 and caveolin-3 had IC_{50} values of 2.7 and 1.8 μM, respectively [131]. Although the exact mechanism by which caveolin inhibits GRK1 remains unknown, a recent study provided evidence for co-localization of caveolin with Rho and GRK1 in vertebrate retina [132].

4.3 Small-Molecule Inhibitors of GRKs

The first small-molecule inhibitors of GRK1 were biochemically identified from a family of nucleoside analogs, the most potent being sangivamycin ($K_i = 180$ nM) [133, 134] and toyocamycin [134]. Sangivamycin binds to GRK6 with a dissociation constant of 1 μM, about 30-fold less than its analog, adenosine [72]. The structure of GRK6 in the presence of sangivamycin determined at a 2.7 Å resolution revealed that this inhibitor interacted with GRK6's ATP-binding site located between the small and large lobes of the kinase domain in the canonical ATP binding site [72]. X-ray crystal structures of GRK1 were obtained with a variety of inhibitors [135, 136]. Paroxetine, a specific GRK2 inhibitor, was found to bind to GRK1 and GRK5 with 16- and 13-fold lower affinities than to GRK2 [137]. A specific inhibitor of GRK2 and GRK5 denoted as CCG215022 was found to have nanomolar IC_{50} values and selectivity against both GRK1 and PKA. The X-ray structure of the GRK5·CCG215022 complex also was recently solved [70]. The kinase domain in this complex was similar to that of GRK6-sangivamycin with only the C-terminal region adopting a different orientation that could interact with the membrane [70].

5 Future Directions

During the past decade there has been much progress in deciphering the molecular basis of GRKs activation, inhibition, and interactions with their molecular targets, such as activated GPCRs (see review [49] for a 30 years progress report up to 2003). This field has advanced greatly from structural studies done on four members of the GRK family, i.e., GRK1, GRK2, GRK5 and GRK6. This research area would benefit greatly from any structure of an activated GRK. Although much has been accomplished with lower-resolution methods used to characterize the GRK1-Rho* complex, high-resolution structures are still needed to provide a molecular view of the interaction between a GRK and its substrate GPCR.

Acknowledgements

We thank Drs. Leslie T. Webster Jr., and members of Palczewski laboratory for helpful comments on this manuscript. This work was supported by funding from the National Institutes of Health EY009339 (KP), EY025451 (KP), the Arnold and Mabel Beckman Foundation (KP), the Canadian Institute for Advanced Research (CIFAR), and the Foundation Fighting Blindness (KP). K.P. is John H. Hord Professor of Pharmacology.

References

1. Palczewski K, Benovic JL (1991) G-protein-coupled receptor kinases. Trends Biochem Sci 16(10):387–391

2. Benovic JL, Mayor F Jr, Somers RL, Caron MG, Lefkowitz RJ (1986) Light-dependent phosphorylation of rhodopsin by beta-adrenergic receptor kinase. Nature 321(6073):869–872

3. Felder RA, Sanada H, Xu J, Yu PY, Wang Z, Watanabe H, Asico LD, Wang W, Zheng SP, Yamaguchi I, Williams SM, Gainer J, Brown NJ, Hazen-Martin D, Wong LJC, Robillard JE, Carey RM, Eisner GM, Jose PA (2002) G protein-coupled receptor kinase 4 gene variants in human essential hypertension. Proc Natl Acad Sci U S A 99(6):3872–3877

4. Gold JI, Gao EH, Shang XY, Premont RT, Koch WJ (2012) Determining the absolute requirement of G protein-coupled receptor kinase 5 for pathological cardiac hypertrophy. Circ Res 111(8):1048–1053

5. Dryja TP (2000) Molecular genetics of Oguchi disease, fundus albipunctatus, and other forms of stationary night blindness: LVII Edward Jackson Memorial Lecture. Am J Ophthalmol 130(5):547–563

6. Lymperopoulos A, Rengo G, Koch WJ (2012) GRK2 inhibition in heart failure: something old, something new. Curr Pharm Design 18(2):186–191

7. Gurevich EV, Premont RT, Gainetdinov RR (2015) G protein-coupled receptor kinases: from molecules to diseases. FASEB J 29(2):361–364

8. Purves D, Augustine GJ, Fitzpatrick D, Katz L, LaMantia A-S, McNamara J, Williams S (2001) The retina. Neuroscience. 2nd edition. Sunderland (MA): Sinauer Associates; 2001. The Retina. Available from: http://www.ncbi.nlm.nih.gov/books/NBK10885/

9. Euler T, Haverkamp S, Schubert T, Baden T (2014) Retinal bipolar cells: elementary building blocks of vision. Nat Rev Neurosci 15(8):507–519

10. Baylor DA, Lamb TD, Yau KW (1979) Responses of retinal rods to single photons. J Physiol 288(Mar):613–634

11. Baylor DA (1987) Photoreceptor signals and vision. Invest Ophth Vis Sci 28(1):34–49

12. Fain GL, Matthews HR, Cornwall MC, Koutalos Y (2001) Adaptation in vertebrate photoreceptors. Physiol Rev 81(1):117–151

13. Palczewski K (2006) G protein-coupled receptor rhodopsin. Annu Rev Biochem 75:743–767

14. Kiser PD, Golczak M, Palczewski K (2014) Chemistry of the retinoid (visual) cycle. Chem Rev 114(1):194–232

15. Kiser PD, Zhang J, Badiee M, Li Q, Shi W, Sui X, Golczak M, Tochtrop GP, Palczewski K (2015) Catalytic mechanism of a retinoid isomerase essential for vertebrate vision. Nat Chem Biol 11(6):409–415

16. Kiser PD, Golczak M, Maeda A, Palczewski K (2012) Key enzymes of the retinoid (visual) cycle in vertebrate retina. Biochim Biophys Acta 1821(1):137–151

17. Krupnick JG, Gurevich VV, Benovic JL (1997) Mechanism of quenching of phototransduction. Binding competition between arrestin and transducin for phosphorhodopsin. J Biol Chem 272(29):18125–18131

18. Hofmann KP, Pulvermuller A, Buczylko J, Van Hooser P, Palczewski K (1992) The role of arrestin and retinoids in the regeneration pathway of rhodopsin. J Biol Chem 267(22):15701–15706

19. Wilden U, Kuhn H (1982) Light-dependent phosphorylation of rhodopsin: number of phosphorylation sites. Biochemistry 21(12):3014–3022

20. Kuhn H, Wilden U (1987) Deactivation of photoactivated rhodopsin by rhodopsin-

kinase and arrestin. J Recept Res 7(1-4):283–298

21. Kuhn H, Dreyer WJ (1972) Light dependent phosphorylation of rhodopsin by ATP. FEBS Lett 20(1):1–6

22. Miller JA, Brodie AE, Bownds MD (1975) Light-activated rhodopsin phosphorylation may control light sensitivity in isolated rod outer segments. FEBS Lett 59(1):20–23

23. Weller M, Virmaux N, Mandel P (1975) Light-stimulated phosphorylation of rhodopsin in the retina: the presence of a protein kinase that is specific for photobleached rhodopsin. Proc Natl Acad Sci U S A 72(1):381–385

24. Bownds D, Dawes J, Miller J, Stahlman M (1972) Phosphorylation of frog photoreceptor membranes induced by light. Nat New Biol 237(73):125–127

25. Hurley JB, Spencer M, Niemi GA (1998) Rhodopsin phosphorylation and its role in photoreceptor function. Vision Res 38(10):1341–1352

26. Baylor DA, Burns ME (1998) Control of rhodopsin activity in vision. Eye 12:521–525

27. Stryer L (1986) Cyclic GMP cascade of vision. Annu Rev Neurosci 9:87–119

28. Sitaramayya A, Liebman PA (1983) Phosphorylation of rhodopsin and quenching of cyclic GMP phosphodiesterase activation by ATP at weak bleaches. J Biol Chem 258(20):12106–12109

29. Kennedy MJ, Lee KA, Niemi GA, Craven KB, Garwin GG, Saari JC, Hurley JB (2001) Multiple phosphorylation of rhodopsin and the in vivo chemistry underlying rod photoreceptor dark adaptation. Neuron 31(1):87–101

30. Ohguro H, Van Hooser JP, Milam AH, Palczewski K (1995) Rhodopsin phosphorylation and dephosphorylation in vivo. J Biol Chem 270(24):14259–14262

31. Ohguro H, RudnickaNawrot M, Buczylko J, Zhao XY, Taylor JA, Walsh KA, Palczewski K (1996) Structural and enzymatic aspects of rhodopsin phosphorylation. J Biol Chem 271(9):5215–5224

32. Mendez A, Burns ME, Roca A, Lem J, Wu LW, Simon MI, Baylor DA, Chen J (2000) Rapid and reproducible deactivation of rhodopsin requires multiple phosphorylation sites. Neuron 28(1):153–164

33. Azevedo AW, Doan T, Moaven H, Sokal I, Baameur F, Vishnivetskiy SA, Homan KT, Tesmer JJ, Gurevich VV, Chen J, Rieke F (2015) C-terminal threonines and serines play distinct roles in the desensitization of rhodopsin, a G protein-coupled receptor. Elife 4:e05981

34. Fredericks ZL, Pitcher JA, Lefkowitz RJ (1996) Identification of the G protein-coupled receptor kinase phosphorylation sites in the human beta(2)-adrenergic receptor. J Biol Chem 271(23):13796–13803

35. Palczewski K, Hargrave PA, Mcdowell JH, Ingebritsen TS (1989) The catalytic subunit of phosphatase 2a dephosphorylates phosphoopsin. Biochemistry 28(2):415–419

36. Palczewski K, McDowell JH, Hargrave PA (1988) Purification and characterization of rhodopsin kinase. J Biol Chem 263(28):14067–14073

37. Weiss ER, Raman D, Shirakawa S, Ducceschi MH, Bertram PT, Wong F, Kraft TW, Osawa S (1998) The cloning of GRK7, a candidate cone opsin kinase, from cone- and rod-dominant mammalian retinas. Mol Vis 4:27

38. Hisatomi O, Matsuda S, Satoh T, Kotaka S, Imanishi Y, Tokunaga F (1998) A novel subtype of G-protein-coupled receptor kinase, GRK7, in teleost cone photoreceptors. FEBS Lett 424(3):159–164

39. Weiss ER, Ducceschi MH, Horner TJ, Li A, Craft CM, Osawa S (2001) Species-specific differences in expression of G-protein-coupled receptor kinase (GRK) 7 and GRK1 in mammalian cone photoreceptor cells: implications for cone cell phototransduction. J Neurosci 21(23):9175–9184

40. Wada Y, Sugiyama J, Okano T, Fukada Y (2006) GRK1 and GRK7: unique cellular distribution and widely different activities of opsin phosphorylation in the zebrafish rods and cones. J Neurochem 98(3):824–837

41. Liu P, Osawa S, Weiss ER (2005) M opsin phosphorylation in intact mammalian retinas. J Neurochem 93(1):135–144

42. Osawa S, Weiss ER (2012) A tale of two kinases in rods and cones. Adv Exp Med Biol 723:821–827

43. Shimauchi-Matsukawa Y, Aman Y, Tachibanaki S, Kawamura S (2005) Isolation and characterization of visual pigment kinase-related genes in carp retina: polyphyly in GRK1 subtypes, GRK1A and 1B. Mol Vis 11:1220–1228

44. Zhao XY, Huang J, Khani SC, Palczewski K (1998) Molecular forms of human rhodopsin kinase (GRK1). J Biol Chem 273(9):5124–5131

45. Tachibanaki S, Arinobu D, Shimauchi-Matsukawa Y, Tsushima S, Kawamura S (2005) Highly effective phosphorylation by G protein-coupled receptor kinase 7 of light-

activated visual pigment in cones. Proc Natl Acad Sci U S A 102(26):9329–9334

46. Rinner O, Makhankov YV, Biehlmaier O, Neuhauss SCF (2005) Knockdown of cone-specific kinase GRK7 in larval zebrafish leads to impaired cone response recovery and delayed dark adaptation. Neuron 47(2):231–242

47. Vogalis F, Shiraki T, Kojima D, Wada Y, Nishiwaki Y, Jarvinen JLP, Sugiyama J, Kawakami K, Masai I, Kawamura S, Fukada Y, Lamb TD (2011) Ectopic expression of cone-specific G-protein-coupled receptor kinase GRK7 in zebrafish rods leads to lower photosensitivity and altered responses. J Physiol 589(9):2321–2348

48. Khani SC, Abitbol M, Yamamoto S, MaravicMagovcevic I, Dryja TP (1996) Characterization and chromosomal localization of the gene for human rhodopsin kinase. Genomics 35(3):571–576

49. Maeda T, Imanishi Y, Palczewski K (2003) Rhodopsin phosphorylation: 30 years later. Prog Retin Eye Res 22(4):417–434

50. Yamamoto S, Sippel KC, Berson EL, Dryja TP (1997) Defects in the rhodopsin kinase gene in the Oguchi form of stationary night blindness. Nat Genet 15(2):175–178

51. Khani SC, Nielsen L, Vogt TM (1998) Biochemical evidence for pathogenicity of rhodopsin kinase mutations correlated with the oguchi form of congenital stationary night blindness. Proc Natl Acad Sci U S A 95(6):2824–2827

52. Fuchs S, Nakazawa M, Maw M, Tamai M, Oguchi Y, Gal A (1995) A homozygous 1-base pair deletion in the arrestin gene is a frequent cause of Oguchi disease in Japanese. Nat Genet 10(3):360–362

53. Huang LL, Li W, Tang WL, Zhu XH, Ou-yang PB, Lu GX (2012) A Chinese family with Oguchi's disease due to compound heterozygosity including a novel deletion in the arrestin gene. Mol Vis 18(57–59):528–536

54. Waheed NK, Qavi AH, Malik SN, Maria M, Riaz M, Cremers FP, Azam M, Qamar R (2012) A nonsense mutation in S-antigen (p.Glu306*) causes Oguchi disease. Mol Vis 18:1253–1259

55. Zhang Q, Zulfiqar F, Riazuddin SA, Xiao X, Yasmeen A, Rogan PK, Caruso R, Sieving PA, Riazuddin S, Hejtmancik JF (2005) A variant form of Oguchi disease mapped to 13q34 associated with partial deletion of GRK1 gene. Mol Vis 11:977–985

56. Cideciyan AV, Zhao X, Nielsen L, Khani SC, Jacobson SG, Palczewski K (1998) Null mutation in the rhodopsin kinase gene slows recovery kinetics of rod and cone phototransduction in man. Proc Natl Acad Sci U S A 95(1):328–333

57. Hayashi T, Gekka T, Takeuchi T, Goto-Omoto S, Kitahara K (2007) A novel homozygous GRK1 mutation (P391H) in 2 siblings with Oguchi disease with markedly reduced cone responses. Ophthalmology 114(1):134–141

58. Oishi A, Akimoto M, Kawagoe N, Mandai M, Takahashi M, Yoshimura N (2007) Novel mutations in the GRK1 gene in Japanese patients with Oguchi disease. Am J Ophthalmol 144(3):475–477

59. Azam M, Collin RW, Khan MI, Shah ST, Qureshi N, Ajmal M, den Hollander AI, Qamar R, Cremers FP (2009) A novel mutation in GRK1 causes Oguchi disease in a consanguineous Pakistani family. Mol Vis 15:1788–1793

60. Chen CK, Burns ME, Spencer M, Niemi GA, Chen J, Hurley JB, Baylor DA, Simon MI (1999) Abnormal photoresponses and light-induced apoptosis in rods lacking rhodopsin kinase. Proc Natl Acad Sci U S A 96(7):3718–3722

61. Lyubarsky AL, Chen C, Simon MI, Pugh EN Jr (2000) Mice lacking G-protein receptor kinase 1 have profoundly slowed recovery of cone-driven retinal responses. J Neurosci 20(6):2209–2217

62. Fan J, Sakurai K, Chen CK, Rohrer B, Wu BX, Yau KW, Kefalov V, Crouch RK (2010) Deletion of GRK1 causes retina degeneration through a transducin-independent mechanism. J Neurosci 30(7):2496–2503

63. Cideciyan AV, Jacobson SG, Gupta N, Osawa S, Locke KG, Weiss ER, Wright AF, Birch DG, Milam AH (2003) Cone deactivation kinetics and GRK1/GRK7 expression in enhanced S cone syndrome caused by mutations in NR2E3. Invest Ophthalmol Vis Sci 44(3):1268–1274

64. Yetemian RM, Brown BM, Craft CM (2010) Neovascularization, enhanced inflammatory response, and age-related cone dystrophy in the Nrl-/-Grk1-/- mouse retina. Invest Ophthalmol Vis Sci 51(12):6196–6206

65. Whitcomb T, Sakurai K, Brown BM, Young JE, Sheflin L, Dlugos C, Craft CM, Kefalov VJ, Khani SC (2010) Effect of g protein-coupled receptor kinase 1 (Grk1) overexpres-

sion on rod photoreceptor cell viability. Invest Ophthalmol Vis Sci 51(3):1728–1737

66. Sakurai K, Young JE, Kefalov VJ, Khani SC (2011) Variation in rhodopsin kinase expression alters the dim flash response shut off and the light adaptation in rod photoreceptors. Invest Ophthalmol Vis Sci 52(9):6793–6800

67. Orban T, Jastrzebska B, Palczewski K (2014) Structural approaches to understanding retinal proteins needed for vision. Curr Opin Cell Biol 27:32–43

68. Lodowski DT, Pitcher JA, Capel WD, Lefkowitz RJ, Tesmer JJ (2003) Keeping G proteins at bay: a complex between G protein-coupled receptor kinase 2 and Gbetagamma. Science 300(5623):1256–1262

69. Komolov KE, Bhardwaj A, Benovic JL (2015) Atomic structure of G protein-coupled receptor kinase 5 (GRK5) reveals distinct structural features novel for GRKs. J Biol Chem 290(34):20629–20647

70. Homan KT, Waldschmidt HV, Glukhova A, Cannavo A, Song J, Cheung JY, Koch WJ, Larsen SD, Tesmer JJ (2015) Crystal structure of G protein-coupled receptor kinase 5 in complex with a rationally designed inhibitor. J Biol Chem 290(34):20649–20659

71. Singh P, Wang B, Maeda T, Palczewski K, Tesmer JJ (2008) Structures of rhodopsin kinase in different ligand states reveal key elements involved in G protein-coupled receptor kinase activation. J Biol Chem 283(20):14053–14062

72. Boguth CA, Singh P, Huang CC, Tesmer JJ (2010) Molecular basis for activation of G protein-coupled receptor kinases. EMBO J 29(19):3249–3259

73. Lodowski DT, Tesmer VM, Benovic JL, Tesmer JJ (2006) The structure of G protein-coupled receptor kinase (GRK)-6 defines a second lineage of GRKs. J Biol Chem 281(24):16785–16793

74. Mushegian A, Gurevich VV, Gurevich EV (2012) The origin and evolution of G protein-coupled receptor kinases. Plos One 7(3)

75. Tesmer JJ, Nance MR, Singh P, Lee H (2012) Structure of a monomeric variant of rhodopsin kinase at 2.5 Å resolution. Acta Crystallogr 68(Pt 6):622–625

76. Palczewski K, Buczylko J, Lebioda L, Crabb JW, Polans AS (1993) Identification of the N-terminal region in rhodopsin kinase involved in its interaction with rhodopsin. J Biol Chem 268(8):6004–6013

77. Orban T, Huang CC, Homan KT, Jastrzebska B, Tesmer JJ, Palczewski K (2012) Substrate-induced changes in the dynamics of rhodopsin kinase (G protein-coupled receptor kinase 1). Biochemistry 51(16):3404–3411

78. Boguth CA, Singh P, Huang CC, Tesmer JJ (2010) Molecular basis for activation of G protein-coupled receptor kinases. EMBO J 29(19):3249–3259

79. Huang CC, Yoshino-Koh K, Tesmer JJ (2009) A surface of the kinase domain critical for the allosteric activation of G protein-coupled receptor kinases. J Biol Chem 284(25):17206–17215

80. Pao CS, Barker BL, Benovic JL (2009) Role of the amino terminus of G protein-coupled receptor kinase 2 in receptor phosphorylation. Biochemistry 48(30):7325–7333

81. Ni Q, Shaffer J, Adams JA (2000) Insights into nucleotide binding in protein kinase A using fluorescent adenosine derivatives. Protein Sci 9(9):1818–1827

82. Xu H, Jiang X, Shen K, Fischer CC, Wedegaertner PB (2014) The regulator of G protein signaling (RGS) domain of G protein-coupled receptor kinase 5 (GRK5) regulates plasma membrane localization and function. Mol Biol Cell 25(13):2105–2115

83. Vishnivetskiy SA, Ostermaier MK, Singhal A, Panneels V, Homan KT, Glukhova A, Sligar SG, Tesmer JJ, Schertler GF, Standfuss J, Gurevich VV (2013) Constitutively active rhodopsin mutants causing night blindness are effectively phosphorylated by GRKs but differ in arrestin-1 binding. Cell Signal 25(11):2155–2162

84. Pulvermuller A, Palczewski K, Hofmann KP (1993) Interaction between photoactivated rhodopsin and its kinase: stability and kinetics of complex formation. Biochemistry 32(51):14082–14088

85. Palczewski K, McDowell JH, Hargrave PA (1988) Rhodopsin kinase: substrate specificity and factors that influence activity. Biochemistry 27(7):2306–2313

86. Shi W, Osawa S, Dickerson CD, Weiss ER (1995) Rhodopsin mutants discriminate sites important for the activation of rhodopsin kinase and Gt. J Biol Chem 270(5):2112–2119

87. Palczewski K, Buczylko J, Kaplan MW, Polans AS, Crabb JW (1991) Mechanism of rhodopsin kinase activation. J Biol Chem 266(20):12949–12955

88. Kelleher DJ, Johnson GL (1990) Characterization of rhodopsin kinase purified from bovine rod outer segments. J Biol Chem 265(5):2632–2639

89. Bayburt TH, Vishnivetskiy SA, McLean MA, Morizumi T, Huang CC, Tesmer JJG, Ernst

OP, Sligar SG, Gurevich VV (2011) Monomeric rhodopsin is sufficient for normal rhodopsin kinase (GRK1) phosphorylation and arrestin-1 binding. J Biol Chem 286(2):1420–1428

90. Hanson SM, Gurevich EV, Vishnivetskiy SA, Ahmed MR, Song XF, Gurevich VV (2007) Each rhodopsin molecule binds its own arrestin. Proc Natl Acad Sci U S A 104(9):3125–3128

91. Jastrzebska B, Orban T, Golczak M, Engel A, Palczewski K (2013) Asymmetry of the rhodopsin dimer in complex with transducin. FASEB J 27(4):1572–1584

92. Jastrzebska B, Ringler P, Lodowski DT, Moiseenkova-Bell V, Golczak M, Muller SA, Palczewski K, Engel A (2011) Rhodopsin-transducin heteropentamer: three-dimensional structure and biochemical characterization. J Struct Biol 176(3):387–394

93. Jastrzebska B, Ringler P, Palczewski K, Engel A (2013) The rhodopsin-transducin complex houses two distinct rhodopsin molecules. J Struct Biol 182(2):164–172

94. Jastrzebska B, Fotiadis D, Jang GF, Stenkamp RE, Engel A, Palczewski K (2006) Functional and structural characterization of rhodopsin oligomers. J Biol Chem 281(17):11917–11922

95. Huang CC, Orban T, Jastrzebska B, Palczewski K, Tesmer JJG (2011) Activation of G protein-coupled receptor kinase 1 involves interactions between its N-terminal region and its kinase domain. Biochemistry 50(11):1940–1949

96. Gan X, Ma Z, Deng N, Wang J, Ding J, Li L (2004) Involvement of the C-terminal proline-rich motif of G protein-coupled receptor kinases in recognition of activated rhodopsin. J Biol Chem 279(48):49741–49746

97. Binder BM, Biernbaum MS, Bownds MD (1990) Light activation of one rhodopsin molecule causes the phosphorylation of hundreds of others. A reaction observed in electropermeabilized frog rod outer segments exposed to dim illumination. J Biol Chem 265(25):15333–15340

98. Chen CK, Inglese J, Lefkowitz RJ, Hurley JB (1995) Ca(2+)-dependent interaction of recoverin with rhodopsin kinase. J Biol Chem 270(30):18060–18066

99. Clarke S (1992) Protein isoprenylation and methylation at carboxyl-terminal cysteine residues. Annu Rev Biochem 61:355–386

100. Zhao X, Yokoyama K, Whitten ME, Huang J, Gelb MH, Palczewski K (1999) A novel form of rhodopsin kinase from chicken retina and pineal gland. FEBS Lett 454(1–2):115–121

101. Inglese J, Koch WJ, Caron MG, Lefkowitz RJ (1992) Isoprenylation in regulation of signal transduction by G-protein-coupled receptor kinases. Nature 359(6391):147–150

102. Rando RR (1996) Chemical biology of protein isoprenylation/methylation. Biochim Biophys Acta 1300(1):5–16

103. Kutuzov MA, Andreeva AV, Bennett N (2012) Regulation of the methylation status of G protein-coupled receptor kinase 1 (rhodopsin kinase). Cell Signal 24(12):2259–2267

104. Lee RH, Brown BM, Lolley RN (1982) Autophosphorylation of rhodopsin kinase from retinal rod outer segments. Biochemistry 21(14):3303–3307

105. Buczylko J, Gutmann C, Palczewski K (1991) Regulation of rhodopsin kinase by autophosphorylation. Proc Natl Acad Sci U S A 88(6):2568–2572

106. Palczewski K, Buczylko J, Van Hooser P, Carr SA, Huddleston MJ, Crabb JW (1992) Identification of the autophosphorylation sites in rhodopsin kinase. J Biol Chem 267(26):18991–18998

107. Horner TJ, Osawa S, Schaller MD, Weiss ER (2005) Phosphorylation of GRK1 and GRK7 by cAMP-dependent protein kinase attenuates their enzymatic activities. J Biol Chem 280(31):28241–28250

108. Osawa S, Jo R, Xiong Y, Reidel B, Tserentsoodol N, Arshavsky VY, Iuvone PM, Weiss ER (2011) Phosphorylation of G protein-coupled receptor kinase 1 (GRK1) is regulated by light but independent of phototransduction in rod photoreceptors. J Biol Chem 286(23):20923–20929

109. Klenchin VA, Calvert PD, Bownds MD (1995) Inhibition of rhodopsin kinase by recoverin. Further evidence for a negative feedback system in phototransduction. J Biol Chem 270(27):16147–16152

110. Calvert PD, Klenchin VA, Bownds MD (1995) Rhodopsin kinase inhibition by recoverin. Function of recoverin myristoylation. J Biol Chem 270(41):24127–24129

111. Senin II, Dean KR, Zargarov AA, Akhtar M, Philippov PP (1997) Recoverin inhibits the phosphorylation of dark-adapted rhodopsin more than it does that of bleached rhodopsin: a possible mechanism through which rhodopsin kinase is prevented from participation in a side reaction. Biochem J 321(Pt 2):551–555

112. Kawamura S (1999) Calcium-dependent regulation of rhodopsin phosphorylation.

Novartis Found Symp 224:208–218, discussion 218–224

113. Makino CL, Dodd RL, Chen J, Burns ME, Roca A, Simon MI, Baylor DA (2004) Recoverin regulates light-dependent phosphodiesterase activity in retinal rods. J Gen Physiol 123(6):729–741

114. Chen CK, Woodruff ML, Chen FS, Chen Y, Cilluffo MC, Tranchina D, Fain GL (2012) Modulation of mouse rod response decay by rhodopsin kinase and recoverin. J Neurosci 32(45):15998–16006

115. Sakurai K, Chen J, Khani SC, Kefalov VJ (2015) Regulation of mammalian cone phototransduction by recoverin and rhodopsin kinase. J Biol Chem 290(14):9239–9250

116. Higgins MK, Oprian DD, Schertler GF (2006) Recoverin binds exclusively to an amphipathic peptide at the N terminus of rhodopsin kinase, inhibiting rhodopsin phosphorylation without affecting catalytic activity of the kinase. J Biol Chem 281(28):19426–19432

117. Ames JB, Levay K, Wingard JN, Lusin JD, Slepak VZ (2006) Structural basis for calcium-induced inhibition of rhodopsin kinase by recoverin. J Biol Chem 281(48):37237–37245

118. Torisawa A, Arinobu D, Tachibanaki S, Kawamura S (2008) Amino acid residues in GRK1/GRK7 responsible for interaction with S-modulin/recoverin. Photochem Photobiol 84(4):823–830

119. Chen CKJ (2002) Recoverin and rhodopsin kinase. Photoreceptors Calcium 514:101–107

120. Zernii EY, Komolov KE, Permyakov SE, Kolpakova T, Dell'Orco D, Poetzsch A, Knyazeva EL, Grigoriev II, Permyakov EA, Senin II, Philippov PP, Koch KW (2011) Involvement of the recoverin C-terminal segment in recognition of the target enzyme rhodopsin kinase. Biochem J 435:441–450

121. Komolov KE, Zinchenko DV, Churumova VA, Vaganova SA, Weiergraber OH, Senin II, Philippov PP, Koch KW (2005) One of the Ca2+ binding sites of recoverin exclusively controls interaction with rhodopsin kinase. Biol Chem 386(3):285–289

122. Iacovelli L, Sallese M, Mariggio S, De Blasi A (1999) Regulation of G-protein-coupled receptor kinase subtypes by calcium sensor proteins. FASEB J 13(1):1–8

123. Senin II, Zargarov AA, Alekseev AM, Gorodovikova EN, Lipkin VM, Philippov PP (1995) N-myristoylation of recoverin enhances its efficiency as an inhibitor of rhodopsin kinase. FEBS Lett 376(1-2):87–90

124. Tachibanaki S, Nanda K, Sasaki K, Ozaki K, Kawamura S (2000) Amino acid residues of S-modulin responsible for interaction with rhodopsin kinase. J Biol Chem 275(5):3313–3319

125. Levay K, Satpaev DK, Pronin AN, Benovic JL, Slepak VZ (1998) Localization of the sites for Ca2+-binding proteins on G protein-coupled receptor kinases. Biochemistry 37(39):13650–13659

126. Pronin AN, Satpaev DK, Slepak VZ, Benovic JL (1997) Regulation of G protein-coupled receptor kinases by calmodulin and localization of the calmodulin binding domain. J Biol Chem 272(29):18273–18280

127. Chuang TT, Paolucci L, DeBlasi A (1996) Inhibition of G protein-coupled receptor kinase subtypes by Ca2+/calmodulin. J Biol Chem 271(45):28691–28696

128. Grigoriev II, Senin II, Tikhomirova NK, Komolov KE, Permyakov SE, Zernii EY, Koch KW, Philippov PP (2012) Synergetic effect of recoverin and calmodulin on regulation of rhodopsin kinase. Front Mol Neurosci 5:28

129. Arinobu D, Tachibanaki S, Kawamura S (2010) Larger inhibition of visual pigment kinase in cones than in rods. J Neurochem 115(1):259–268

130. Bruel C, Cha K, Niu L, Reeves PJ, Khorana HG (2000) Rhodopsin kinase: two mAbs binding near the carboxyl terminus cause time-dependent inactivation. Proc Natl Acad Sci U S A 97(7):3010–3015

131. Carman CV, Lisanti MP, Benovic JL (1999) Regulation of G protein-coupled receptor kinases by caveolin. J Biol Chem 274(13):8858–8864

132. Berta AI, Boesze-Battaglia K, Magyar A, Szel A, Kiss AL (2011) Localization of caveolin-1 and c-src in mature and differentiating photoreceptors: raft proteins co-distribute with rhodopsin during development. J Mol Histol 42(6):523–533

133. Lebioda L, Hargrave PA, Palczewski K (1990) X-ray crystal-structure of sangivamycin, a potent inhibitor of protein-kinases. FEBS Lett 266(1-2):102–104

134. Palczewski K, Kahn N, Hargrave PA (1990) Nucleoside inhibitors of rhodopsin kinase. Biochemistry 29(26):6276–6282

135. Homan KT, Larimore KM, Elkins JM, Szklarz M, Knapp S, Tesmer JJ (2015) Identification and structure-function analysis of subfamily selective g protein-coupled receptor kinase inhibitors. ACS Chem Biol 10(1):310–319

136. Homan KT, Wu E, Cannavo A, Koch WJ, Tesmer JJ (2014) Identification and charac-

terization of amlexanox as a G protein-coupled receptor kinase 5 inhibitor. Molecules 19(10):16937–16949

137. Thal DM, Homan KT, Chen J, Wu EK, Hinkle PM, Huang ZM, Chuprun JK, Song J, Gao E, Cheung JY, Sklar LA, Koch WJ, Tesmer JJ (2012) Paroxetine is a direct inhibitor of g protein-coupled receptor kinase 2 and increases myocardial contractility. ACS Chem Biol 7(11):1830–1839

138. Rasmussen SG, DeVree BT, Zou Y, Kruse AC, Chung KY, Kobilka TS, Thian FS, Chae PS, Pardon E, Calinski D, Mathiesen JM, Shah ST, Lyons JA, Caffrey M, Gellman SH, Steyaert J, Skiniotis G, Weis WI, Sunahara RK, Kobilka BK (2011) Crystal structure of the beta2 adrenergic receptor-Gs protein complex. Nature 477(7366):549–555

Chapter 3

Visual G Protein-Coupled Receptor Kinases

Chih-Chun Hsu and Ching-Kang Jason Chen

Abstract

Discovered in the 1970s, cloned in the 1990s, and extensively studied both biochemically and genetically over the past four decades, G protein-coupled receptor kinase 1 (GRK1), and a close homolog GRK7, are indispensable for timely phototransduction recovery and dark adaptation of retinal rod and cone photoreceptors. By phosphorylating activated visual pigments, these GRKs enable the binding of visual arrestins to photoexcited pigments to stop phototransduction at the receptor level. Mutations in the GRK1 gene cause a form of stationary night blindness in humans called *Oguchi* disease, with peculiar physiological and anatomical symptoms. Whereas the importance of these visual GRKs is well established, many questions remain unanswered with regard to expression, posttranslational modifications, substrate specificity, enzymatic actions, intracellular targeting, and regulation by other proteins. This chapter summarizes the current state of knowledge, discusses the relationship between GRK1 and GRK7 in the context of *Oguchi* disease, and pinpoints fruitful future directions for advancement of the vision research field.

Key words G protein-coupled receptor kinase 1 (GRK1), G protein-coupled receptor kinase 7 (GRK7), Retina, Photoreceptors, Phototransduction, Visual pigment, Recoverin/S-modulin, *Oguchi* disease

1 Introduction

G protein-coupled receptors (GPCRs) are the largest group of membrane receptors in eukaryotes. These receptors act through heterotrimeric G proteins to regulate intracellular second messenger levels in response to extracellular stimuli. They participate in a wide range of physiological processes such as hormonal action, neurotransmission, and sensation of light, smell, and taste. Efficient GPCR signaling requires that the lifetime of activated receptor be tightly controlled. Rapid termination of activated GPCRs involves the concerted actions of GPCR kinases (GRKs) and arrestins. GRKs catalyze phosphorylation of Ser/Thr residues located in intracellular loops and C-terminal tail of activated GPCRs to promote binding of arrestins, which prevents further G-protein activation [1]. Members of the GRK family are single unit kinases [2], which can be divided into three subgroups based on sequence

Vsevolod V. Gurevich et al. (eds.), *G Protein-Coupled Receptor Kinases*, Methods in Pharmacology and Toxicology,
DOI 10.1007/978-1-4939-3798-1_3, © Springer Science+Business Media New York 2016

homology and function. The ubiquitously expressed GRK2-like subfamily contains GRK2 and GRK3. The GRK4-like subfamily consists of GRK4, GRK5, and GRK6, with the latter two being ubiquitously expressed and the former one with a restricted expression pattern in testis and cerebellum. The two members of the GRK1-like subfamily: GRK1 and GRK7, are expressed specifically in retinal photoreceptors [3]. All GRKs have a similar structural organization with an N-terminal helical region of about 20 amino acids [4], followed by a Regulator of G-protein Signaling (RGS) homology (RH) domain [5–7], a conserved serine/threonine kinase domain, and a variable and long carboxyl-terminal domain unique to each of the three subfamilies. The N-terminal regions of GRK4, GRK5, and GRK6 interact with phosphatidylinositol 4,5-bisphosphate (PIP_2) [8]. GRK2 also interacts with $G\alpha_q$ family members through its RH domain [5, 6]. The C-terminal regions contain different protein motifs that contribute to the diversity of GRK function, regulation, and interaction. GRK2 and GRK3 contain a pleckstrin homology (PH) domain required for interactions with PIP_2 and $G\beta\gamma$ subunits [9]. GRK4-like members have palmitoylation sites at certain cysteine residues, along with other membrane targeting motifs [2]. The two visual GRKs (GRK1 and GRK7) have the so-called CaaX boxes, which are sites for protein prenylation and subsequent modifications [10]. The importance and regulation of GRK2- and GRK4-like GRKs are covered in accompanying chapters, whereas this chapter focuses on GRK1 and GRK7, the so-called visual GRKs.

Historically, enzymatic activities capable of phosphorylating visual pigment in a light-dependent manner in vertebrate retinal extracts were noted in the early 1970s [11, 12]. However, despite efforts from many laboratories over subsequent decades, pinpointing the exact identity of the responsible protein(s) and isolating it in sufficient purity and quantity proved to be challenging (for a review, see [13]). A key advance was made by the cloning of GRK1 [14], which came shortly after the cloning of GRK2 [15]. Subsequently, principal findings were made regarding the function of GRK1 in timely termination of phototransduction in mammalian retinal photoreceptors [16–19]. The realization of the existence of an additional visual GRK dates back to the cloning of OIGRK-C in medaka fish, *Oryzias latipes* in 1998 [20]. The first mammalian GRK7, with 59 % sequence identity to OIGRK-C, was described soon after in two cone dominant animals: eastern chipmunk and 13-line ground squirrel [21]. Different from GRK1, which is expressed primarily in rods and occasionally in cones of certain species, GRK7 is expressed primarily in cones [3, 20, 21]. A detailed expression study later revealed that various species use GRK1 and GRK7 differently. For instance, rodents express GRK1 in both rods and cones, as there appears to be no GRK7 expression in their retinas [3, 22]. Carp, zebrafish, and human express GRK1 in rods and both GRK1 and GRK7 in cones [23–25]. The intrinsic differences between GRK1 and GRK7 as well as their expression patterns contributes to diversity in visual responses and to disparity in pathophysiologies among different species with similar gene mutations. This chapter will summarize current studies on GRK1 and GRK7, and conclude with pathological mechanisms of human *Oguchi* disease.

2   Established Roles of GRK1 and GRK7 in Phototransduction

Retinal photoreceptors convert light into electric signals by a process called phototransduction [26, 27]. In rod cells, this process is initiated by light-induced isomerization of 11-*cis*-retinal to the all-*trans* form while it is covalently attached to a lysine residue in rhodopsin. The formation of all-*trans* retinal inside the rhodopsin core induces a series of conformational changes that results in an active intermedate called metarhodopsin II (Rho*), which can catalyze the exchange of GDP for GTP on visual G-protein (transducin) α subunit, $G\alpha_t$. The GTP-bound form of transducin ($G\alpha_t$ GTP) activates phosphodiesterase 6 (Pde6) by binding and sequestering its inhibitory γ subunit, unleashing the catalytic activity of this very efficient enzyme [28]. This leads to rapid reduction of intracellular cGMP levels and closure of cGMP-gated cation channels located on the plasma membranes of rod outer segment (ROS). The reduction of cation influx leads to membrane hyperpolarization and decreased release of the neurotransmitter glutamate at the rod's synaptic terminal. Retinal photoreceptors come in different sizes in species with different body temperatures. A mathematical model factoring in these two variables [29] could approximate the activation phase of rhodopsin signaling in rods of different species and therefore activation of phototransduction was considered solved in the early 1990s. The research focus then shifted to the less-understood recovery phase of phototransduction, whose efficiency conceivably limits the temporal resolution of vision. Under this consideration, the minute-long decay time found for metarhodopsin II in vitro became glaringly incompatible with most people's living experiences and indicated the existence of fast and robust mechanisms in vivo that deactivate Rho* and other active intermediates generated during activation. In mouse ROS, timely Rho* deactivation is initiated via rapid phosphorylation by GRK1, which triggers binding of arrestin to prevent further transducin activation [16, 30]. Transgenic mice with truncated rhodopsin lacking GRK1 phosphorylation sites have greatly prolonged rod single-photon responses with an exponentially distributed duration [31, 32]. In GRK1-KO rods, both the amplitude and the duration of single-photon response are similarly increased [16]. GRK7 seems also to be essential for phototransduction recovery in cone cells because knocking down GRK7 in zebrafish slowed recovery of the cone-driven electroretinogram (ERG) response. This retinal defect seems to result in reduction of temporal contrast sensitivity under light-adapted conditions, as assayed by optokinetic response, thus establishing a role for GRK7 in the recovery phase of cone phototransdution [33]. Biochemically, GRK7 was reported to have better catalytic efficiency than GRK1 on light-dependent visual pigment phosphorylation in several systems studied [23, 24, 34]. In one study, however, recombinant GRK7 and GRK1 were found to have similar catalytic activity in phosphorylating rhodopsin with a V_{max} of 920 and 1130 nmol/min/mg kinase, respectively. GRK7 had a K_m for ATP (21.4 μM) that was twice as much as GRK1 (10.6 μM) [35]. In contrast, a study in carp showed that native GRK7 has a much higher activity than GRK1. In isolated carp cone membrane preparations, the total rate of phosphate incorporation into visual pigment increased as the bleaching level increased, while the total rate remained unchanged when the bleach level went beyond 3.9% in rod membrane preparations. This dramatic difference lead to speculations that GRK7's high catalytic activity is responsible for the much shorter cone photoresponses and the broader dynamic range of carp cone vs. rod cells without apparent saturation under very bright stimulus conditions [23]. In an attempt to compare GRK7 and GRK1 in vivo, *Vogalis et al.* generated transgenic zebrafish overexpressing either GRK1 or GRK7 in rods [36]. Results from their study, however, were a bit challenging to interpret as for unknown reasons GRK7 overexpression specifically reduced transducin level, which may have contributed to the observed lower rod sensitivity in those animals.

It is worth noting that the robust Rho* phosphorylation by GRKs does not dominate the time course of rod recovery under normal conditions in species such as mice and human, which have slenderer photoreceptors [37]. In species such as salamander with larger photoreceptors, visual pigment deactivation is rate-limiting for recovery [38]. Indeed, transgenic mouse rods with GRK1 overexpression showed no changes in the activation, and only moderately accelerated rod recovery despite dramatic enhancement of light-dependent rhodopsin phosphorylation [39]. When compared to WT rods, and those with overexpressed transducin GTPase accelerating protein (GAP), it seems that mouse rod recovery is instead rate-limited by transducin deactivation [37].

A unique property of GRKs is their selectivity for activated GPCRs. Different from other kinases, which often have multiple targets in cells, GRK1 phosphorylated C-terminal Ser/Thr residues of rhodopsin only in the presence of bleached rhodopsin [40–43]. Studies using rhodopsin C-terminal peptide showed Ser338, Ser343, and Thr336 to be the preferred GRK1 phosphorylation sites, with Ser338 and Ser343 being the major sites during recovery of phototransduction [44, 45]. Further in vivo studies found that a single phosphate group is incorporated into rhodopsin in a light-dependent manner, primarily at Ser338 under flashes but expand to Ser334 upon continuous illumination. Interestingly, dephosphorylation of Ser338 was complete within 30 min, whereas dephosphorylation of Ser334 required up to 60 min [46]. Later studies painted a somewhat different picture, with Ser343 being phosphorylated the most rapidly, followed by Ser338, and then by Ser334 [47]. Cone opsin phosphorylation sites are less scrutinized, but one study demonstrated in zebrafish blue pigment that residues at 339 or 340, 341 or 342, 348, and 349 could be phosphorylated, and in green cone cells that positions 333, 334, 344, and 341 could be phosphorylated [48]. Much less is known about the dynamics and preferred sites of mammalian cone pigment phosphorylation by visual GRKs. A systematic proteomic survey and/or generation of phospho-specific antibodies to putative Ser/Thr sites may therefore be useful for further insights.

3   Regulation of Visual GRKs

In vertebrates, GRK1 is localized to the outer segment of photoreceptors where phototransduction takes place [16, 25]. To target GRK1 to such a specialized locale, a prenyl binding protein, PrBP/δ, encoded by the *Pde6d* gene, was shown to play an important role [49, 50]. However, the best-known inhibitory regulation of visual GRKs is the calcium-dependent binding of recoverin or S-modulin to GRK1 [51–54]. This interaction occurs in solution at sub-μM range of Ca^{2+} [51]. It was reported that GRK1 and recoverin form a ternary complex with Rho* [55, 56], where the N-terminal domain of GRK1 interacted with recoverin [57] and prevented the conformational changes that move the rhodopsin C-terminal tail into the GRK1's catalytic groove, hence blocking Rho* phosphorylation [58]. The physiological relevance of this recoverin/GRK1 interaction is best demonstrated during light adaptation in recoverin knockout rods where a background light-induced acceleration of phototransduction recovery was effectively eliminated [39]. This effect was later determined not to proceed through accelerated Rho* phosphorylation, but through a yet-to-be identified mechanism on PDE deactivation [59]. Whereas background light was shown to accelerate GRK1-mediated Rho* deactivation in mouse rods in a recoverin-dependent manner [60], GRK1 could apparently affect additional phototransduction step(s). A candidate mechanism is through its N-terminal RH domain, given the precedence that the RH domain of GRK2 has weak GAP activity on $G\alpha_q$ [5]. However, when the transducin GAP complex (the complex of transducin with RGS9/Gβ5-L and γ subunit of Pde6 that enhances GTPase activity of transducin and accelerates its inactivation [61]) was inactivated, GRK1 overexpression did not rescue the delay of rod recovery [39]. Furthermore, when transducin deactivation was made not rate-limiting in rod recovery (by overexpressing transducin GAP), overexpressing GRK1 had no acceleratory effect on recovery. These data suggest that GRK1 may have other substrates than Rho* in ROS, and identifying them may shed important light onto this puzzle.

The regulation of GRK7 is less understood. The prenyl-binding protein PrBP/δ can interact with GRK7 in vitro [50]. However, the function of PrBP in GRK7 targeting to photoreceptor outer segment has not been characterized in vivo. A 20-residue N-terminal peptide derived from carp GRK7 binds and impedes S-modulin/recoverin's inhibition of kinase activity in carp cone membrane [62], suggesting that the physiological function identified for GRK1 and S-modulin/recoverin in mouse rods may be extended to photoreceptors of species where GRK7 is the primary visual GRK, e.g. in cones of pigs and dogs [22]. Visinin, a Ca^{2+} sensor similar to recoverin, is known to inhibit GRK7 activity in cone. In isolated carp rod and cone membrane preparations, S-modulin/recoverin and visinin are functionally indistinguishable. In the dark, however, the inhibition of GRK activity by visinin is 2.5 times higher in cones than that by S-modulin/recoverin in rods because the concentration of visinin (1.2 mM) is higher than S-modulin (53 μM). Not surprisingly, the N-terminal peptide of carp GRK7 also binds visinin, implying a direct interaction between the two proteins [58]. Another potentially important aspect of GRK1 and GRK7 regulation is that Ser residues in the N-terminal domain of both visual GRKs are substrates of protein kinase A (PKA), and that phosphorylation by PKA attenuates their catalytic activity [35]. The physiological relevance of this in vitro finding has not been scrutinized, but it potentially allows PKA to alter the recovery kinetics of phototransduction by slowing down deactivation of visual pigment and making it rate-limiting. Finally, GRK1 and GRK7 undergo autophosphorylation at unique C-terminal Ser residues (e.g. S488/S489 on GRK1 [63] and S490 on GRK7 [3]). The function of autophosphorylation has not been established but a report replacing endogenous GRK1 with a transgenic chimeric GRK1 without the two autophosphorylation sites found normal kinetics of rod recovery, suggesting that it is not needed for GRK activity [60]. The finding is consistent with structural studies of GRK1 which revealed that autophosphorylation is not a prerequisite for GRK1 to be active [64].

4   Posttranslational Modifications and Visual GRK Structure

The presence of a C-terminal CaaX box in both visual GRKs indicates that these kinases are isoprenylated, endoproteolyzed, and contain a terminal carboxy-methylated cysteine [65]. In an ectopic system, these isoprenylation-related modifications were needed for full kinase activity, and the length of the isoprene moiety controls GRK's membrane affinity [10]. There is no report yet on the exact state of CaaX box-mediated modification in native GRKs, but in another ectopic system, these modifications were found to be heterogeneous [66]. In mice lacking the prenyl-binding protein PrBP/δ, GRK1 transportation to the outer segment is impaired but not completely eliminated, suggesting that in addition to being needed for full kinase activity and membrane affinity, these modifications may have a role in targeting GRK1 to the outer segment [49]. Carboxyl methylation of GRK1 was found to increase in the dark-adapted retinas due to higher level of Ca^{2+}, which inhibits demethylation by recoverin. The demethylation can be stimulated by low-affinity nucleotide binding such as ATP [67]. Thus, CaaX box modification may also have a role in GRK stability in vivo.

Crystal structures of a truncated from of GRK1 and some other mutants without the CaaX box have been available since 2008 [64, 68]. This truncated recombinant GRK1 contains catalytic activity toward Rho* in vitro. In this structure, the kinase domain is comprised of a small lobe (residues 181–268) and a large lobe (residues 269–454), with the active site situated in a cleft between them. Basic residues located on surface of the large lobe are required for binding peptide substrates. The small lobe contains a phosphate-binding loop, which directly interacts with the triphosphate tail of ATP and helps to stabilize the phosphorylation transition state. Residues 455–511 are the C-terminal extension of the GRK1 kinase domain, which is composed of three critical regions: the C-terminal large lobe tether (residues 455–571), active site tether (AST; residues 472–480), and N-terminal small lobe tether (residues 498–511). C-terminal and N-terminal lobe tethers form extensive interaction with the large and small lobes, respectively, while AST contributes residues directly to the nucleotide binding site. Along with other elements in the kinase C-terminal extension, the AST is thought to coordinate nucleotide and peptide binding within GRK1. Evolutionarily speaking, GRKs appear to come from inserting a protein kinase domain within an RH domain. The RH domain of GRK1 is composed of nine typical RGS domain-like α-helices, with two additional GRK-specific helices. Because the N-terminus of GRK1 is involved in the interaction with recoverin [57] and activated receptors [69], further structural study, preferably that of a complex between GRK1 and visual pigment, will help clarify how the extreme N-terminus of GRK1 is involved in recognition of activated receptors [70]. There is currently no structural information on GRK7. However, it is noteworthy that the GRK1 and GRK7 CaaX box sequences are distinct in a way that GRK1 is supposedly farnesylated and GRK7 geranylgeranylated [65]. In an ectopic system, the isoprene moiety affects membrane affinity of recombinant GRK1 [10]. However, the majority of endogenous GRK1 in mouse retina is membrane associated in the dark and site-directed mutagenesis designed to make GRK1 geranylgeranylated did not alter the fraction of mutant GRK1 associated with membranes [39]. Targeting of GRK1 is facilitated by PrBP/δ, which has much higher affinity for farnesyl than geranylgeranyl groups [50]. It will be interesting to see whether PrBP/δ helps target GRK7 to outer segments in vivo. Despite these differences, the high sequence homology (85%) between the two visual GRKs suggests that what is found for GRK1 is likely applicable to GRK7 [3, 22].

5   *Oguchi* Disease

Described by *Chuta Oguchi* more than a century ago, *Oguchi* disease is a rare form of autosomal recessive congenital stationary night blindness characterized by slow dark adaptation and a peculiar fundus discoloration in human [19]. The fundus discoloration can be reverted upon prolonged dark adaptation. This reversal is known as the *Mizuo-Nakamura* phenomenon, and is a diagnostic hallmark for this rare form of night blindness [71]. Genetic defects underlying this disease have been found in genes essential for rhodopsin deactivation, namely, arrestin [72] and GRK1 [19, 73]. To effectively evade saturation in slenderer mammalian rods, GRK1 and arrestin work together to shorten Rho* lifetime. Mutations in either gene thus leave Rho* shutoff to its natural decay, with a time constant of minutes instead of milliseconds. To date, nine mutations in human GRK1 gene [19, 74–79] and five in arrestin gene [71, 72, 76, 80, 81] have been identified. All *Oguchi* patients are night blind and with markedly slow dark adaptation. However, their color vision and daytime visual acuity appear normal. When modeled by targeted deletion in mice, rod activities of mutant mice are in line with *Oguchi* patient symptoms. However, the severe recovery delay seen in the cone-derived ERG responses in GRK1$^{-/-}$ mice is contradictory to normal daytime vision found in most patients [18]. The disparity between human and mouse GRK7 expression offers the most parsimonious explanation why human *Oguchi* patients possess normal daytime vision [3, 73]. GRK1 is expressed in both rod and cone photoreceptors in human and mouse [18, 25]. GRK7 is expressed in human cones, but mouse cones have only GRK1 [22]. In this scenario, GRK7 is expected to substitute or compensate for the loss of GRK1 in human but not in mouse because it is not present in retina of the latter species [3, 22]. This hypothesis is supported by biochemical studies demonstrating the ability of GRK7 to phosphorylate visual pigments, and in most cases GRK7 is a superior enzyme to GRK1 [22–24, 34]. Genetic studies demonstrating the ability of GRK7 to substitute for GRK1 is currently underway in at least two laboratories, as are studies aiming at exploring the more interesting question of whether having both visual GRKs in one photoreceptor type confer any additional advantage. A published transgenic study in zebrafish to the latter effect is available [36], but results therein must be interpreted with caution due to an unexpected reduction of G protein expression in the transgenic animals used. Finally, it would be interesting to determine whether the hallmark of human *Oguchi* disease, namely, the *Mizuo-Nakamura* phenomenon, can be recapitulated in animal models. Fundus coloration reflects mostly the level of unbleached visual pigment (typically rhodopsin) in the retina. The discoloration in fundi of *Oguichi* disease patients suggests somewhat compromised pigment regeneration ability under normal light-adapted conditions. Mechanistic investigations may therefore be launched if a similar phenomenon can be ascertained in animal models.

6   Future Research Opportunities in Visual GRKs

Current research efforts on visual GRKs merely characterize their roles in vision in the context of visual pigment phosphorylation, physiological function, and to some extent pathophysiological consequences among the relatively few *Oguchi* disease patients. Although probing the fundamental properties of visual GRKs may advance the field, especially its activation mechanism and role of CaaX box modifications, developing the visual system as an in vivo and noninvasive platform to test potential drugs that preferably target one GRK over the other, or direct GRKs toward a preferred GPCR, may be equally if not more impactful. Given the readiness commercial turnkey devices currently available, such should be easy to implement. For example, one can ectopically express GRK2- or GRK4-like kinases in GRK1$^{-/-}$ background in rod or cone photoreceptor and then test whether conditions or drugs can be found to alter these GRKs' ability to substitute for GRK1. A more immediate breakthrough in visual GRK studies may be to figure out to what extent and under what conditions visual GRK activity can be modulated by other proteins such as protein kinase A [35], because reducing GRK1 levels or its catalytic activity will change the rate-limiting step of photoreceptor recovery and the duration of the photoresponse [16, 60]. It is likely that this particular form of GRK regulation contributes to the incredible dynamic range of the visual system. Finally, it is now apparent that GRK1 has additional substrates in rod outer segment [59, 82]. Identifying these substrate(s) should lead to a better understanding of GRK function in the visual system as well as in other signal transduction systems.

Acknowledgement

Ching-Kang Jason Chen is the Alice McPherson Retina Research Foundation Endowed Chair at the Baylor College of Medicine. The Department of Ophthalmology receives an unrestricted grant from Research to Prevent Blindness, Inc.

References

1. Reiter E, Lefkowitz RJ (2006) GRKs and beta-arrestins: roles in receptor silencing, trafficking and signaling. Trends Endocrinol Metab 17(4):159–165

2. Pitcher JA, Freedman NJ, Lefkowitz RJ (1998) G protein-coupled receptor kinases. Annu Rev Biochem 67:653–692

3. Chen CK, Zhang K, Church-Kopish J, Huang W, Zhang H, Chen YJ, Frederick JM, Baehr W (2001) Characterization of human GRK7 as a potential cone opsin kinase. Mol Vis 7:305–313

4. Lodowski DT, Pitcher JA, Capel WD, Lefkowitz RJ, Tesmer JJ (2003) Keeping G proteins at bay: a complex between G protein-coupled receptor kinase 2 and Gbetagamma. Science 300:1256–1262

5. Carman CV, Parent JL, Day PW, Pronin AN, Sternweis PM, Wedegaertner PB, Gilman AG, Benovic JL, Kozasa T (1999) Selective regulation of Galpha(q/11) by an RGS domain in the G protein-coupled receptor kinase, GRK2. J Biol Chem 274:34483–34492

6. Ribas C, Penela P, Murga C, Salcedo A, García-Hoz C, Jurado-Pueyo M, Aymerich I, Mayor FJ (2007) The G protein-coupled receptor kinase (GRK) interactome: role of GRKs in GPCR regulation and signaling. Biochim Biophys Acta 1768:913–922

7. Soundararajan M, Willard FS, Kimple AJ, Turnbull AP, Ball LJ, Schoch GA, Gileadi C, DE Fedorov OY, Higman VA, Hutsell SQ, Sundström M, Doyle DA, Siderovski DP (2008) Structural diversity in the RGS domain and its interaction with heterotrimeric G protein alpha-subunits. Proc Natl Acad Sci U S A 105(17):6457–6462

8. Willets JM, Challiss RA, Nahorski SR (2003) Non-visual GRKs: are we seeing the whole picture? Trends Pharmacol Sci 24:626–633

9. Pitcher JA, Touhara K, Payne ES, Lefkowitz RJ (1995) Pleckstrin homology domain-mediated membrane association and activation of the beta-adrenergic receptor kinase requires coordinate interaction with G beta gamma subunits and lipid. J Biol Chem 270:11707–11710

10. Inglese J, Glickman JF, Lorenz W, Caron MG, Lefkowitz RJ (1992) Isoprenylation of a protein kinase. Requirement of farnesylation/alpha-carboxyl methylation for full enzymatic activity of rhodopsin kinase. J Biol Chem 267(3):1422–1425

11. Frank RN, Cavanagh HD, Kenyon KR (1973) Light-stimulated phosphorylation of bovine visual pigments by adenosine triphosphate. J Biol Chem 248(2):596–609

12. Kühn H, Dreyer WJ (1972) Light dependent phosphorylation of rhodopsin by ATP. FEBS Lett 20:1–6

13. Maeda T, Imanishi Y, Palczewski K (2003) Rhodopsin phosphorylation: 30 years later. Prog Retin Eye Res 22(4):417–434

14. Lorenz W, Inglese J, Palczewski K, Onorato JJ, Caron MG, Lefkowitz RJ (1991) The receptor kinase family: primary structure of rhodopsin kinase reveals similarities to the beta-adrenergic receptor kinase. Proc Natl Acad Sci U S A 88:8715–8719

15. Benovic JL, Strasser RH, Caron MG, Lefkowitz RJ (1986) Beta-adrenergic receptor kinase: identification of a novel protein kinase that phosphorylates the agonist-occupied form of the receptor. Proc Natl Acad Sci U S A 83:2797–2801

16. Chen CK, Burns ME, Spencer M, Niemi GA, Chen J, Hurley JB, Baylor DA, Simon MI (1999) Abnormal photoresponses and light-induced apoptosis in rods lacking rhodopsin kinase. Proc Nat Acad Sci U S A 96:3718–3722

17. Khani SC, Abitbol M, Yamamoto S, Maravic-Magovcevic I, Dryja TP (1996) Characterization and chromosomal localization of the gene for human rhodopsin kinase. Genomics 35(3):571–576

18. Lyubarsky AL, Chen C-K, Simon MI, Pugh EN (2000) Mice lacking G-protein receptor kinase 1 have profoundly slowed recovery of cone-driven retinal responses. J Neurosci 20:2209–2217

19. Yamamoto S, Sippel KC, Berson EL, Dryja TP (1997) Defects in the rhodopsin kinase gene in the Oguchi form of stationary night blindness. Nat Genet 15:175–178

20. Hisatomi O, Matsuda S, Satoh T, Kotaka S, Imanishi Y, Tokunaga F (1998) A novel subtype of G-protein-coupled receptor kinase, GRK7, in teleost cone photoreceptors. FEBS Lett 424:159–164

21. Weiss ER, Raman D, Shirakawa S, Ducceschi MH, Bertram PT, Wong F, Kraft TW, Osawa S (1998) The cloning of GRK7, a candidate cone opsin kinase, from cone- and rod-dominant mammalian retinas. Mol Vis 4:27

22. Weiss ER, Ducceschi MH, Horner TJ, Li A, Craft CM, Osawa S (2001) Species-specific differences in expression of G-protein-coupled receptor kinase (GRK) 7 and GRK1 in mammalian cone photoreceptor cells: implications for cone cell phototransduction. J Neurosci 21:9175–9184

23. Tachibanaki S, Arinobu D, Shimauchi-Matsukawa Y, Tsushima S, Kawamura S (2005) Highly effective phosphorylation by G protein-coupled receptor kinase 7 of light-activated visual pigment in cones. Proc Natl Acad Sci U S A 102:9329–9334

24. Wada Y, Sugiyama J, Okano T, Fukada Y (2006) GRK1 and GRK7: unique cellular distribution and widely different activities of opsin phosphorylation in the zebrafish rods and cones. J Neurochem 98:824–837

25. Zhao X, Huang J, Khani SC, Palczewski K (1998) Molecular forms of human rhodopsin kinase (GRK1). J Biol Chem 273(9): 5124–5131

26. Chen CK (2005) The vertebrate phototransduction cascade: amplification and termination mechanisms. Rev Physiol Biochem Pharmacol 154:101–121

27. Stryer L (1986) Cyclic GMP cascade of vision. Annu Rev Neurosci 9(87-119)

28. Leskov IB, Klenchin VA, Handy JW, Whitlock GG, Govardovskii VI, Bownds MD, Lamb TD, Pugh ENJ, Arshavsky VY (2000) The gain of rod phototransduction: reconciliation of biochemical and electrophysiological measurements. Neuron 27(3):525–537

29. Lamb TD, Pugh ENJ (1992) A quantitative account of the activation steps involved in phototransduction in amphibian photoreceptors. J Physiol 449:719–758

30. Xu J, Dodd RL, Makino CL, Simon MI, Baylor DA, Chen J (1997) Prolonged photoresponses in transgenic mouse rods lacking arrestin. Nature 389:505–509

31. Chen J, Makino CL, Peachey NS, Baylor DA, Simon MI (1995) Mechanisms of rhodopsin inactivation in vivo as revealed by a COOH-terminal truncation mutant. Science 267(5196):374–377

32. Mendez A, Burns ME, Roca A, Lem J, Wu LW, Simon MI, Baylor DA, Chen J (2000) Rapid and reproducible deactivation of rhodopsin requires multiple phosphorylation sites. Neuron 28(1):153–164

33. Rinner O, Makhankov YV, Biehlmaier O, Neuhauss SC (2005) Knockdown of cone-specific kinase GRK7 in larval zebrafish leads to impaired cone response recovery and delayed dark adaptation. Neuron 47:231–242

34. Liu P, Osawa S, Weiss ER (2005) M opsin phosphorylation in intact mammalian retinas. J Neurochem 93:135–144

35. Horner TJ, Osawa S, Schaller MD, Weiss ER (2005) Phosphorylation of GRK1 and GRK7 by cAMP-dependent protein kinase attenuates their enzymatic activities. J Biol Chem 280:28241–28250

36. Vogalis F, Shiraki T, Kojima D, Wada Y, Nishiwaki Y, Jarvinen JL, Sugiyama J, Kawakami K, Masai I, Kawamura S, Fukada Y, Lamb TD (2011) Ectopic expression of cone-specific G-protein-coupled receptor kinase GRK7 in zebrafish rods leads to lower photosensitivity and altered responses. J Physiol 589(Pt 9):2321–2348

37. Krispel CM, Chen D, Melling N, Chen YJ, Martemyanov KA, Quillinan N, Arshavsky VY, Wensel TG, Chen CK, Burns ME (2006) RGS expression rate-limits recovery of rod photoresponses. Neuron 51(4):409–416

38. Matthews HR, Sampath AP (2010) Photopigment quenching is Ca2+ dependent and controls response duration in salamander L-cone photoreceptors. J Gen Physiol 135(4): 355–366

39. Chen CK, Woodruff ML, Chen FS, Chen Y, Cilluffo MC, Tranchina D, Fain GL (2012) Modulation of mouse rod response decay by rhodopsin kinase and recoverin. J Neurosci 32(45):15998–16006

40. Brown NG, Fowles C, Sharma R, Akhtar M (1992) Mechanistic studies on rhodopsin kinase. Light-dependent phosphorylation of C-terminal peptides of rhodopsin. Eur J Biochem 208(3):659–667

41. McCarthy NE, Akhtar M (2002) Activation of rhodopsin kinase. Biochem J 363(Pt 2):359–364

42. Palczewski K, Buczylko J, Kaplan MW, Polans AS, Crabb JW (1991) Mechanism of rhodopsin kinase activation. J Biol Chem 266: 12949–12955

43. Shi GW, Chen J, Concepcion F, Motamedchaboki K, Marjoram P, Langen R, Chen J (2005) Light causes phosphorylation of nonactivated visual pigments in intact mouse rod photoreceptor cells. J Biol Chem 280:41184–41191

44. Ohguro H, Palczewski K, Ericsson LH, Walsh KA, Johnson RS (1993) Sequential phosphorylation of rhodopsin at multiple sites. Biochemistry 32(21):5718–5724

45. Papac DI, Oatis JEJ, Crouch RK, Knapp DR (1993) Mass spectrometric identification of phosphorylation sites in bleached bovine rhodopsin.Biochemistry 32(23):5930–5934

46. Ohguro H, Van Hooser JP, Milam AH, Palczewski K (1995) Rhodopsin phosphorylation and dephosphorylation in vivo. J Biol Chem 270(24):14259–14262

47. Kennedy MJ, Lee KA, Niemi GA, Craven KB, Garwin GG, Saari JC, Hurley JB (2001) Multiple phosphorylation of rhodopsin and the in vivo chemistry underlying rod photoreceptor dark adaptation. Neuron 31(1): 87–101

48. Kennedy MJ, Dunn FA, Hurley JB (2004) Visual pigment phosphorylation but not transducin translocation can contribute to light adaptation in zebrafish cones. Neuron 41(6):915–928

49. Zhang H, Li S, Doan T, Rieke F, Detwiler PB, Frederick JM, Baehr W (2007) Deletion of PrBP/delta impedes transport of GRK1 and PDE6 catalytic subunits to photoreceptor outer segments. Proc Natl Acad Sci U S A 104(21):8857–8862

50. Zhang H, Liu XH, Zhang K, Chen CK, Frederick JM, Prestwich GD, Baehr W (2004) Photoreceptor cGMP phosphodiesterase delta subunit (PDEdelta) functions as a prenylbinding protein. J Biol Chem 279(1): 407–413

51. Chen C-K, Inglese J, Lefkowitz RJ, Hurley JB (1995) Ca2+-dependent interaction of recoverin with rhodopsin kinase. J Biol Chem 270:18060–18066

52. Kawamura S (1993) Rhodopsin phosphorylation as a mechanism of cyclic GMP phosphodiesterase regulation by S-modulin. Nature 362(6423):855–857

53. Kawamura S, Takamatsu K, Kitamura K (1992) Purification and characterization of S-modulin, a calcium-dependent regulator on cGMP phosphodiesterase in frog rod photoreceptors. Biochem Biophys Res Commun 186(1): 411–417

54. Klenchin VA, Calvert PD, Bownds MD (1995) Inhibition of rhodopsin kinase by recoverin. Further evidence for a negative feedback system in phototransduction. J Biol Chem 270:16147–16152

55. Iacovelli L, Sallese M, Mariggiò S, de Blasi A (1999) Regulation of G-protein-coupled receptor kinase subtypes by calcium sensor proteins. FASEB J 13(1):1–8

56. Senin I, Koch KW, Philippov PP (2002) Ca2+-dependent control of rhodopsin phosphorylation: recoverin and rhodopsin kinase. Adv Exp Med Biol 514:69–99

57. Ames JB, Levay K, Wingard JN, Lusin JD, Slepak VZ (2006) Structural basis for calcium-induced inhibition of rhodopsin kinase by recoverin. J Biol Chem 281(48):37234–37245

58. Arinobu D, Tachibanaki S, Kawamura S (2010) Larger inhibition of visual pigment kinase in cones than in rods. J Neurochem 115(1):259–268

59. Chen CK, Woodruff ML, Fain GL (2015) Rhodopsin kinase and recoverin modulate phosphodiesterase during mouse photoreceptor light adaptation. J Gen Physiol 145(3):213–224

60. Chen CK, Woodruff ML, Chen FS, Chen D, Fain GL (2010) Background light produces a recoverin-dependent modulation of activated-rhodopsin lifetime in mouse rods. J Neurosci 30:1213–1220

61. Makino ER, Handy JW, Li T, Arshavsky VY (1999) The GTPase activating factor for transducin in rod photoreceptors is the complex between RGS9 and type 5G protein beta subunit. Proc Natl Acad Sci U S A 96(5): 1947–1952

62. Torisawa A, Arinobu D, Tachibanaki S, Kawamura S (2008) Amino acid residues in GRK1/GRK7 responsible for interaction with S-modulin/recoverin. Photochem Photobiol 84(4):823–830

63. Palczewski K, Buczyłko J, Van Hooser P, Carr SA, Huddleston MJ, Crabb JW (1992) Identification of the autophosphorylation sites in rhodopsin kinase. J Biol Chem 267(26): 18991–18998

64. Singh P, Wang B, Maeda T, Palczewski K, Tesmer JJ (2008) Structures of rhodopsin kinase in different ligand states reveal key elements involved in G protein-coupled receptor kinase activation. J Biol Chem 283: 14053–14062

65. Lane KT, Beese LS (2006) Thematic review series: lipid posttranslational modifications. Structural biology of protein farnesyltransferase and geranylgeranyltransferase type I. J Lipid Res 47(4):681–699

66. Bruel C, Cha K, Reeves PJ, Getmanova E, Khorana HG (2000) Rhodopsin kinase: expression in mammalian cells and a two-step purification. Proc Natl Acad Sci U S A 97(7): 3004–3009

67. Kutuzov MA, Andreeva AV, Bennett N (2012) Regulation of the methylation status of G protein-coupled receptor kinase 1 (rhodopsin kinase). Cell Signal 24(12):2259–2267

68. Tesmer JJ, Nance MR, Singh P, Lee H (2012) Structure of a monomeric variant of rhodopsin kinase at 2.5 A resolution. Acta Crystallogr Sect F Struct Biol Cryst Commun 68(Pt 6):622–625

69. Huang CC, Orban T, Jastrzebska B, Palczewski K, Tesmer JJ (2011) Activation of G protein-coupled receptor kinase 1 involves interactions between its N-terminal region and its kinase domain. Biochemistry 50:1940–1949

70. Homan KT, Wu E, Wilson MW, Singh P, Larsen SD, Tesmer JJG (2014) Structural and functional analysis of G protein-coupled receptor kinase inhibition by paroxetine and a rationally designed analog. Mol Pharmacol 85(2):237–248

71. Sonoyama H, Shinoda K, Ishigami C, Tada Y, Ideta H, Ideta R, Takahashi M, Miyake Y (2011) Oguchi disease masked by retinitis pigmentosa. Doc Ophthalmol 123(2):127–133

72. Fuchs S, Nakazawa M, Maw M, Tamai M, Oguchi Y, Gal A (1995) A homozygous 1-base pair deletion in the arrestin gene is a frequent cause of Oguchi disease in Japanese. Nat Genet 10(3):360–362

73. Cideciyan AV, Zhao X, Nielsen L, Khani SC, Jacobson SG, Palczewski K (1998) Null mutation in the rhodopsin kinase gene slows recovery kinetics of rod and cone phototransduction in man. Proc Natl Acad Sci U S A 95(1):328–333

74. Azam M, Collin RW, Khan MI, Shah ST, Qureshi N, Ajmal M, den Hollander AI, Qamar R, Cremers FP (2009) A novel mutation in GRK1 causes Oguchi disease in a consanguineous Pakistani family. Mol Vis 15:1788–1793

75. Hayashi T, Gekka T, Takeuchi T, Goto-Omoto S, Kitahara K (2007) A novel homozygous GRK1 mutation (P391H) in 2 siblings with Oguchi disease with markedly reduced cone responses. Ophthalmology 114:134–141

76. Huang L, Li W, Tang W, Zhu X, Ou-Yang P, Lu G (2012) A Chinese family with Oguchi's disease due to compound heterozygosity including a novel deletion in the arrestin gene. Mol Vis 18:528–536

77. Oishi A, Akimoto M, Kawagoe N, Mandai M, Takahashi M, Yoshimura N (2007) Novel mutations in the GRK1 gene in Japanese patients with Oguchi disease. Am J Ophthalmol 144:475–477

78. Skorczyk-Werner AJ, Kociecki J, Wawrocka A, Wicher K, Krawczyński MR (2015) The first case of Oguchi disease, type 2 in a Polish patient with confirmed GRK1 gene mutation. Klin Oczna 117(1):27–30

79. Zhang Q, Zulfiqar F, Riazuddin SA, Xiao X, Yasmeen A, Rogan PK, Caruso R, Sieving PA, Riazuddin S, Hejtmancik JF (2005) A variant form of Oguchi disease mapped to 13q34 associated with partial deletion of GRK1 gene. Mol Vis 11:977–985

80. Nakamura M, Miyake Y (2004) Molecular genetic study of congenital stationary night blindness. Nippon Ganka Gakkai Zasshi 108(11):665–673

81. Waheed NK, Qavi AH, Malik SN, Maria M, Riaz M, Cremers FP, Azam M, Qamar R (2012) A nonsense mutation in S-antigen (p.Glu306*) causes Oguchi disease. Mol Vis 18:1253–1259

82. Gurevich EV, Tesmer JJ, Mushegian A, Gurevich VV (2012) G protein-coupled receptor kinases: more than just kinases and not only for GPCRs. Pharmacol Ther 133:40–69

Chapter 4

Molecular Basis for Targeting, Inhibition, and Receptor Phosphorylation in the G Protein-Coupled Receptor Kinase 4 Subfamily

Tyler S. Beyett, Sumit J. Bandekar, and John J.G. Tesmer

Abstract

G protein-coupled receptor (GPCR) kinases (GRKs) regulate many physiological processes by serving as a feedback mechanism that dampens extracellular signals during stress. The seven human GRKs belong to three subfamilies with distinct structural features and membrane targeting mechanisms. Although crystal structures representing each subfamily have now been reported, a recent series of GRK4 subfamily structures provide new information about how these enzymes interact with membranes and how they might be regulated. This review highlights these advances and discusses why GRK4 subfamily members may be more predisposed than other GRKs to phosphorylate both active and inactive forms of GPCRs.

Key words Ca^{2+}·calmodulin, Desensitization, G-protein-coupled receptors (GPCRs), GPCR kinases (GRKs), Hypertension, Hypertrophy, Inhibition, Membrane targeting, Parkinson's disease, Phosphorylation, PIP_2

1 Introduction

G protein-coupled receptors (GPCRs) constitute a large family of cell-surface receptors that contribute to three of the five primary senses and are involved in a host of other key physiological processes such as regulation of heart contractility and neurotransmission [1]. GPCR signaling is initiated upon the binding of an extracellular cue, which elicits a conformational change in the receptor that promotes its ability to bind and catalyze the exchange of bound GDP for GTP on the Gα subunit of heterotrimeric G proteins. The heterotrimeric G protein then dissociates into Gα·GTP and Gβγ components, which in turn instigate downstream intracellular signaling events [2].

GPCR signaling is rapidly desensitized at multiple levels to allow for adaptation and to avoid cellular damage. Desensitization at the level of the receptor is primarily instigated by a family of

Vsevolod V. Gurevich et al. (eds.), *G Protein-Coupled Receptor Kinases*, Methods in Pharmacology and Toxicology, DOI 10.1007/978-1-4939-3798-1_4, © Springer Science+Business Media New York 2016

GPCR kinases (GRKs), which phosphorylate activated GPCRs on serine or threonine residues in their extended third cytoplasmic loops or C-terminal tails, which primes these receptors for binding arrestins. The arrestin–GPCR complex is unable to couple with additional heterotrimeric G proteins and targeted to clathrin-coated pits for receptor endocytosis. Internalized receptors are then either degraded or recycled back to the membrane [3].

GRKs are grouped into three subfamilies [4] that differ most obviously in the structure of their C-termini, which encode different modes of membrane targeting. The GRK1/7 subfamily is comprised of the rhodopsin and cone opsin kinases and are prenylated at their C-termini. The GRK2/3 subfamily has a C-terminal pleckstrin homology (PH) domain that binds PIP_2 and free $G\beta\gamma$ subunits. The GRK4/5/6 subfamily contains a membrane-binding amphipathic helix (αCT) and, in GRK4 and GRK6, palmitoylation sites just C-terminal to this helix (Fig. 1). With the exception of GRK1 and 7, which are primarily expressed in retinal rod and cone cells, respectively, and GRK4, which is expressed in the testes and kidney, GRKs are ubiquitously expressed and regulate a wide variety of GPCRs [3]. Although important for maintaining cellular homeostasis, excess GRK activity has been implicated in the progression of many diseases [5]: GRK2 and 5 in heart failure and cardiac hypertrophy [6], GRK4 in hypertension [6, 7], and GRK6 in Parkinson's disease [8] and multiple myeloma [9]. Loss of GRK1 activity, on the other hand, leads to a rare form of stationary night blindness [10–12].

2   GRK Structure and GPCR Interaction Models

Since 2003, multiple crystal structures have been reported for each of the three GRK subfamilies. The models all reveal a highly conserved configuration for the catalytic core, which can be thought of as a protein kinase A (PKA), G, and C (AGC) kinase domain inserted into a loop of a regulatory of G-protein signaling homology (RH) domain (Fig. 1a). The RH domain plays a scaffolding role for the various functional elements of the enzyme as well as providing a binding site for $G\alpha_q$ in the GRK2 subfamily [13] and phosphatidylinositides in the GRK4 subfamily [14]. The GRK kinase domain is characterized by small and large lobes as well as by other features characteristic of the AGC kinase family [15], including an extended "C tail" that crosses over and contributes to the active site as it spans the two lobes [16]. The GRK large lobe contains the binding site for disordered extended loops or C-termini of GPCRs that contain phosphoacceptor sites. Consistent with the broad selectivity exhibited by GRKs for GPCRs, there does not seem to be a consensus sequence other than a general preference for acidic residues preceding the phosphorylation site in peptide

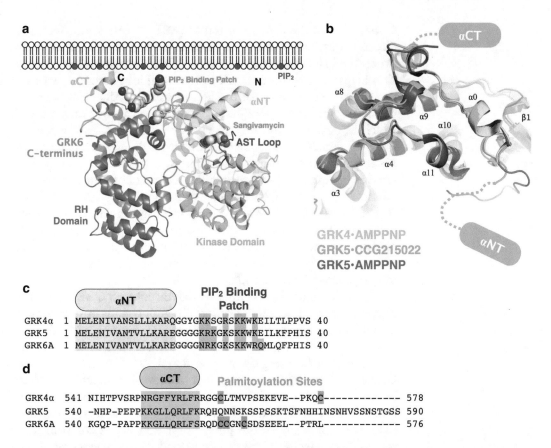

Fig. 1 GRK4 subfamily structure and membrane interaction sites. (**a**) A model of GRK5 associated with a membrane. The αNT and αCT helices from GRK6 (PDB entry 3NYN) were modeled onto GRK5 (4WNK) such that the terminal helices and basic PIP₂ binding patch were along the same plane. The C-terminus of chain B of the GRK6·sangivamycin complex is shown as it interacts with chain A. (**b**) A view of GRK4 family member structures from the perspective of the membrane, highlighting the close proximity of the termini. This is in contrast to the GRK6·sangivamycin structure where the C-terminus is far removed from the membrane (see panel **a**). The recent GRK4 and GRK5 structures may therefore represent a more membrane-associated conformation, as their termini would reside in the same plane. Primary sequences of the N-terminal (**c**) and C-terminal (**d**) regions of human GRK4 subfamily members

substrates [17–19], opposite from other AGC kinases. This likely reflects the fact that GRKs generate clusters of phosphorylated residues in GPCRs to prime them for arrestin binding. Unlike most AGC kinases, GRKs have an activation loop that does not contain phosphorylation sites. Despite this, in all crystal structures reported to date, the GRK activation loop adopts a conformation similar to those of activated canonical AGC kinase domains.

The C-tail of the kinase domain is a key regulatory element in AGC kinases [16], and typically only becomes well ordered when the two lobes of the kinase domain approach an active conformation wherein catalytic residues from both lobes are properly aligned for phosphotransfer. In activated PKA, the central region of the

C-tail, termed the active site tether (AST), spans both lobes and directly contributes to the nucleotide binding site [20]. In many other AGC kinases, phosphorylation of the C-tail at two conserved sites helps to anchor the C-tail to the small lobe, thereby favoring the active configuration of the kinase domain. Most GRKs retain the first of these phosphorylation sites, known as the "turn motif," which is located in the AST [15]. The GRK AST, however, contains a significantly shorter domain-bridging loop near its N-terminus than in other AGC kinases, and thus has been postulated as being insufficient to stabilize a closed conformation of the kinase domain on its own, even upon addition of excess ATP or ATP analogs (Fig. 2a) [3]. In most previously reported GRK structures, the AST is either poorly ordered or completely unresolved, consistent with the inactive conformations of their kinase domains. When segments of the AST are observed, they are typically involved in strong crystal contacts [21].

In addition to the RH-kinase catalytic core, all GRKs contain a highly conserved helical region of ~20 amino acids at their amino terminus strongly implicated in direct interactions with GPCRs (Fig. 1a, c) [22–27]. In all but two GRK crystal structures, this N-terminal helical region is disordered. The structure of the GRK1·ATP complex was the first to reveal a nearly complete N-terminal region, which was unexpectedly phosphorylated and bound to the cleft formed between the kinase and RH domains [21]. It is not known if this phosphorylation site or conformation is physiologically meaningful. The second structure was that of the GRK6·sangivamycin complex [25], which features a kinase domain conformation more similar to that of the transition state structure of PKA than any GRK published to date. The large and small lobes in the GRK6·sangivamycin complex are only 7° more "open" than those of PKA, key catalytic residues are close to being in the correct configuration for the phosphotransfer reaction, and most of the AST is ordered. In this complex, the N-terminal region of GRK6 forms a single helix (αNT) that packs alongside the AST, together forming a bridge between the small and large lobes and interacting with residues known to be required for kinase activity [28]. Despite the shorter loop at the amino terminus of the AST, the GRK6 AST otherwise adopts a trajectory across the kinase domain similar to that observed in the transition-state structure of PKA (Fig. 2a).

The interaction between αNT and the AST, positioned immediately over the hinge of the kinase domain, suggests a model for how activated GPCRs allosterically control the degree of domain closure and GRK activity. Although the αNT helix in the GRK6·sangivamycin complex is stabilized by a non-physiological crystal contact with a symmetry-related αNT helix, this lattice contact may mimic the interaction of the αNT helix with a GPCR substrate, or at least with an environment that stabilizes the active

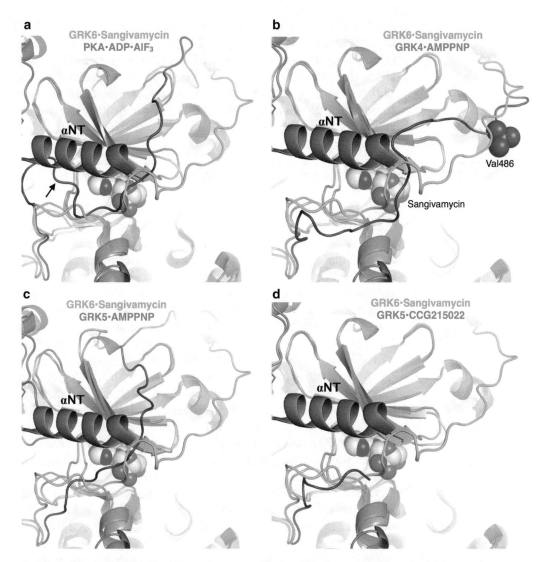

Fig. 2 Different configurations of the AST region in GRK4 subfamily members. The AST of GRK6·sangivamycin (PDB entry 3NYN) compared with those in (**a**) transition-state PKA (1L3R), (**b**) GRK4-A486V·AMPPNP (4YHJ), (**c**) GRK5·AMPPNP (4TND), and (**d**) GRK5·CCG215022 (4WNK). The GRK6 AST is colored *green*, and those of PKA, GRK4, and GRK5 are magenta. All proteins were aligned using the small lobe of the kinase omitting the P-loop. PKA has a more extended loop near the N-terminus of the AST, as indicated by the arrow in panel **a**, which may aid in kinase closure and activation. The loop is shorter in GRKs, thereby helping to create the αNT binding site. The AST of GRK4·AMPPNP (chain A) and GRK5·AMPPNP are relatively well ordered, but take different routes across the surface of the small lobe of the kinase. The AST loop in the GRK5·CCG215022 structure is not resolved beyond residue 473

conformation of the kinase. Indeed, GRKs are not very specific for their GPCR substrates other than the fact that they favor the agonist-bound form, and any close packing environment with complementary physicochemical features to the αNT/AST surface may be sufficient to activate the kinase domain. Mutational studies of αNT in GRK6 [25], GRK1 [26], and most recently GRK2 [27] support a model wherein exposed hydrophobic residues at the tip of the helix are important for GPCR phosphorylation, whereas those that pack against the kinase domain are important for the phosphorylation of both receptors and soluble substrates because these latter interactions help stabilize a catalytically competent configuration of the kinase domain.

3   New GRK4 Subfamily Structures and Kinase Domain Activation

In 2015, three different structural analyses of GRK4 subfamily members were published, providing significant insights into the structure and function of this GRK subfamily, in particular about its possible mechanisms of membrane association. One paper describes human GRK5 complexes with the nucleoside analog sangivamycin and the non-hydrolyzable ATP analog β,γ-imidoadenosine 5′-triphosphate (AMPPNP) [29]. Both represent the same crystal form. The second reports the structure of bovine GRK5 co-crystallized with a rationally designed ATP-competitive inhibitor CCG215022 [30]. The third reports the structure of the A486V mutant of human GRK4 in complex with AMPPNP [31]. Interestingly, none of these structures exhibit an RH domain-mediated domain-swapped dimer similar to those observed in prior structures of GRK6 and wild-type GRK1 [21, 25, 32]. GRK4 instead crystallized as a distinct homodimer that buries ~5000 Å^2 of accessible surface area involving the activation loop of one sub-unit packing against the RH and kinase domains of another. The physiological significance of this novel dimer interface is not clear. Sedimentation equilibrium analysis demonstrated that GRK4 is a monomer in solution [31], and although residues in the interface are somewhat conserved throughout the GRK4 subfamily, they are primarily hydrophilic in nature and unlikely to persist under physiological conditions.

The AST is well ordered in chain A (but not chain B) of the GRK4·AMPPNP structure, and also in the GRK5·sangivamycin/AMPPNP structures. Whereas the AST region in GRK4 packs over the active site similarly to the AST in the GRK6·sangivamycin structure and in other active AGC kinases (Fig. 2b), those of GRK5 adopt a dramatically different path (Fig. 2c) (although similar in its C-terminal region to the AST of PKA, cf. Fig. 2a). The AST of the GRK5·CCG215022 complex is only resolved up to residue Tyr473, an extent similar to what is observed in previous GRK1 and GRK4 subfamily structures, including chain B of the new GRK4 structure (Fig. 2d). Does the presence of an ordered AST region indicate that some of these new structures represent active configurations?

To help answer this question, the relative orientation of the small and large lobes can be compared to that of the transition state structure of PKA (Fig. 3). The GRK6·sangivamycin complex remains the most active-like structure by this criterion, as its lobes are rotated apart by only 7° from that of PKA. Those of GRK5·CCG215022 are ~11° more open than that of PKA, those of GRK5 in the AMPPNP/sangivamycin bound state are ~15° more open, and those of GRK4·AMPPNP are ~17° more open and most closely resemble that of the previously determined GRK6·AMPPNP structure [32]. Thus, all three new GRK4 subfamily structures exhibit relatively inactive kinase domain conformations irrespective of the degree of order in their AST regions. AST ordering in these structures is most easily explained by the fact that AST residues 476–488 in chain A of GRK4, and residues 470–475 and 487–493 in GRK5 are involved in extensive crystal lattice contacts, which likely dictate both the structure and trajectory of their AST loops.

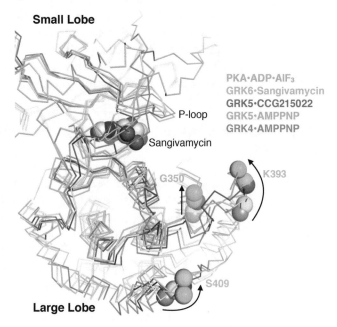

Fig. 3 Comparison of GRK4 subfamily member structures with the transition-state model of PKA, showing changes in the relative orientation of the large and small lobes associated with activation. Shown are PKA (*green*, 1L3R), GRK6·sangivamycin (*cyan*, 3NYN), GRK5·CCG215022 (*magenta*, 4WNK), GRK5·AMPPNP (*yellow*, 4TND), and GRK4 A486V (*salmon*, 4YHJ). All kinases were aligned to the small lobe of PKA. Three positions in the kinase large lobe are highlighted with a sphere to help highlight the degree of closure in the large lobe. The corresponding residues in the GRK6·sangivamycin complex are noted beside each set of spheres for reference. The GRK6·sangivamycin complex exhibits the closest degree of domain closure to that of transition state PKA

Interestingly, the human GRK4 structure contains the point mutant A486V, which in the context of the GRK4γ splice variant is associated with human hypertension [7]. The A486V mutation is located in the turn motif of the AST, immediately adjacent to the Ser485 autophosphorylation site (Fig. 2a). Based on the phosphorylation of peptides derived from the dopamine D_1 receptor, the A486V mutation seems to promote kinase autophosphorylation, which in turn increases GRK4 activity on receptors [31]. Although the side chain of Val486 is disordered in Chain A of the GRK4 crystal structure, modeling indicates that the side chain would not be in an orientation that could make intramolecular contacts with the small lobe. Thus the simplest molecular explanation for the kinetic effects of the A486V mutation is that it enhances the interaction of the AST region with the GRK4 kinase large lobe during the process of autophosphorylation. However, it should be noted that this region of the GRK4 AST is ordered by a nearby crystal contact and thus could be in a non-physiological configuration. Interestingly, threonine and valine are found at the analogous position of GRK4 from other species, including other primates. Thus, although described as a "constitutively active" mutant, it may simply be a polymorphism that restores activity to an otherwise partially disabled kinase. Humans may therefore have evolved a GRK4 with Ala486 to repress its activity in cellular contexts that are unique to our species.

4   New GRK4 Subfamily Structures Refine Mechanisms of Membrane Localization

GRK4 family members are believed to be in equilibrium with the plasma membrane due to their ability to bind negatively charged phospholipids via two regions: a basic patch formed by residues from the RH domain and small lobe near the N-terminus of the enzyme [33], and a basic C-terminal region containing αCT (Fig. 1) [34, 35]. In the GRK6·sangivamycin structure, several sulfate anions are observed bound to the basic patch. These anions may mimic the binding of phosphates in the head groups of phosphatidylinositides, which are found predominantly in the inner leaflet of the plasma membrane. The close proximity of this patch to αNT is consistent with the proposed role of αNT in binding receptors, and would help explain why receptors and negatively charged membrane lipids are required for full activation of GRK4 subfamily members.

The C-terminal lipid-binding region is also well resolved in the GRK6·sangivamycin structure, but its configuration represents a bit of a conundrum. The αCT helix is far removed from the expected membrane plane as defined by the αNT helix and the

N-terminal PIP_2 binding site, and the hydrophobic residues in the C-terminal helix that presumably interact with the acyl phase of the membrane are sequestered (Fig. 1a). Furthermore, the C-terminal region of GRK6 is domain swapped across a crystallographic dimer interface formed by the RH domain. A similar domain-swapped dimer is also observed in all wild-type GRK1 structures and that of the GRK6·AMPPNP complex, although not as much of the C-terminus is ordered in these structures. Size exclusion chromatography and sedimentation equilibrium analyses are consistent with GRK6 being in a monomeric state in solution, and mutational disruption of residues in the dimer interface did not significantly affect in vitro phosphorylation of receptor substrates [32]. However, the residues that form the RH-mediated dimer interface are highly conserved among GRK1 and 4 subfamily members, suggesting that it could still represent a physiologically relevant protein–protein interaction site. Indeed, cell-based studies of GRK5 suggest that oligomerization mediated by this surface is important for its constitutive membrane association and ultimately for full activity. In this study, it was further suggested that the membrane binding motifs of an individual GRK5 subunit are insufficient for persistent membrane association [36].

The two new GRK5 structures may help resolve this C-terminal conundrum. In both unique crystal forms, GRK5 crystallized as a monomer with its C-termini forming consistent, novel structures that pack against the conserved residues of the RH domain that were involved in the previously observed RH-mediated dimer interface (Fig. 1a, b). These C-terminal structures are also free of obfuscating crystal contacts or domain swaps, which supports their physiological significance. Based on sequence conservation, it seems likely that the C-terminus of GRK6 could also form this structure if it were not for competition with the crystallographic dimer. An analogous C-terminal structure, however, was not observed in the GRK4 structure, perhaps due to relatively low sequence conservation with GRK5 and 6 in this region. Perturbation of the interface between the C-terminus and the RH domain of GRK5 led to decreased catalytic activity on receptors both in vitro and in cells [30, 36], suggesting that integrity of this interface is important for membrane-specific functions of GRK5. However, analogous mutations in GRK1 and 6 did not lead to defects, at least in vitro [21, 32]. Thus, there may be important functional differences among GRK4 subfamily members that depend on subtle changes in membrane targeting by their C-termini.

Recently, we determined a low-resolution 4 Å structure of the $GRK5_{531}$·CCG215022 complex (Bandekar, Beyett, & Tesmer, unpublished data), in which the GRK5 terminus was truncated after residue 531—thus analogous to the ordered portions of the

GRK4 structure. The overall conformation of $GRK5_{531}$ closely resembles that of the GRK5·CCG215022 structure, demonstrating that absence of the C-terminus does not influence overall conformation. Indeed, deletion of the C-terminal helix in GRK5 reduces receptor phosphorylation while having no effect on soluble substrate phosphorylation, consistent with a specific role in membrane localization [34].

It is possible that the C-termini of GRK5 and 6 can switch between an αCT sequestered (either dimeric or perhaps with the domain swap resolved) as in the GRK6·sangivamycin structure, and a monomeric membrane-competent state, as in the new structures of GRK5 (Fig. 1a). In support of this model, mutations of residues in GRK5 analogous to those in GRK6 that would interact with a sequestered C-terminus decrease thermal stability of the soluble enzyme [30]. It has also been observed that GRK6 can be orders of magnitude less efficient at phosphorylating receptor substrates than other GRKs, but just as efficient at phosphorylating peptides [18, 28], and is less strongly associated with membranes than GRK5 [37, 38]. Thus, GRK6 may more readily adopt a C-terminal sequestered state. However, there are factors that confound interpretation. The unique presence of acidic residues in the C-terminus of the GRK6A isoform relative to GRK5 and other GRK6 splice variants may lead to electrostatic repulsion of the enzyme from the inner leaflet of the membrane [37, 39]. There is also evidence that dimerization of GRK5 through its RH domain (analogous to that observed in wild-type GRK1 structures and the GRK6·sangivamycin complex) is important for dictating the membrane localization of GRK5, and hence its activity on GPCRs—in particular because the activity of variants with mutations in the putative dimerization interface can be rescued by appending additional membrane targeting motifs to the C-terminus [36].

5   Differential Roles of the N- and C-Terminal Phospholipid Binding Sites in the GRK4 Subfamily

The activities of all GRK4 subfamily members are dependent on anionic phospholipids: they not only aid in membrane recruitment, but also act as allosteric activators. Both N- and C-terminal regions of these kinases have been proposed to play a role in membrane targeting of GRK5. Recent studies employing sum frequency generation (SFG) spectroscopy attempted to better define the specific roles of these elements [40]. A peptide corresponding to residues 2–31 of GRK5 bound to model membranes constitutively, but only becomes partially helical in the presence of trifluoroethanol (TFE), a helix-inducing solvent. As this region would form the αNT helix in the full-length enzyme, addition of TFE may emulate conformational changes induced by GPCR binding. However, membrane binding of this peptide seems entirely due to the basic residues in positions 25–31, which constitute most of the proposed N-terminal PIP$_2$ binding site in GRK5 [33]. A peptide corresponding to the αCT helix of GRK5, spanning residues 546–565, also binds to membranes but adopts a partially helical configuration even in the absence of TFE. Both N- and C-terminal peptides bind membranes irrespective of the presence of PIP$_2$, but neither peptide in isolation is likely to have enough structure to dictate specific interactions with PIP$_2$. In other words, amino acids 2–31 are probably unresponsive to PIP$_2$ because their conformation is not constrained by the fold of the RH-kinase core.

SFG studies of full-length GRK5 are consistent with its adoption of a specific orientation on highly charged membrane surfaces [41]. Truncation of the C-terminal lipid binding domain had no effect, suggesting that the N-terminal patch is alone responsible for mandating a specific membrane-bound orientation compatible with GPCR binding. When the N-terminal PIP$_2$ binding patch was ablated by site-directed mutagenesis, GRK5 still bound to membranes but exhibited no specific orientation, consistent with the C-terminal αCT helix of GRK5 being attached to the rest of the kinase by a flexible tether. Thus, both lipid-binding sites in GRK5 contribute to membrane binding, but only the N-terminal site seems to mandate a specific orientation of the catalytic core.

Given the functional importance of the lipid binding sites in GRK4 subfamily members, it is not surprising that they have emerged as key regulatory sites. As noted above, acidic residues near αCT in GRK6 have profound effects on GRK6 activity [37, 39], and phosphorylation of GRK5 by PKC in its C-terminus is thought to be inhibitory due to similar electrostatic effects [42]. Calmodulin (CaM) is an intracellular Ca^{2+} sensor that binds and inhibits most GRKs, but has strong preference for GRK4 subfamily members [43, 44]. Ca^{2+}·CaM binds to both the N- and C-terminal membrane phospholipid binding motifs, consistent with the observation that Ca^{2+}·CaM can strip the 2–31 and 546–565 GRK5 peptides from lipid bilayers [40]. In cells, Ca^{2+}·CaM disrupts membrane association of GRK5 [45] and allows a nuclear localization motif in the large lobe of the kinase domain to target GRK5 to the nucleus [46, 47]. The two new GRK5 structures demonstrate that the N- and C-terminal lipid binding sites are in close proximity to each other, and thus it is possible that Ca^{2+}·CaM can bind both regions simultaneously (Fig. 1a, b). Palmitoylation also plays a role in the membrane targeting of GRK4 and GRK6 isoforms, and because palmitoylation is reversible it represents another mechanism by which to regulate the activity of GRK4 and GRK6.

6   Conclusions and Remaining Questions

With a complete set of structures now available for the GRK4 subfamily, our understanding of the structure and function is now greater than ever. This information provides hypotheses for some recent surprising biochemical observations. The paradigm of GRKs being specific for agonist-bound GPCRs has been challenged previously (see [48]), but a more comprehensive assessment has now shown that GRK5 and 6, but not GRK2, are capable of constitutive phosphorylation of a panel of GPCRs in cells [49, 50]. This phenomenon did not extend to all GPCRs, as inactive D_2 dopamine receptors were not phosphorylated by GRK5 or 6. The crystal structures for GRK4, 5, and 6 demonstrate that their kinase domains can exist in a wide range of conformations, including those anticipated to be nearly fully activated (Fig. 3). GRK2, on the other hand, has not yet been observed a similarly closed/active state. Thus, the constitutive activity of GRK4 subfamily kinases on some GPCRs may reflect their propensity to assume an active configuration on their own, perhaps simply via their interactions with phospholipids. An evolutionary explanation for constitutive activity would be to promote arrestin-mediated recycling/degradation or signaling for receptors in their basal state [49].

Crystal structures of active GPCRs in complex with nanobodies, heterotrimeric G proteins, and most recently arrestin have recently been reported [51–53]. However, an analogous GPCR–GRK structure remains elusive and is one of the most important structural targets left in the field. Such a structure would provide insights into the specific interactions formed between GPCRs and GRKs, how specificity for particular GPCRs might be achieved (e.g. for the D_2 dopamine receptor [49]), confirm what the active configuration of a GRK looks like, and provide additional hypotheses about how allosteric activation of the kinase is achieved. What are the prospects? Crystals of a GRK–GPCR complex will likely require that PIP_2 or an analogous negatively charged lipid to be reconstituted with the complex, as it has for other integral membrane protein complexes like the inwardly rectifying potassium channel [54]. The fact that GRK4 subfamily members seem to have activity against inactive receptors opens the door to using both agonist and inverse agonist stabilized forms of GPCRs as crystallographic targets (a caveat being that in this scenario GRKs may only interact with the long, flexible cytoplasmic loops and tails of inactivated receptors). The structure of G_s in complex with the β_2AR receptor was facilitated by a nanobody raised against the chemically cross-linked complex. However, the affinity of GRKs for GPCRs is comparatively much lower, and agonist-specific chemical crosslinking or the formation of an engineered disulfide bridge between GPCR and GRK has not yet been convincingly demonstrated.

The arrestin complex with a constitutively active variant of rhodopsin was achieved via the use of a constitutively active variant of arrestin predisposed for binding. Although constitutively active mutants of GRK4 like A486V have been reported, these variants seem to simply revert the sequence of the human enzyme back to those found in most other GRK4 subfamily members. Thus, a crystallographic approach remains very challenging.

Another important structurally uncharacterized GRK interaction is that of the $Ca^{2+} \cdot CaM$-GRK complex, which is of particular importance for the regulation of GRK4 subfamily members during cardiac hypertrophy [47]. Although purification of $Ca^{2+} \cdot CaM$ complexes with GRK4 subfamily members is readily achieved [44], crystallization has not yet proven successful, perhaps because $Ca^{2+} \cdot CaM$ interacts with flexible regions of the kinase, rendering the complex structurally heterogeneous. The fact that $Ca^{2+} \cdot CaM$ may interact simultaneously with two different regions of the kinase domain also suggests a non-canonical interaction, or perhaps multiple interaction modes. Despite these hurdles, we now know that all members of the GRK4 subfamily are accessible for structural analysis, and the recent structural work may provide useful information for designing new GRK variants that would facilitate crystallization of GRK-$Ca^{2+} \cdot CaM$ complexes.

Acknowledgments

This work was supported in part by NIH grants HL086865 and HL122416 to J.T., and a Pharmacological Sciences Training Program fellowship (T32-GM007767) to T.B. Use of the Advanced Photon Source, an Office of Science User Facility operated for the U.S. Department of Energy (DOE) Office of Science by Argonne National Laboratory, was supported by the U.S. DOE under Contract No. DE-AC02-06CH11357. Use of the LS-CAT Sector 21 was supported by the Michigan Economic Development Corporation and the Michigan Technology Tri-Corridor (Grant 085P1000817).

References

1. Pierce KL, Premont RT, Lefkowitz RJ (2002) Seven-transmembrane receptors. Nat Rev Mol Cell Biol 3(9):639–650

2. Gilman AG (v1987) G proteins: transducers of receptor-generated signals. Annu Rev Biochem 56:615–649

3. Gurevich EV, Tesmer JJ, Mushegian A, Gurevich VV (2012) G protein-coupled receptor kinases: more than just kinases and not only for GPCRs. Pharmacol Ther 133(1):40–69

4. Mushegian A, Gurevich VV, Gurevich EV (2012) The origin and evolution of G protein-coupled receptor kinases. PloS One 7(3): e33806

5. Metaye T, Gibelin H, Perdrisot R, Kraimps JL (2005) Pathophysiological roles of G-protein-coupled receptor kinases. Cell Signal 17(8): 917–928

6. Sato PY, Chuprun JK, Schwartz M, Koch WJ (2015) The evolving impact of G protein-

coupled receptor kinases in cardiac health and disease. Physiol Rev 95(2):377–404

7. Yang J, Villar VA, Jones JE, Jose PA, Zeng C (2015) G protein-coupled receptor kinase 4: role in hypertension. Hypertension 65(6): 1148–1155

8. Gainetdinov RR, Bohn LM, Sotnikova TD, Cyr M, Laakso A, Macrae AD, Torres GE, Kim KM, Lefkowitz RJ, Caron MG, Premont RT (2003) Dopaminergic supersensitivity in G protein-coupled receptor kinase 6-deficient mice. Neuron 38(2):291–303

9. Tiedemann RE, Zhu YX, Schmidt J, Yin H, Shi CX, Que Q, Basu G, Azorsa D, Perkins LM, Braggio E, Fonseca R, Bergsagel PL, Mousses S, Stewart AK (2010) Kinome-wide RNAi studies in human multiple myeloma identify vulnerable kinase targets, including a lymphoid-restricted kinase, GRK6. Blood 115(8): 1594–1604

10. Hayashi T, Gekka T, Takeuchi T, Goto-Omoto S, Kitahara K (2007) A novel homozygous GRK1 mutation (P391H) in 2 siblings with Oguchi disease with markedly reduced cone responses. Ophthalmology 114(1):134–141

11. Yamamoto S, Sippel KC, Berson EL, Dryja TP (1997) Defects in the rhodopsin kinase gene in the Oguchi form of stationary night blindness. Nat Genet 15(2):175–178

12. Zhang Q, Zulfiqar F, Riazuddin SA, Xiao X, Yasmeen A, Rogan PK, Caruso R, Sieving PA, Riazuddin S, Hejtmancik JF (2005) A variant form of Oguchi disease mapped to 13q34 associated with partial deletion of GRK1 gene. Mol Vis 11:977–985

13. Tesmer VM, Kawano T, Shankaranarayanan A, Kozasa T, Tesmer JJ (2005) Snapshot of activated G proteins at the membrane: the $G\alpha_q$-GRK2-G$\beta\gamma$ complex. Science 310(5754): 1686–1690

14. Homan KT, Glukhova A, Tesmer JJ (2013) Regulation of g protein-coupled receptor kinases by phospholipids. Curr Med Chem 20(1):39–46

15. Pearce LR, Komander D, Alessi DR (2010) The nuts and bolts of AGC protein kinases. Nat Rev Mol Cell Biol 11(1):9–22

16. Kannan N, Haste N, Taylor SS, Neuwald AF (2007) The hallmark of AGC kinase functional divergence is its C-terminal tail, a cis-acting regulatory module. Proc Natl Acad Sci U S A 104(4):1272–1277

17. Onorato JJ, Palczewski K, Regan JW, Caron MG, Lefkowitz RJ, Benovic JL (1991) Role of acidic amino acids in peptide substrates of the b-adrenergic receptor kinase and rhodopsin kinase. Biochemistry 30(21):5118–5125

18. Loudon RP, Benovic JL (1994) Expression, purification, and characterization of the G protein-coupled receptor kinase GRK6. J Biol Chem 269(36):22691–22697

19. Kunapuli P, Onorato JJ, Hosey MM, Benovic JL (1994) Expression, purification, and characterization of the G protein-coupled receptor kinase GRK5. J Biol Chem 269(2): 1099–1105

20. Madhusudan, Akamine P, Xuong NH, Taylor SS (2002) Crystal structure of a transition state mimic of the catalytic subunit of cAMP-dependent protein kinase. Nat Struct Biol 9(4):273–277

21. Singh P, Wang B, Maeda T, Palczewski K, Tesmer JJ (2008) Structures of rhodopsin kinase in different ligand states reveal key elements involved in G protein-coupled receptor kinase activation. J Biol Chem 283(20): 14053–14062

22. Palczewski K, Buczylko J, Lebioda L, Crabb JW, Polans AS (1993) Identification of the N-terminal region in rhodopsin kinase involved in its interaction with rhodopsin. J Biol Chem 268(8):6004–6013

23. Noble B, Kallal LA, Pausch MH, Benovic JL (2003) Development of a yeast bioassay to characterize G protein-coupled receptor kinases. Identification of an NH_2-terminal region essential for receptor phosphorylation. J Biol Chem 278(48):47466–47476

24. Pao CS, Barker BL, Benovic JL (2009) Role of the amino terminus of G protein-coupled receptor kinase 2 in receptor phosphorylation. Biochemistry 48(30):7325–7333

25. Boguth CA, Singh P, Huang CC, Tesmer JJ (2010) Molecular basis for activation of G protein-coupled receptor kinases. EMBO J 29(19):3249–3259

26. Huang CC, Orban T, Jastrzebska B, Palczewski K, Tesmer JJ (2011) Activation of G protein-coupled receptor kinase 1 involves interactions between its N-terminal region and its kinase domain. Biochemistry 50(11):1940–1949

27. Beautrait A, Michalski KR, Lopez TS, Mannix KM, McDonald DJ, Cutter AR, Medina CB, Hebert AM, Francis CJ, Bouvier M, Tesmer JJ, Sterne-Marr R (2014) Mapping the putative G protein-coupled receptor (GPCR) docking site on GPCR kinase 2: insights from intact cell phosphorylation and recruitment assays. J Biol Chem 289(36):25262–25275

28. Huang CC, Yoshino-Koh K, Tesmer JJ (2009) A surface of the kinase domain critical for the allosteric activation of G protein-coupled receptor kinases. J Biol Chem 284(25): 17206–17215

29. Komolov KE, Bhardwaj A, Benovic JL (2015) Atomic structure of G protein-coupled receptor kinase 5 (GRK5) reveals distinct structural features novel for GRKs. J Biol Chem 290(34):20629–20647

30. Homan KT, Waldschmidt HV, Glukhova A, Cannavo A, Song J, Cheung JY, Koch WJ, Larsen SD, Tesmer JJ (2015) Crystal structure of G protein-coupled receptor kinase 5 in complex with a rationally designed inhibitor. J Biol Chem 290(34):20649–20659

31. Allen SJ, Parthasarathy G, Darke PL, Diehl RE, Ford RE, Hall DL, Johnson SA, Reid JC, Rickert KW, Shipman JM, Soisson SM, Zuck P, Munshi SK, Lumb KJ (2015) Structure and function of the hypertension variant A486V of G protein-coupled receptor kinase 4. J Biol Chem 290(33):20360–20373

32. Lodowski DT, Tesmer VM, Benovic JL, Tesmer JJ (2006) The structure of G protein-coupled receptor kinase (GRK)-6 defines a second lineage of GRKs. J Biol Chem 281(24):16785–16793

33. Pitcher JA, Fredericks ZL, Stone WC, Premont RT, Stoffel RH, Koch WJ, Lefkowitz RJ (1996) Phosphatidylinositol 4,5-bisphosphate (PIP_2)-enhanced G protein-coupled receptor kinase (GRK) activity. Location, structure, and regulation of the PIP_2 binding site distinguishes the GRK subfamilies. J Biol Chem 271(40):24907–24913

34. Pronin AN, Carman CV, Benovic JL (1998) Structure-function analysis of G protein-coupled receptor kinase-5. Role of the carboxyl terminus in kinase regulation. J Biol Chem 273(47):31510–31518

35. Thiyagarajan MM, Stracquatanio RP, Pronin AN, Evanko DS, Benovic JL, Wedegaertner PB (2004) A predicted amphipathic helix mediates plasma membrane localization of GRK5. J Biol Chem 279(17):17989–17995

36. Xu H, Jiang X, Shen K, Fischer CC, Wedegaertner PB (2014) The regulator of G protein signaling (RGS) domain of G protein-coupled receptor kinase 5 (GRK5) regulates plasma membrane localization and function. Mol Biol Cell 25(13):2105–2115

37. Jiang X, Benovic JL, Wedegaertner PB (2007) Plasma membrane and nuclear localization of G protein coupled receptor kinase 6A. Mol Biol Cell 18(8):2960–2969

38. Tran TM, Jorgensen R, Clark RB (2007) Phosphorylation of the β_2-adrenergic receptor in plasma membranes by intrinsic GRK5. Biochemistry 46(50):14438–14449

39. Vatter P, Stoesser C, Samel I, Gierschik P, Moepps B (2005) The variable C-terminal extension of G-protein-coupled receptor kinase 6 constitutes an accessorial autoregulatory domain. FEBS J 272(23):6039–6051

40. Ding B, Glukhova A, Sobczyk-Kojiro K, Mosberg HI, Tesmer JJ, Chen Z (2014) Unveiling the membrane-binding properties of N-terminal and C-terminal regions of G protein-coupled receptor kinase 5 by combined optical spectroscopies. Langmuir 30(3):823–831

41. Yang P, Glukhova A, Tesmer JJ, Chen Z (2013) Membrane orientation and binding determinants of G protein-coupled receptor kinase 5 as assessed by combined vibrational spectroscopic studies. PLoS One 8(11):e82072

42. Pronin AN, Benovic JL (1997) Regulation of the G protein-coupled receptor kinase GRK5 by protein kinase C. J Biol Chem 272(6):3806–3812

43. Pronin AN, Satpaev DK, Slepak VZ, Benovic JL (1997) Regulation of G protein-coupled receptor kinases by calmodulin and localization of the calmodulin binding domain. J Biol Chem 272(29):18273–18280

44. Levay K, Satpaev DK, Pronin AN, Benovic JL, Slepak VZ (1998) Localization of the sites for Ca2+-binding proteins on G protein-coupled receptor kinases. Biochemistry 37(39):13650–13659

45. Chuang TT, Paolucci L, De Blasi A (1996) Inhibition of G protein-coupled receptor kinase subtypes by Ca2+/calmodulin. J Biol Chem 271(45):28691–28696

46. Johnson LR, Scott MG, Pitcher JA (2004) G protein-coupled receptor kinase 5 contains a DNA-binding nuclear localization sequence. Mol Cell Biol 24(23):10169–10179

47. Gold JI, Martini JS, Hullmann J, Gao E, Chuprun JK, Lee L, Tilley DG, Rabinowitz JE, Bossuyt J, Bers DM, Koch WJ (2013) Nuclear translocation of cardiac g protein-coupled receptor kinase 5 downstream of select gq-activating hypertrophic ligands is a calmodulin-dependent process. PLoS One 8(3):e57324

48. Felder RA, Sanada H, Xu J, Yu PY, Wang Z, Watanabe H, Asico LD, Wang W, Zheng S, Yamaguchi I, Williams SM, Gainer J, Brown NJ, Hazen-Martin D, Wong LJ, Robillard JE, Carey RM, Eisner GM, Jose PA (2002) G protein-coupled receptor kinase 4 gene variants in human essential hypertension. Proc Natl Acad Sci U S A 99(6):3872–3877

49. Li L, Homan KT, Vishnivetskiy SA, Manglik A, Tesmer JJ, Gurevich VV, Gurevich EV (2015) G protein-coupled receptor kinases of the GRK4 protein subfamily phosphorylate inactive G protein-coupled receptors (GPCRs). J Biol Chem 290(17):10775–10790

50. Inagaki S, Ghirlando R, Vishnivetskiy SA, Homan KT, White JF, Tesmer JJ, Gurevich VV, Grisshammer R (2015) G protein-coupled receptor kinase 2 (GRK2) and 5 (GRK5) exhibit selective phosphorylation of the neurotensin receptor in vitro. Biochemistry 54(28):4320–4329

51. Rasmussen SG, Choi HJ, Fung JJ, Pardon E, Casarosa P, Chae PS, Devree BT, Rosenbaum DM, Thian FS, Kobilka TS, Schnapp A, Konetzki I, Sunahara RK, Gellman SH, Pautsch A, Steyaert J, Weis WI, Kobilka BK (2011) Structure of a nanobody-stabilized active state of the beta(2) adrenoceptor. Nature 469(7329):175–180

52. Rasmussen SG, DeVree BT, Zou Y, Kruse AC, Chung KY, Kobilka TS, Thian FS, Chae PS, Pardon E, Calinski D, Mathiesen JM, Shah ST, Lyons JA, Caffrey M, Gellman SH, Steyaert J, Skiniotis G, Weis WI, Sunahara RK, Kobilka BK (2011) Crystal structure of the β_2 adrenergic receptor-G_s protein complex. Nature 477(7366):549–555

53. Kang Y, Zhou XE, Gao X, He Y, Liu W, Ishchenko A, Barty A, White TA, Yefanov O, Han GW, Xu Q, de Waal PW, Ke J, Tan MH, Zhang C, Moeller A, West GM, Pascal BD, Van Eps N, Caro LN, Vishnivetskiy SA, Lee RJ, Suino-Powell KM, Gu X, Pal K, Ma J, Zhi X, Boutet S, Williams GJ, Messerschmidt M, Gati C, Zatsepin NA, Wang D, James D, Basu S, Roy-Chowdhury S, Conrad CE, Coe J, Liu H, Lisova S, Kupitz C, Grotjohann I, Fromme R, Jiang Y, Tan M, Yang H, Li J, Wang M, Zheng Z, Li D, Howe N, Zhao Y, Standfuss J, Diederichs K, Dong Y, Potter CS, Carragher B, Caffrey M, Jiang H, Chapman HN, Spence JC, Fromme P, Weierstall U, Ernst OP, Katritch V, Gurevich VV, Griffin PR, Hubbell WL, Stevens RC, Cherezov V, Melcher K, Xu HE (2015) Crystal structure of rhodopsin bound to arrestin by femtosecond X-ray laser. Nature 523(7562):561–567

54. Whorton MR, Mackinnon R (2013) X-ray structure of the mammalian GIRK2-betagamma G-protein complex. Nature 498(7453):190–197

Chapter 5

"Barcode" and Differential Effects of GPCR Phosphorylation by Different GRKs

Kunhong Xiao and Hongda Liu

Abstract

As the largest known family of cell surface receptors and the most common therapeutic drug targets, G protein-coupled receptors (GPCRs) are at the center of modern medicine. Multiple site phosphorylation of GPCRs by G protein-coupled receptor kinases (GRKs) plays an essential role in the regulation of various functions and signaling cascades of a receptor. Research in recent years has elucidated a common mechanism by which different ligand-bound GPCRs engage different GRKs, which in turn phosphorylate distinct sites or overlapping sets of sites on the receptor. These different patterns of phosphorylation (the "barcode") result in distinct consequences in receptor function and signaling. Here, we review these recent findings and discuss the ramifications of this phenomenon in biology and medicine.

Key words G protein-coupled receptor, GPCR, G protein-coupled receptor kinases, GRK, Phosphorylation, Barcode, Arrestin, β-arrestin

1 Introduction

G protein-coupled receptors (GPCRs), also referred to as seven transmembrane-spanning receptors (7TMRs), constitute the largest known family of cell surface receptors. The human genome encodes more than 800 GPCRs, responding to a diverse array of extracellular stimuli including light, odorants, chemoattractants, neurotransmitters, and hormones [1–5]. These receptors regulate virtually all known physiological processes in humans. The clinical significance of GPCRs is reflected by the facts that compounds targeting these receptors, directly or indirectly, as agonists or antagonists, account for about 60 % of all prescription drug sales worldwide [6].

Despite the exceptional diversity of GPCR functions, the molecular components, dynamic behavior, and regulatory mechanism of their signaling pathways appear to be well conserved. As the name implies, classic GPCR signaling is conducted primarily through activation of heterotrimeric G proteins. When an external

Vsevolod V. Gurevich et al. (eds.), *G Protein-Coupled Receptor Kinases*, Methods in Pharmacology and Toxicology, DOI 10.1007/978-1-4939-3798-1_5, © Springer Science+Business Media New York 2016

ligand molecule binds to a GPCR, it induces a conformational change in the receptor, causing the activation of cognate G proteins. The exchange of GDP for GTP then triggers the dissociation of the Gα subunit from the Gβγ dimer, which subsequently activates a series of intercellular signaling cascades and ultimately leads to changes in cellular physiology [7]. The dynamic sensitivity of GPCR function and signaling is in large part a function of their regulation by the G protein-coupled receptor kinase (GRK)/β-arrestin system [8–10]. This regulation is accomplished by a two-step process involving the phosphorylation of the carboxyl terminus and/or intracellular loops of the receptor by the GRKs, and the subsequent binding of β-arrestins. β-Arrestin binding uncouples the G protein and terminates G protein-mediated signaling (desensitization) and facilitates clathrin-mediated endocytosis (internalization) of the receptor [10].

This classic mechanism of regulating GPCR signaling via the GRK/β-arrestin system provides the foundation to understanding how the GPCR functions are regulated. However, it does not offer mechanistic details to explain certain new observations in the field of GPCR biology and pharmacology. For example, research in recent years has revealed that the GRK/β-arrestin system not only desensitizes the G protein-dependent signaling, but also leads to stimulus-dependent recruitment of β-arrestin (β-arrestin1 and 2) to the activated receptor and nucleates formation and activation of multi-protein signaling complexes that initiate G protein-independent signaling [8, 11–13]. This multifunctional G-protein-independent signaling is ligand-specific. A detailed and unifying mechanism has been lacking to explain the ligand specificity and multifunctionality of this G protein-independent, β-arrestin-mediated signaling. In addition, recent studies using "loss-of-function" techniques, such as siRNA, to delete individual GRKs or combinations of GRKs have revealed that distinct GRKs contribute differently to the processes of receptor desensitization, endocytosis, and signaling. For example, both the V2 vasopressin receptor (V2R) and angiotensin II type 1A receptor (AT1aR), prototypical G_s- and G_q-coupled receptors, respectively, engage different GRKs for different functional purposes [14, 15]. GRK2 and 3 are responsible for the majority of agonist-stimulated receptor phosphorylation, β-arrestin recruitment, and internalization; however, GRK6 is the primary player responsible for dictating β-arrestin-mediated signaling to extracellular-signal-regulated kinases 1/2 (ERK 1/2). Similarly, the β2 adrenergic receptor (β2AR) mimics both the V2R and AT1AR in its selective use of GRK2 or 6, leading to distinct functional outcomes [14–16]. The most obvious hypothesis to explain such findings would be that different ligand-bound GPCRs engage different GRKs, which phosphorylate distinct sites or overlapping sets of sites on a given receptor. The patterns of phosphorylation (the "barcode") direct distinct signaling and functional consequences (Fig. 1). This GPCR phosphorylation "barcode"

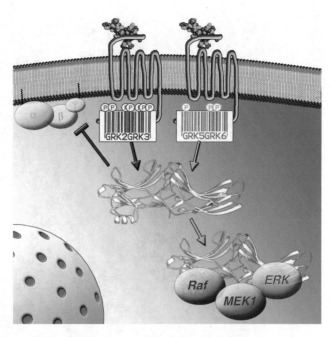

Fig. 1 GPCR phosphorylation barcode hypothesis. Different ligands promote the engagement of different GRKs, which in turn phosphorylate distinct sites or overlapping sets of sites on a given GPCR. These different patterns of phosphorylation (the "barcode") induce functionally distinct conformations of the receptor-bound β-arrestin, thus leading to distinct functional consequences

hypothesis is supported by accumulating experimental evidence and has proven to be a unifying mechanism for GPCR functions and signaling. This chapter will summarize recent studies that elucidate the GPCR "barcode" mechanism and discuss the ramifications of this phenomenon in the fields of biology and medicine.

2   GPCR Phosphorylation by GRKs

2.1   Different GRKs

GRKs are serine/threonine protein kinases that regulate the activity of GPCRs by phosphorylating their intracellular loops and carboxyl terminal tails after receptor and G protein activation. In stark contrast to the great multiplicity of GPCRs, there are only seven members in the GRK family. These GRKs can be divided into the following three subfamilies based on sequence and functional homology: 1) the rhodopsin kinase subfamily (GRK1[17] and GRK7[18]), 2) the β-adrenergic receptor (βAR) kinase subfamily (GRK2 [19] and GRK3 [20]), and 3) the GRK4 subfamily (GRK4 [21], GRK5 [22, 23], and GRK6 [24–29]) (Table 1). All GRKs share about 50–90% sequence similarity, with a conserved tripartite structural architecture: a central serine/threonine kinase domain (~270 amino acids) flanked by an NH_2-terminal domain of

Table 1
The GRK family

GRK name	Gene symbol	Size (kDa)	PTMs	Subfamily	Tissue distribution	Notes
G protein-coupled receptor kinase 1	*GRK1*	63	Farnesylation	Rhodopsin-kinase subfamily	Retina>>pineal	Rhodopsin kinase
G protein-coupled receptor kinase 2	*ADRBK1* (GRK2)	79		βAR kinase subfamily	Leukocytes>front cortex of brain>heart>lung>kidney, thyroid nodules	β-Adrenergic receptor kinase 1 (BARK1)
G protein-coupled receptor kinase 3	*ADRBK2* (GRK3)	80		βAR kinase subfamily	Brain>spleen>heart, lung, kidney, thyroid nodules	β-Adrenergic receptor kinase 2 (BARK2)
G protein-coupled receptor kinase 4	*GRK4*	66	Palmitoylation	GRK4 subfamily	Testis>>>brain, thyroid nodules	Has been associated with regulation of kidney tubule function
G protein-coupled receptor kinase 5	*GRK5*	68		GRK4 subfamily	Heart, placenta, lung>skeletal muscle>brain, liver, pancreas>kidney, thyroid nodules	Knockout mice have altered core body temperature
G protein-coupled receptor kinase 6	*GRK6*	66	Palmitoylation	GRK4 subfamily	Brain, skeletal muscle>pancreas>heart, lung, kidney, placenta>liver, thyroid nodules	Knockout mice are supersensitive to dopaminergics
G protein-coupled receptor kinase 7	*GRK7*	62	Geranylgeranylation	Rhodopsin-kinase subfamily	Retina, particularly cones	Cone opsin kinase

Table 2
Distinct GRK phosphorylation sites on the β2AR differentially encode distinct β-arrestin functions

	Desensitization	Internalization	ERK activation
GRK2	++++	++++	–(inhibitory)
GRK6	+++	++	++++

approximately 185 amino acids (containing a short proximal NH_2-terminal region), followed by an RH domain (regulator of G protein signaling (RGS) homology domain) and a COOH-terminal domain of varying length (~105–230 amino acids) [22, 27–30]. The kinase domain is shared by the βAR kinases and the GRK4 subfamilies. The NH_2 terminus is unique to the GRK family of protein kinases and important for receptor recognition, whereas the COOH terminus is the most diverse region among GRK subfamilies [27, 28, 30]. A unique feature of the βAR kinase subfamily is a COOH-terminal pleckstrin homology (PH) domain for phospholipid and Gβγ binding. The kinases in the GRK4 subfamily (GRK4, GRK5, and GRK6) use other mechanisms for membrane targeting, such as palmitoylation and patches of positively charged residues [31–34].

2.2 Tissue- and/or Cell-Specific Expression of GRKs

Previous studies have suggested that GRKs have little or no receptor specificity [35]. The small number of kinases in the GRK family appears to be involved in phosphorylating hundreds of GPCR substrates. However, the functional specificity of GRKs was revealed in vivo by studying the GRK transgenic and/or knockout mice. For example, it was reported that GRK2 mainly phosphorylates β-adrenergic receptors and angiotensin II type 1 receptors [36], while GRK3 primarily targets olfactory receptors and α-adrenergic receptors [37–39]. On the other hand, knocking out GRK5 and 6 individually displayed selectively impaired desensitization of muscarinic and dopaminergic receptors, respectively [40, 41]. Although the molecular mechanisms remain largely unknown, it is reasonable to speculate that the in vivo functional specificity of GRKs is related to their subcellular location, cell-specific expression patterns, and tissue-specific expression levels.

The two members in the rhodopsin-kinase subfamily, GRK1 (rhodopsin kinase) and GRK7, are generally confined to retinal rods and cones [26, 27, 34, 42–45] (Table 1). GRK4 shows only very localized expression in testes, the cerebellum, kidneys, and the uterus myometrium [46–50]. GRK2, 3, 5, and 6 are ubiquitously expressed at varying levels depending on tissue types [27, 42]. For example, although GRK2, 3, 5, and 6 are all expressed in the heart, the most prominent GRKs in the human heart are GRK2 and 5

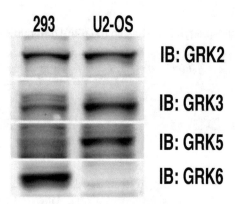

Fig. 2 Distinct expression patterns of GRKs in different cell types. Immunoblotting reveals that HEK293 cells predominantly express GRK2 and 6 (*left lane*), while U2-OS osteosarcoma cells express relatively more GRK3 and 5 than HEK293 cells and little to no GRK6. For each GRK, an immunoblot is shown of equal amounts of total protein from each cell line [55]

[51, 52]. The expression levels of GRK3 and 6 are relatively low [52–54].

GRKs are also expressed at different levels in different cell types. For example, it is reported that, compared to HEK293 cells, U2-OS osteosarcoma cells express more GRK3 and GRK5 but no GRK6 (Fig. 2) [55]. Fluorescence resonance energy transfer (FRET) assay in live cells revealed that U2-OS and HEK293 cells utilize different subsets of their expressed GRKs to phosphorylate β2AR and promote β-arrestin recruitment to the receptor [55]. GRK knockdown by RNA interference (RNAi) technology in U2-OS cells suggested that GRK3 is most efficacious in promoting β-arrestin recruitment to the β2AR. In HEK293 cells, simultaneous knockdown of both GRK2 and GRK3 has an additive effect. This finding revealed that cells could use cell type-specific expression patterns of GRKs to regulate GPCR function and signaling.

2.3 The Roles of GRK-Mediated GPCR Phosphorylation

2.3.1 The Roles of GRKs in GPCR Desensitization

Phosphorylation of GPCRs on the carboxyl terminus and intracellular loops by GRKs is important for receptor desensitization, internalization, trafficking, and β-arrestin-mediated signaling. GRKs were first discovered through their roles in GPCR desensitization. The primary function of GRKs is to desensitize activated GPCRs, a negative regulation that includes phosphorylating the activated receptor, uncoupling the receptor from G protein, and initiating the receptor internalization. The first description of GPCR phosphorylation in a stimulus-dependent manner was reported for rhodopsin in 1972 [56, 57]. Then the enzyme, "opsin kinase" (modern name GRK1), which can selectively phosphorylate the active form of rhodopsin, was identified and isolated in 1975 [58–61]. Later it was discovered that rhodopsin phosphorylation by GRK1 is necessary for the rapid deactivation of the receptor [62]. This discovery led to a speculation that receptor phosphorylation may be a general molecular mechanism for GPCR deactivation or homologous desensitization when a cell's response to a special agonist decreases. This hypothesis was quickly confirmed in the β2AR system with the demonstration that catecholamine-induced desensitization of the β2AR was tightly associated with receptor phosphorylation [63–65]. The role of GRKs in GPCR desensitization was later elucidated in many other receptors as a general regulatory mechanism [66]. GRK2 (βARK), an enzyme responsible for this desensitization process, was soon identified during the study of βAR phosphorylation [19]. GRK2 has many similar properties to GRK1. Both kinases were found to be associated with a reduction in the function of corresponding receptors [67, 68]. In 1990s, several other GRKs, such as GRK3 [18], GRK4 [21], GRK5 [69], GRK6 [70], and GRK7 [71] were identified as regulators of GPCR desensitization.

Later it was discovered that GRK phosphorylation of the agonist-activated receptor alone can only attenuate GPCR signaling by up to 30 % [72–74]. Arrestins, a new family of regulatory proteins, were soon shown to be required to achieve substantial desensitization [75–77]. The arrestin family includes four members. Arrestin1 (visual arrestin) and arrestin 4 (X arrestin) are expressed in retinal rods and cones, respectively [8, 78]. Arrestin 2 and 3 (hereafter referred to as β-arrestin1 and 2, respectively) are ubiquitously expressed and recruited by almost all GPCRs in a receptor phosphorylation-dependent manner [8]. The role of GRKs in this process is that they phosphorylate the activated (agonist-occupied) GPCRs, promoting the recruitment of arrestins to sterically block the activation of G protein, therefore leading to rapid homologous desensitization.

2.3.2 The Roles of GRKs in GPCR Trafficking (Internalization, Recycling, and Resensitization)

In addition to their roles in GPCR desensitization, GRKs also play key roles in receptor trafficking, a process that classically serves to internalize, resensitize, and recycle receptors back to the plasma membrane [12, 79–81]. In response to agonist stimulation, GPCRs are sequestered and internalized from the plasma membrane so that they will not be available for persistent agonist stimulation at the cell surface [82]. This ensures that extracellular stimuli are transduced into cells with appropriate magnitude. As a result of the arrestin binding, GRK-phosphorylated receptors are targeted for clathrin-mediated endocytosis. The carboxyl-terminal tails of arrestins contain binding sites for both the β2-adaptin of the AP-2 adaptor complex and clathrin, which links the receptors to clathrin-coated pits (CCPs) [83–85]. Disruption of the AP-2 or clathrin binding sites on the arrestin carboxyl-terminal tails ablates receptor sequestration and internalization [86]. Many GPCRs undergo this clathrin-mediated endocytosis. Subsequently, the CCPs gradually invaginate and finally leave the plasma membrane as free clathrin-coated-vesicles (CCVs) [87]. The CCVs then fuse with early endosomes, whereupon GPCRs are either recycled back to the cell surface or directed to late endosomes or lysosomes for degradation.

The role of GRKs in GPCR trafficking is that GRKs phosphorylate clusters of serine and threonine residues in the intracellular loops and/or carboxyl-terminal tail, and the phosphorylation status of a receptor dictates arrestin interaction. Two patterns of agonist activation-dependent receptor–arrestin interaction were discovered with respect to arrestin's endocytic adaptor function and the stability of the receptor–arrestin complexes [88]. Class A receptors, such as the β2AR, interact with β-arrestins transiently and with low-affinity binding. After targeting GPCRs to CCPs, β-arrestin dissociates from the GPCR and the receptor internalizes without the arrestin. On the other hand, class B receptors, such as the V2R, bind to β-arrestin tightly. Following recruitment to CCPs, β-arrestin remains bound to the receptor on the surface of endocytic vesicles. The stability of the receptor/arrestin complex is the determining factor regulating the profile of GPCR trafficking, including the process of internalization, recycling, and resensitization. Impairment of the phosphorylation status of a receptor by mutating the key serine and threonine residues generally leads to impaired receptor internalization and resensitization, demonstrating the close correlation between GRK-mediated phosphorylation and receptor trafficking [89–92].

2.3.3 The Roles of GRKs in G Protein-Independent, β-Arrestin-Mediated GPCR Signaling

Recent studies have shown that, in addition to their role in desensitizing G protein-mediated signaling and facilitating the endocytosis of GPCRs, β-arrestin molecules (β-arrestin1 and 2) also serve as multifunctional adaptors and signal transducers, linking GPCRs to a growing list of signaling molecules (e.g., MAPK, Src, and Akt) [8, 9, 11, 12, 80, 81, 93–98]. The discovery of β-arrestin as a signaling molecule originated from a study that revealed β-arrestin-dependent formation of β2AR-Src protein kinase complexes, resulting in the activation of MAP kinases ERK1 and ERK2 [99]. Later, β-arrestins were found to recruit a growing list of signaling molecules to the receptor–β-arrestin complexes to initiate a new wave of cellular signaling, independent of G protein activation. These signaling molecules include MAP kinases, AKT, phosphatidylinositol 3-kinase (PI3-kinase), E3 ubiqutin ligases, phosphodiesterases, small GTPases, guanine nucleotide exchange factors, and transcription factors [12, 13, 77, 78, 90–96]. Using mass spectrometry-based proteomics as a tool, it was discovered that more than 300 proteins interact with β-arrestin1 and 2 [100]. This study provides evidence of significant specialization in the functions of β-arrestin in G protein-independent, β-arrestin-mediated GPCR signaling. The large and diverse set of proteins obtained in the global proteomics screen also underscores the potential broad regulatory roles of the newly discovered, G protein-independent, β-arrestin-mediated GPCR signaling in mammalian cellular physiology [100].

It is now clear that GPCRs use two parallel signaling pathways to translate extracellular stimuli to intracellular signals; one is mediated by G proteins and referred to as G protein-mediated signaling, while the other is mediated by β-arrestins and referred to as β-arrestin-mediated signaling. The discovery of β-arrestin-mediated signaling has led to an exciting new field in GPCR drug discovery—the development of "biased agonists". A biased agonist is a ligand that stabilizes a particular active receptor conformation, thus stimulating certain responses but not others. Classical agonists usually stimulate both G protein- and β-arrestin-mediated signaling. However, a G protein-biased agonist selectively activates the G protein-mediated signaling, whereas a β-arrestin-biased agonist selectively activates β-arrestin-mediated signaling. This concept of biased agonists opens a new door for GPCR drug discovery in which one could differentiate and possibly separate the side effects of the activation of some receptors from their beneficial effects. For a particular GPCR, if the therapeutic effect of a drug comes mainly through one signaling pathway, while the side effects come mainly through the other pathway, a biased agonist could be developed into a more effective drug that can maximize the therapeutic effects, at the same time minimizing the side-effect profiles. For example, carvedilol (Coreg®), a β-blocker, was recently demonstrated to selectively stimulate β-arrestin-mediated signaling [101, 102]. Therefore, carvedilol is a prototype for a new generation of therapeutic β2AR ligands.

GPCR phosphorylation by GRKs plays critical role in regulating G protein-independent, β-arrestin-mediated GPCR signaling. It was speculated that the phosphorylation status of the agonist-occupied receptor might regulate the conformation of β-arrestin recruited to the receptor–β-arrestin complexes. The conformational changes in β-arrestins dictate their protein–protein interaction capabilities, and thus the β-arrestin-mediated GPCR signaling. Given the plethora of phosphorylation states of numerous receptors, the precise mechanism by which GRK phosphorylation regulates the magnitude and specificity of G protein-mediated and β-arrestin-mediated signaling remains to be elucidated.

3 Different GRKs Contribute Differentially to Distinct GPCR Functional and Signaling Consequences: Experimental Evidence Supporting the "Barcode" Hypothesis for GPCR Signaling

Since the discovery of GRKs, it was speculated that different GRKs may contribute differently to GPCR function and signaling. Over the past several decades, extensive studies in a number of GPCRs provided accumulating experimental evidence that supports this hypothesis. In a number of GPCRs, the use of a "loss-of-function" strategy by siRNAs to knockdown individual GRKs or combinations of GRKs provided experimental evidence to support the notion that distinct GRKs contribute differently to the processes of receptor desensitization, trafficking, and signaling [14–16, 103]. In Table 3, we summarize the different roles of GRKs in a number of GPCRs and below discuss detailed experimental evidence derived from several representative receptors.

3.1 β2-Adrenergic Receptor (β2AR)

In 1990s, monoclonal antibodies (mAbs) against different GRKs were generated. By using these antibodies, it was discovered that among the GRKs (GRK2-6) that phosphorylated the G_s-coupled β2AR, GRK2 was the predominant GRK responsible for β2AR phosphorylation and desensitization in HEK293 cells [19]. A later study using PKA inhibitor H-89 and β-arrestin siRNA in the β2AR system revealed that β2AR signaling to ERK1/2 could be resolved into two separate pathways: an H-89-sensitive, PKA-dependent G protein-mediated pathway and a β-arrestin-mediated pathway [16]. The G protein/PKA-dependent signaling was rapid and peaked within 2–5 min. The β-arrestin-mediated signaling was slower and peaked at around 5–10 min. Overexpression of GRK5 or 6 increased receptor phosphorylation, β-arrestin recruitment, and agonist-stimulated ERK1/2 activation [16]. On the other hand, GRK2 was ineffective, and β-arrestins recruited to GRK2-phosphorylated receptors appeared not to be involved in ERK1/2 activation. A β-arrestin-biased β2AR mutant, β2AR[T68F,Y132G,Y219A] (β2AR[TYY]), which is incapable of G protein activation, recruited β-arrestins to initiate β-arrestin-dependent internalization and ERK1/2 activation. It was observed that although agonist-induced receptor phosphorylation was weak for β2AR[TYY], the β-arrestin recruitment was moderate and ERK1/2 activation robust [16]. This lack of correlation between receptor phosphorylation, β-arrestin recruitment, and β-arrestin-mediated ERK1/2 activation indicated that the specific constellation of phosphorylation sites on a receptor targeted by the different GRKs may form a "barcode" that "instructs" the bound β-arrestins as to which functions to perform by virtue of inducing specific conformational changes.

3.2 V2-Vasopressin Receptor 2 (V2R)

The notion of GPCR phosphorylation barcoding was also suggested by the study of another G_s-coupled receptor, V2R. It was demonstrated that the V2R also regulates ERK1/2 activation via either G_s or β-arrestin [15]. The G_s-dependent ERK1/2 activation is rapid and transient while the β-arrestin-dependent phosphorylation of ERK1/2 is slower and more sustained. GRK2 and 3 contribute to almost all the GRK-mediated phosphorylation and consequent β-arrestin recruitment to the V2R, whereas GRK5 and 6 are less effective. Although GRK5 and 6 mediated much less

Table 3
Different GRKs act on various GPCRs and mediate different functions

GRK	Receptor	Functions	Cell types	Phosphorylation sites	Reference
GRK2/3	AT1aR	Desensitization and internalization	HEK293		[14, 104, 167]
GRK2/3	AT1aR	Inhibit β-arrestin-mediated ERK activation			[14, 168]
GRK2	α1BAR	Desensitization	COS-7	S404, S408, S410	[169]
GRK2/3	α2BAR	Agonist-induced downregulation	NG-108		[170, 171]
GRK2	β2AR	β-arrestin2 recruitment	HEK293 U2-OS		[12]
GRK2/3/5/6	β2AR	Receptor desensitization and internalization	HEK293 COS-7	S355,356	[1, 2, 4, 129, 172]
GRK2	β2AR	Inhibit β-arrestin-mediated ERK activation; Inhibit GRK6 phosphorylation		T360, S364, S396, S401, S407, S411	[150, 173]
GRK2	β2AR	Increase translocation of GLUT4			[174]
GRK2	β2AR	Changes receptor to G_i-biased signaling	Cardiomyocytes and in vivo mice		[175]
GRK2	V(1A)R	GRK2/β-arrestin1-dependent ERK signaling	H9c2 cells		[176]
GRK2/3	V2R	Phosphorylation and desensitization of receptor, recruitment of β-arrestins	HEK293		[15]
GRK2	CXCR1	Phosphorylation, desensitization, and internalization, CXCL8-induced phosphoinositide hydrolysis and exocytosis; ERK1/2 phosphorylation	RBL-2H3		[108]

(continued)

Table 3
(continued)

GRK	Receptor	Functions	Cell types	Phosphorylation sites	Reference
GRK2/6	CXCR2	Phosphorylation, desensitization, and internalization; CXCL8-induced phosphoinositide hydrolysis and exocytosis	RBL-2H3		[108]
GRK2/3	CXCR4	CXCL12-promoted phosphorylation at S324/325 and S338/339, internalization, inhibition of calcium mobilization, and desensitization	HEK293 Neuroblastoma		[107, 177, 178]
GRK2	CXCR4	Negatively regulate calcium mobilization; inhibit ERK1/2 activation	HEK293	S346-348S351/352	[106]
GRK2/3/6	CXCR5	Agonist-induced phosphorylation and desensitization	RBL-2H3 COS-7 HEK293	336, 337, 342, 349	[151, 152]
GRK2	CXCR7	Induce activation of ERK1/2 and AKT	Astrocytes		[109]
GRK2	CXCR9	Internalization	CD4+ T cells from patients		[179]
GRK2/3	D1R	Rightward shift of the dopamine dose–response curve with little effect on maximal activation	HEK293		[180]
GRK2/3	D2R	Phosphorylation affects recycling without effect on internalization or desensitization	HEK293	S285/286, T287, S288, T293, S311, S317, S321	[181]
GRK2	D2R	Phosphorylation and sequestration	HEK293		[123]
GRK2	D2R	Internalization and resensitization	HEK293 SH-SY5Y	T225	[125]

Kinase	Receptor	Function	Cell type	Phosphosite	Ref.
GRK2	D2R	Regulate internalization and signaling of D2R in a phosphorylation-independent manner. Enzymatic activity was required for enhancement of internalization but not for the inhibition of signaling. Agonist-induced phosphorylation of D2R accelerates the recycling of internalized receptor proteins	HEK293	T225	[124]
GRK2/3	D3R	Reduce interaction between the D3R and filamin	HEK293		[182]
GRK2	FSH-R	Promote both desensitization and internalization, but negatively regulate β-arrestin-dependent ERK activation	HEK293	Five Ser/Thr residues in the C terminus of the receptor (638–644)	[183]
GRK2/3	H1R	Desensitization	ULTR		[184]
GRK2	H2R	Desensitization	COS-7 CHO-K1		[185, 186]
GRK2	H2R	Phosphorylation-independent desensitization of H2R, but phosphor-dependent receptor internalization and resensitization	HEK293		[186]
GRK2	IGF-1R	Promote AKT signaling, inhibit ERK activation, reduce ligand-induced degradation of IGF-1R	HEK293	S1248	[187]
GRK2	IGF-1R	Inhibit Tyr phosphorylation of IGF1R by other kinases	HepG2		[188]
GRK2	LPA-1R	Desensitization	FRTL-5 HEK293		[189, 190]

(continued)

Table 3
(continued)

GRK	Receptor	Functions	Cell types	Phosphorylation sites	Reference
GRK2	LPA-1R	Inhibit activation of ERK	FRTL-5 PC12		[190–192]
GRK2	LPA-1R	Abolish inhibitory effect of LPA on ERK5	PC12		[193]
GRK2	LPA-1R	RalA-GRK2-LPA1R complex	HEK293		[189]
GRK2	LPA-2R	Receptor desensitization	HEK293		[189]
GRK2	Delta-opioid receptor	GRK2 is required for delta-opioid receptor internalization in neurons but not in HEK293			[138]
GRK2	Delta-opioid receptor	DPDPE, instead of TIPP, could activate GRK2, and induce internalization	CHO cells		[194, 195]
GRK2	Delta-opioid receptor	GRK2 phosphorylation-dependent internalization mediated by β-arrestin1/2 leads to recycling, whereas GRK2-independent internalization mediated by β-arrestin2 alone leads to receptor degradation	HEK293		[110]
GRK2	Delta-opioid receptor	Etorphine-induced receptor desensitization but no effect was observed with peptidic agonists	Neuroblastoma SK-N-BE	S363, but no correlation between desensitization and phosphorylation of this amino acid	[196]
GRK2/6	Delta-opioid receptor	DPDPE-induced receptor desensitization	NG108-15		[197]
GRK2/3	Kappa-opioid receptor	Desensitization and internalization	AtT-20 HEK293	S369	[141, 198]

GRK	Receptor	Effect/function	Cell/tissue	Site	References
GRK2	Kappa-opioid receptor	Desensitization and phosphorylation of the human kappa opioid receptor after (−)U50,488H pretreatment, but not rat kappa opioid receptor	CHO		[147–149]
GRK2/3	Mu-opioid receptor	Internalization	BHK; lumber of the spinal cord; locus ceruleus (LC) neurons; hippocampus Sf9 cell		[199–202]
GRK2	Mu-opioid receptor	No effect on ERK1/2 activity	HEK293	S375	[203]
GRK2	Mu-opioid receptor	Activate cSrc, stimulate tyrosine phosphorylation of $G\alpha_{i2}$, induce $G\alpha_{i2}$-RGS12 association	Smooth muscle cell		[204]
GRK2	Mu-opioid receptor	Increase the affinity of agonists, but not antagonists	U2-OS		[119]
GRK2	Mu-opioid receptor	Activated by DAMGO or etorphine but not morphine	HEK293		[111–113, 115, 116]
GRK2	Mu-opioid receptor	There is a difference in the GRK requirement for initial ligand-induced internalization compared to subsequent rounds of reinternalization	HEK293		[205]
GRK2	Mu-opioid receptor	Involved in the short-term regulation of mu-opioid receptors in vivo and relevant role in opiate tolerance, dependence, and withdrawal	Rat brain tissue		[206]
GRK2/3/6	Mu-opioid receptor	Prevent opioid tolerance development and improve the analgesic efficacy of opioid drugs	Brain tissue		[114]

(continued)

Table 3
(continued)

GRK	Receptor	Functions	Cell types	Phosphorylation sites	Reference
GRK2/3	Opioid receptor-like 1 (ORL1) receptor	Desensitization	SH-SY5Y BE(2)-C		[144, 145]
GRK2	PTHR	Phosphorylation, but not required for efficient receptor internalization	HEK293 COS-1	Among 483, 485, 486, 489, 495, and 498	[207]
GRK2	M3 mAChR	Phosphor-independent inhibition of carbachol-mediated calcium mobilization and ERK pathway	HEK293		[208]
GRK2	M4 muscarinic receptor	Desensitization and internalization	NG108-15		[209]
GRK2	Leukotriene B(4) (LTB(4)) receptor (BLT1)	Desensitization	HEK293		[210]
GRK2	Melanocortin 1 receptor (MC1R)	Desensitization	HEK293 Melanoma cells		[211]
GRK2	Endothelin A and B receptors (ETA-R and ETB-R)	Desensitization	HEK293		[212]
GRK2	GIPR	Enhance agonist-induced phosphorylation; internalization not affected	HEK293		[213]
GRK3	α1AR	Decrease agonist-stimulated activation of ERK1/2	Mice		[214]

GRK3	CXCR4	Promote ERK1/2 activation	HEK293	S346-348, S351/352	[106]
GRK3	Delta-opioid receptor	Desensitization	Oocytes	T161 (second intracellular loop)	[215]
GRK3/5	Mu-opioid receptor	Phosphorylation under etonitazene and fentanyl stimulation		T370,S375 T379	[216]
GRK3/5	Mu-opioid receptor	Agonist induced receptor desensitization at a rate dependent on agonist efficacy	HEK293		[146]
GRK3	Nociceptin, orphanin FQ receptor (NOPR)	Mediated JNK but not ERK signaling	HEK293	S363	[217]
GRK3	CRF1 receptors	Desensitization	Y-79		[218]
GRK4	D1R	Desensitization and internalization	HEK293 renal proximal tubule cells IEC-6	T428 and S431	[122, 219, 220]
GRK4	D3R	Phosphorylation and critical for p44/42 phosphorylation after agonist stimulation	Human proximal tubule cells		[49]
GRK4	GABA(B) receptor	Desensitization	BHK		[221]
GRK4	Metabotropic glutamate 1 (mGlu(1)) receptor	Desensitization	Cerebellar Purkinje cells HEK293		[47, 222]

(continued)

Table 3
(continued)

GRK	Receptor	Functions	Cell types	Phosphorylation sites	Reference
GRK5/6	AT1AR	Enhances β-arrestin-mediated ERK activation			[14, 168]
GRK5/6	AT1aR	Receptor phosphorylation and desensitization	HEK293		[223]
GRK5	β1AR	Reduce β1AR association with PSD-95	COS-7 HEK293		[224]
GRK5/6	β2AR	Increase β-arrestin binding, mediate ERK pathway	HEK293		[16]
GRK5/6	V2R	Appeared exclusively to support β-arrestin2-mediated ERK activation	HEK293		[15]
GRK5	Kappa-opioid receptor	Desensitization	Oocytes	S369	[225]
GRK5	IGF-1R	Promote IGF1-mediated ERK and AKT activation	HEK293		[187]
GRK5	D1AR	Induce a rightward shift in the EC$_{50}$ value with an additional 40% reduction in the maximal activation by dopamine	HEK293		[180]
GRK6	βAR	Desensitization	Myometrial cells		[226]
GRK6	CXCR1	Phosphorylation, desensitization, and internalization; CXCL8-induced phosphoinositide hydrolysis and exocytosis	RBL-2H3		[108]

GRK6	Calcitonin gene-related peptide (CGRP) receptor	CGRP-mediated desensitization		HEK293	[227]
GRK6	D1R	Desensitization		IEC-6 HEK293	[228]
GRK6	IGF-1R	Promote IGF1-mediated ERK and AKT activation, enhance ligand-induced degradation of IGF-1R	S1291	HEK293	[187]
GRK6	M3 mAChR	Desensitization		SH-SY5Y cells	[229]
GRK6	Melanocortin 1 receptor (MC1R)	Desensitization and impairment of agonist-dependent signaling and inhibition of agonist-independent constitutive signaling		HEK293 melanoma cells	[211]
GRK6	OTR	Desensitization		Myometrial smooth muscle cells ULTR cells	[230]

V2R phosphorylation and β-arrestin recruitment, they appeared to be responsible for β-arrestin-mediated ERK1/2 activation. It is interesting that depletion of GRK2 from cells by siRNA increased β-arrestin-mediated ERK1/2 activation. This result suggested that there is no simple correlation between the activation level of the β-arrestin2-mediated ERK1/2 activation and the amount of β-arrestin2 recruited to the receptor.

3.3 Angiotensin II Type 1A Receptor (AT1AR)

Further evidence in support of the "barcode" hypothesis was also provided by G_q-coupled receptors such as AT1aR [14]. It was reported that agonist-induced AT1aR phosphorylation was reduced by overexpression of a dominant negative K220R mutant GRK2 [104]. Cellular overexpression of GRK2[K220R] not only inhibited agonist-induced AT1aR phosphorylation, but also prevented receptor desensitization, as assessed by angiotensin II-stimulated GTPase activity in membranes prepared from agonist-treated and control cells. This finding indicated the critical role of GRK2 in the phosphorylation and desensitization of AT1aR. Through siRNA-mediated depletion, GRK2 was found to be a major kinase for AT1aR phosphorylation, contributing mostly to receptor internalization and β-arrestin recruitment in HEK293 cells. In addition, only GRK2 and 3 are associated with β-arrestin-mediated AT1aR internalization. In contrast, β-arrestin-mediated ERK signaling required receptor phosphorylation by GRK5 and 6, even though they account for a small fraction of the total receptor phosphorylation and β-arrestin recruitment. Moreover, depletion of either GRK5 or GRK6 alone by siRNA leads to an almost complete termination of β-arrestin-mediated ERK1/2 activation, suggesting that phosphorylation by both GRKs may be required. This finding suggested that GRK5/6 may phosphorylate distinct sites on the AT1aR and that both contributions were necessary to promote the ERK activation via β-arrestin. Such a mechanism also indicated tight control on β-arrestin-dependent signaling. Interestingly, both depletion of GRK2/3 and overexpression of GRK5/6 can increase the β-arrestin-mediated ERK1/2 activation. To some extent, it is the interplay between GRK2 and GRK5/6 that defines the duration and intensity of the β-arrestin signaling mechanism, thus emphasizing the importance of tight control of the balance between the G-protein- and β-arrestin-mediated pathway by different GRKs. Possible explanations are either a physical competition between GRKs for access to the receptor, or that GRK2/3 phosphorylation may inhibit subsequent receptor phosphorylation by GRK5/6. These findings indicate the distinct functional potentials of β-arrestins bound to AT1aR phosphorylated by different GRKs, and these different functional effects of receptor phosphorylation are induced by the different phosphorylation sites, which can constitute a barcode directing downstream signaling.

3.4 Chemokine Receptors

For the CCR7 chemokine receptor, it was reported that although both endogenous ligands, CCL19 and CCL21, induce G protein activation and subsequent calcium mobilization with equal potency, only activation by CCL19 promotes robust desensitization [105]. Using siRNA technology for GRKs, it was demonstrated that CCL19 and CCL21 result in striking differences in activation of the GRK/β-arrestin system [103]. CCL19 leads to robust CCR7 phosphorylation and β-arrestin recruitment catalyzed by both GRK3 and GRK6. In contrast, CCL21 activates GRK6 alone. This difference in GRK activation leads to distinct functional consequences. While both ligands lead to β-arrestin recruitment, only CCL19 leads to the redistribution of β-arrestin-GFP into endocytic vesicles and classical receptor desensitization. In contrast, both agonists are capable of signaling through GRK6 and β-arrestin to activate ERK1/2 [103].

A recent study of the CXC chemokine receptor CXCR4 used mass spectrometry in conjunction with phospho-specific antibodies to map phosphorylation sites upon SDF1 stimulation [106]. Of the eighteen potential serine/threonine phosphorylation sites on the CXCR4's C-terminus, three sites were mapped via mass spectrometry and four additional sites were localized with phospho-specific antibodies. GRK6 was found to account for the majority of the phosphorylation sites identified while no GRK2/3 sites were found. However, it was demonstrated that multiple GRKs regulate CXCR4 signaling, including GRK2. Silencing of either GRK2 or 6 by siRNA led to increased calcium mobilization, whereas knockdown of GRK3 or 6 led to decreased ERK1/2 activation [106]. This study revealed that site-specific phosphorylation of CXCR4 is tightly regulated by different GRKs. Interestingly, GRK2 knockdown led to enhanced ERK1/2 activation, suggesting coordination among the GRKs in terms of signaling, though no mechanistic explanation could be deduced in the absence of identified GRK2 phosphorylation sites.

By using site-specific phospho-antibodies against CXCR4, it was demonstrated that the endogenous ligand, CXCL12, promotes robust phosphorylation at S346/347 mediated by GRK2/3 [107]. The phosphorylation of S346/347 in the CXCR4 preceded phosphorylation at S324/325 and S338/339. After CXCL12 washout, the phosphorylation levels of S338/339 and S324/325 were rapidly decreased whereas phosphorylation at S346/347 was prolonged. A S346-348A mutant showed strongly impaired CXCL12-promoted phosphorylation at S324/325 and S338/339, defective internalization, increased calcium mobilization, and reduced desensitization. This finding suggested that the triple serine motif S346–S348 contains a major initial CXCR4 phosphorylation site that is prerequisite for subsequent receptor phosphorylation on other sites.

A recent study in CXCR1 and CXCR2 revealed that these two chemokine receptors also couple to distinct GRKs to mediate and regulate leukocyte functions [108]. It was shown that inhibition of GRK2 and GRK6 by shRNA in RBL-2H3 cells decreased CXCR1 and CXCR2 phosphorylation, desensitization, and internalization, respectively. Meanwhile, CXCL8-induced phosphoinositide hydrolysis and exocytosis were enhanced. GRK2 had no significant effect on CXCR2-induced ERK1/2 phosphorylation, whereas depletion of GRK2 diminished CXCR1-induced ERK1/2 activation. Depletion of GRK6 had no effect on CXCR1 function. These results indicated that CXCR1 and CXCR2 couple to distinct GRK isoforms to mediate and regulate inflammatory responses. CXCR1 predominantly couples to GRK2, whereas CXCR2 interacts with GRK6 to negatively regulate receptor sensitization and trafficking, thus affecting cell signaling and angiogenesis.

In addition, it was reported that GRK2 is an essential regulator of CXCR7 signaling in astrocytes [109]. SDF-1/CXCL12-induced activation of ERK1/2 and AKT through CXCR7 was abrogated following the depletion of GRK2 by siRNA, but not by the depletion of GRK3, GRK5, or GRK6. This result suggests that GRK2 plays critical role in mediating the signaling of SDF-1/CXCL12-bound CXCR7.

3.5 Opioid Receptors

For the delta-opioid receptor (DOR), it was shown that receptor internalization followed via two distinct pathways in HEK293 cells [110]. The GRK2 phosphorylation-dependent internalization is mediated by both β-arrestin1/2, leading delta-opioid receptor recycling, whereas the GRK2-independent internalization mediated by β-arrestin2 alone leads to receptor degradation.

Different ligands of the mu-opioid receptor (MOR) also induce distinct responses to GRK2. For example, the activation of GRK2 can be mediated by DAMGO or etorphine, but not morphine [111–118]. GRK2 could increase the affinity of agonists, but not antagonists [119]. MORs could be phosphorylated by GRK5 upon morphine stimulation, which produces different effects compared with those of other GRKs [120]. Activation of GRK2/3 could be mediated by DAMGO, while the same agonist cannot promote the receptor phosphorylation by GRK6 in NG108-15 cells [113], even though experiments showed GRK2/3/6 may be effective in preventing opioid tolerance development and improving the analgesic efficacy of opioid drugs [114]

3.6 Dopamine Receptors

The hypothesis that different GRKs contribute differently to distinct GPCR functional and signaling consequences was also supported by studies of the dopamine receptors. It was reported that different GRKs direct the distinct regulation of D1 dopamine receptor (D1R) [121]. For example, GRK2/3 induced the rightward shift of the dopamine dose–response curve of D1R with little effect on the maximal activation, while GRK5 caused a rightward shift in the EC_{50} value with an additional 40% reduction in the maximal activation of dopamine. In another study, it was demonstrated that homologous desensitization of the D1R in human renal proximal tubules appeared to involve GRKs only in later stages of the process [122]. The early phase of homologous desensitization is regulated by a non-GRK-mediated pathway. In addition, GRK4 was more efficacious than GRK2 in facilitating homologous desensitization of the D1R.

The D2 dopamine receptor (D2R) also exhibited GRK-independent desensitization and internalization. Early in 1999, it was reported that the sequestration of D2R occurs through a GRK2/5-mediated pathway in HEK293 cells [123]. Later it was shown that ligand-induced internalization of D2R can occur in two different manners, one is a phosphorylation-dependent manner, which was mediated by the serine/threonine (Ser/Thr) residues in the second loop and third loop, and the other is a phosphorylation-independent manner [124, 125]. It was suggested that GRK2-mediated internalization and inhibition of the D2R signaling can occur without receptor phosphorylation, however the GRK2-mediated phosphorylation can enhance the former process. Receptor phosphorylation could affect recycling, indicating GRK2/3 can participate in the post-endocytic trafficking of the D2R.

With all this accumulating experimental evidence suggesting that different GRKs contribute differentially to distinct GPCR functional and signaling consequences, it is reasonable to hypothesize that distinct ligands or GRKs may lead to the phosphorylation of distinct sites, or sets of sites, on GPCRs. These distinct phosphorylation patterns on a given receptor induce functionally distinct conformations of the receptor-bound β-arrestin, thus leading to distinct functional consequences.

4   Differential GPCR Phosphorylation by Different GRKs: The "Barcode" Mechanism

4.1 Experimental Proof of the "Barcode" Hypothesis for GPCR Signaling

The "barcode" hypothesis provides an excellent theoretical foundation to explain many new observations in GPCR biology and pharmacology. However, since no defined phosphorylation consensus motifs for GRKs have been identified, little is known about the actual sites of phosphorylation on GPCRs targeted by individual GRKs or induced by different ligands, and how these phosphorylation sites regulate the specific functional consequences of β-arrestin engagement. Whereas phosphorylation sites on a number of GPCRs, such as rhodopsin [126], somatostatin (sst2A) [127], smoothened [128], and β2AR [129–131], have been studied using mutagenesis, phospho-specific antibodies, and/or mass spectrometry (MS), no data were reported on quantitatively mapping GRK-specific phosphorylation sites on a receptor and then correlating the site-specific phosphorylation with GPCR function.

As with many GPCRs, the β2AR has an abundance of serine and threonine residues on the carboxyl tail and the intracellular loops that are potential sites of phosphorylation. It should be noted that although several studies have been directed at the determination of phosphorylation sites on the β2AR [129, 131–134], few were attempted to precisely assign specific sites to different GRKs. Several studies have implicated the cytoplasmic tail of the β2AR as the site of GRK-mediated phosphorylation. Using phosphoserine-specific antibodies, it was reported that overexpression of GRK2 and 5 could increase basal levels of phosphorylation of the putative GRK sites S355, S356, which are not dependent on PKA sites [129]. An earlier study used a purified, recombinant human β2AR in conjunction with purified GRK2 and 5 proteins to delineate overlapping patterns of phosphorylation sites with these two GRKs [131]. The GRK2 and 5 phosphorylation sites were mapped to a 40-amino acid peptide located at the extreme carboxyl-terminal tail of the β2AR. Of the phosphorylatable serine and threonine within this region, six were assigned as GRK5 sites (T384, T393, S396, S401, S407, and S411) and four as GRK2 sites (T384, S396, S401, and S407) [131]. However, the relevance of these studies to the actual events occurring in cells is somewhat uncertain due to the high concentrations of receptors and GRKs utilized in these in vitro experiments. Mutagenesis studies have shown that the mutation of all serine and threonine residues in the C-terminus of the β2AR to alanine and/or glycine prevents agonist stimulated phosphorylation [135], receptor/β-arrestin interaction [133], β-arrestin-mediated desensitization [132], internalization [133], and ERK1/2 activation [80]. However, recent studies have shown that not all phosphorylation sites are required for each of the β-arrestin-mediated functions.

4.1.1 Cell Type-Based Receptor Phosphorylation "Barcode"

The idea of GPCR "barcode" was first suggested based on the studies of tissue-specific GPCR signaling. It was demonstrated that GPCR signaling is a flexible and dynamic process that varies depending on the cell type in which the receptor is expressed [136, 137]. The same receptor can be phosphorylated in distinct manners in different cell types. Later, it was observed that siRNA silencing of GRK2 reduced internalization of the delta-opioid receptor to ~50–70% of normal in neurons [138]. However, GRK2 silencing had virtually no effect on sequestration of the receptor stimulated by agonists in HEK293 cells, although GRK2 was present and actively functioned in the internalization of 5-HT4R in the HEK293 cells. This observation suggested that molecular factors of internalization were different in neurons and HEK293 cells, with β-arrestins contributing to sequestration in both cell types, while GRK2 and PKC activities were only involved in the neurons [138]. Therefore, even with the same receptor, the same agonist can induce distinct signaling patterns in different cell types.

4.1.2 Different Receptor Subtypes Use Different GRKs

As described above, GRK2 could promote the phosphorylation, desensitization, and internalization of CXCR1, and inhibit CXCL8-induced phosphoinositide hydrolysis and exocytosis in vitro. GRK6 functions similarly, but its predominant receptor substrate was CXCR2, not CXCR1. These results indicate that CXCR1 and CXCR2 couple to distinct GRK isoforms to mediate and regulate inflammatory responses, thus affecting cell signaling [139].

The opioid receptors serve as another good example to demonstrate barcode regulation depending on ligand efficiency and receptor subtype. Apart from the normal desensitization and internalization for the delta-opioid receptor [140], the kappa-opioid receptor [32, 141], the mu-opioid receptor [140, 142, 143], and opioid receptor-like 1 [144, 145], the agonist barcode toward GRK3 activation may be different compared with GRK2. For example, mu-opioid receptor desensitization was significantly slower when GRK3 was knocked down [146], while no effect of GRK2 knockdown was observed. Etonitazene and fentanyl were shown to induce receptor phosphorylation at T370, S375, and T379, predominantly by GRK3 in vivo, as indicated by immunoprecipitation and nanoflow liquid chromatography-tandem mass spectrometry analysis [120].

In the study where receptors and kinases were tagged with fluorophores at their respective C terminus, laser scanning microscopy was used to observe co-internalization of delta-opioid receptors with GRK2 or 3. No such co-internalization was observed for mu-receptors in NG108-15 and HEK293 cells [141]. Another opioid receptor family member, the kappa-opioid receptor, also showed differential effects of GRK2: the desensitization and phosphorylation of the human kappa-opioid receptor after (−) U50,488H treatment was observed, whereas the rat kappa-opioid receptor was not phosphorylated and desensitized or internalized by GRK2 upon stimulation by the same agonist [147–149].

4.1.3 Ligand-Specific GPCR Phosphorylation

Technological advances in mass spectrometry-based quantitative proteomics made this research effort possible. As a proof of principle, the β2AR was used as a model receptor to test the "barcode" hypothesis of GPCR signaling [150]. Using mass spectrometry as a tool, thirteen phosphorylation sites (S246, S261, S262, S345, S346, S355, S356, T360, S364, S396, S401, S407, and S411) were identified on β2AR (Fig. 3) [150]. To quantitatively characterize these phosphorylation events, a Stable Isotope Labeling with Amino acids in Cell culture (SILAC) strategy was employed to

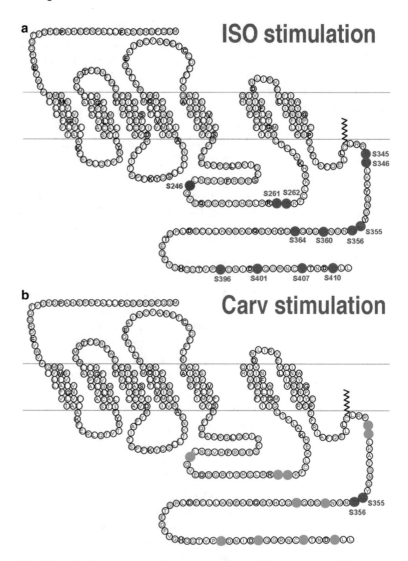

Fig. 3 Quantitative mass spectrometry analysis of isoproterenol (ISO) (**a**) and carvedilol (Carv) (**b**)-stimulated β2AR phosphorylation. Profiling of phosphorylation changes in the β2AR upon isoproterenol or carvedilol treatment by LC/MS/MS in combination with SILAC. The 13 phosphorylation sites identified are shown as *filled circles*. Carvedilol stimulation only induces significant changes in the phosphorylation levels at S355/S356. S246 is the only site whose phosphorylation decreased upon isoproterenol stimulation

detect the difference in the relative levels of phosphorylation of each site before and after agonist stimulation. Upon isoproterenol (a full and unbiased β2AR agonist) stimulation, the phosphorylation of these sites increased by a factor ranging from 7.5 to more than 300 (Fig. 3a) [150]. The only exception is the phosphorylation level of S246, which decreased by 50% upon isoproterenol stimulation. In contrast, β2AR stimulation by 10 μM carvedilol (Coreg®) for 5 min only induced an increase in phosphorylation levels of S355 and S356 (Fig. 3b). Carvedilol is a β-adrenergic antagonist that has recently been shown to selectively activate β-arrestin-mediated signaling, even while blocking G protein-dependent signaling. These data support the concept that different ligands (such as unbiased agonist vs. biased ligand) induce different phosphorylation patterns of specific receptors. The most reasonable explanation for this phenomenon is that different ligands may selectively engage different GRKs, thus leading to distinct receptor phosphorylation patterns.

In addition to adrenergic receptors, the ligand-associated barcode also exists in the chemokine receptor (CXCR). The regulation of CXCRs by GRKs was first characterized in CXCR5 in 1997 [151], showing CXCR5 could be phosphorylated by GRK2, 3, 5, 6 in HEK293 and COS-7 cells. Whereas all four GRKs tested could phosphorylate CXCR5, selectivity of the GRKs was also evident. GRK2 and GRK3 overexpression led to increases in phosphorylation primarily in the presence of agonist, GRK5 and GRK6 phosphorylated CXCR5 even in the absence of agonist stimulation, showing a level of selectivity and agonist independence of GRK phosphorylation. Later, it was reported that GRK2 (possibly together with GRK3) induced CXCR5 phosphorylation, desensitization, and internalization, thus attenuating agonist-induced calcium mobilization by CXCR5 signaling [152]. Using receptor mutants, it was showed that serine residues at positions 336, 337, 342, and 349 represent GRK phosphorylation sites on CXCR5. This study also revealed that chemokines differ in their ability to induce CXCR5 phosphorylation and desensitization.

4.1.4 GRK-Specific GPCR Phosphorylation

Although the GRK phosphorylation sites have been reported on several receptors, there was no systematic report on the β2AR because there are so many possible arrangements of Ser/Thr residues on the different intracellular domains that could be phosphorylated by GRKs [22]. Through MS and other experiments, we successfully mapped the phosphorylation sites targeted by individual GRKs and revealed a detailed mechanism how a "barcode" of phosphorylated Ser/Thr residues of β2AR evoked by different GRKs and read by β-arrestin directs distinct signaling [150].

To quantitatively characterize the actual sites of phosphorylation on GPCRs targeted by individual GRKs, RNAi technology was used to silence the expression of different GRKs individually, and SILAC was then used to quantitatively measure the extent of phosphorylation of each site on the β2AR upon depletion of each individual GRK. It was found that the depletion of GRK6 specifically reduced isoproterenol-promoted phosphorylation of S355 and S356 fivefold (Fig. 4). Depletion of GRK2 reduced the phosphorylation of T360, S364, S396, S401, S407, and S411 by two to threefold (Fig. 4). The extents of phosphorylation of S261, S262, S345, and S346 did not significantly change when either GRK2 or 6 was depleted. Based on these findings, it was concluded

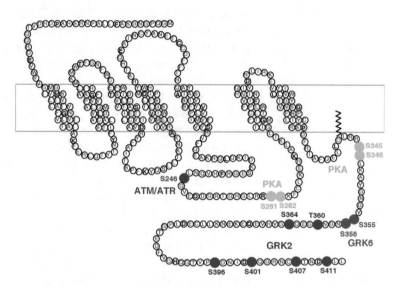

Fig. 4 GRK2 and 6 phosphorylate different sites on the β2AR. GRK2 and GRK6 phosphorylation sites were mapped on the β2AR using RNAi technology and a quantitative mass spectrometry-based proteomic approach. Residues whose phosphorylation levels decreased upon GRK2 or GRK6 siRNA are shown as *red* or *blue filled circles*, respectively. PKA consensus sites are shown. S246 has been previously identified as a consensus site for ATM phosphorylation

that GRK2 is mainly responsible for the phosphorylation of T360, S364, S396, S401, S407, and S411, and that GRK6 is responsible for the phosphorylation of S355 and S356 upon agonist stimulation (Fig. 4). In addition, S261/S262 and S345/S346 were previously reported to be consensus sites for PKA, as shown in Fig. 4. S246 was previously identified as a consensus site for ATM phosphorylation [153]. This study was the first to provide direct experimental evidence for the GPCR phosphorylation barcoding mechanism—the distinct sets of phosphorylation sites targeted by the different GRKs establish a "barcode" that imparts distinct conformations to the recruited β-arrestin, thus potentially regulating its functional activities. These results point toward a new paradigm for understanding how signaling by GPCRs is regulated.

It is interesting that while knockdown of GRK6 led to a fivefold decrease in the phosphorylation of S355 and S356, knockdown of GRK2 led to a 1.5-fold increase in the phosphorylation of the two sites shown in Fig. 4. This finding through MS analysis was verified by immunoprecipitation (IP) of β2AR from HEK293 cells stably expressing receptors that contain an N-terminal FLAG tag and then by probing these β2AR with a phospho-specific antibody directed at these sites. Treatment with a control siRNA and stimulation with isoproterenol led to a rapid, sustained, and robust increase in the phosphorylation of S355/S356 (Fig. 5a, b). Treatment with GRK2 siRNA resulted in increased phosphorylation at these sites over the time period of stimulation with

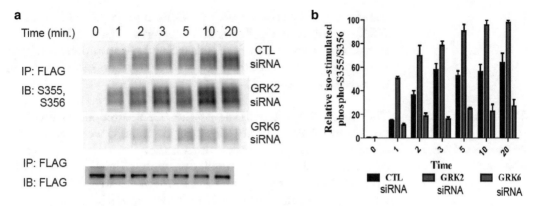

Fig. 5 GRK2 and 6 expression levels alter phosphorylation of the β2AR serines 355 and 356. (**a**) The *top three panels* are western blot analyses with a phospho-specific antibody recognizing pSer355/pSer356 on β2AR immunoprecipitated from stably expressing HEK293 cells (2 pmol/mg) that have been transfected with either control (CTL), GRK2 or GRK6 siRNA, respectively. The *bottom panel* is a FLAG western blot to show equal loading of immunoprecipitated β2AR. (**b**) Quantitation of three independent experiments described in (**a**). The largest signal in each experiment was normalized to 100 % subsequent to normalization via FLAG western blots. Data shown are the mean ± SEM for three independent experiments. The pS355/pS356 data for control (CTL)-siRNA transfected cells is shown in *black*; for GRK2-siRNA transfected cells is shown in *red*; for GRK6-siRNA transfected cells is shown in *blue*

isoproterenol. The largest differences, in comparison to control siRNA, occurred at the earlier time points (Fig. 5b; red bars). Conversely, GRK6 siRNA treatment led to a marked decrease in the phosphorylation of S355/S356 (Fig. 5b; blue bars). Thus, GRK2 appears to inhibit GRK6 phosphorylation of S355/S356.

The GRK phosphorylation may have more patterns since the detailed mechanisms still need to be investigated. For example, S404, S408, and S410 were identified as the phosphorylation sites involved in GRK2-induced desensitization of a subtype of adrenergic receptor, α1B-AR [154]. It was also suggested that these sites could be phosphorylated independently following agonist stimulation of the receptor. Overexpression of GRK2 was able to specifically increase agonist-induced phosphorylation of receptor mutants carrying S404, S408, and S410 individually or in different combinations, meaning that GRK2 can phosphorylate S404, S408, and S410 of the receptor independently. These data argued for a nonsequential mechanism of receptor phosphorylation by GRK2.

4.1.5 Distinct Receptor Phosphorylation Barcodes are Responsible for Distinct GPCR Functions and Signaling

4.1.5.1 Silencing of GRK2 and/or 6 Impairs β2AR Desensitization

To correlate the distinct GPCR phosphorylation barcodes with different receptor functions and signaling, a live cell biosensor, GloSensor, was used to measure β2AR efficacy for stimulating G_s-dependent cAMP generation upon altering its phosphorylation pattern with GRK siRNAs [150]. Endogenous β2ARs in GloSensor HEK stable cells were pre-stimulated with either vehicle (DMSO) or 100 nM isoproterenol for 5 min and then washed and re-challenged with isoproterenol over an entire dose–response curve. This treatment induces a 50 % loss of maximal cAMP signal in cells transfected with control siRNA. Cells transfected with GRK2, GRK6 or GRK2 and 6 siRNA show impairment of this desensitization after restimulation of the cells with 10 μM isoproterenol. This result suggested that both GRK2 and 6 are responsible for β2AR desensitization (Table 2).

4.1.5.2 Internalization of the β2AR is Affected by the Expression of Both GRK2 and 6

The internalization patterns of the β2AR after knockdown of GRK2 and GRK6, either alone or combined, were studied to reveal their roles in receptor internalization [150]. In the presence of a control siRNA and stimulation with 10 μM isoproterenol, internalization is rapid, with a maximum of 50 % of the β2AR being internalized in 30 min. Knockdown of GRK2 slows the initial rate of internalization and significantly reduces the maximum observed internalization to 20 %. GRK6 siRNA also slows the initial rate of β2AR internalization and lowers the maximum observed internalization to 35 %. Ablation of both GRK2 and 6 almost completely blocks receptor internalization. The data suggested that both GRK2 and 6 are responsible for β2AR internalization (Table 2).

To summarize, for the β_2AR, phosphorylation appears to be a prerequisite for β-arrestin recruitment and β-arrestin-mediated signaling, whereas this does not appear to be the case for the AT1AR. Although both the distal and the proximal phosphorylation residues of the β_2AR are important for β-arrestin binding, it is the distal residues (assigned as GRK sites here) that confer high-affinity binding and also coordinate protein–protein interactions that facilitate internalization [133, 150].

4.1.5.3 Effects of GRK siRNA on β2AR-stimulated pERK

To test whether GRK2 or 6 can specifically promote β-arrestin-mediated ERK activation through the β2AR, we stimulated HEK293 cells stably expressing the β2AR with either isoproterenol or carvedilol after they had been treated with GRK-specific siRNAs [150]. The time course of ERK activation was recorded to determine the effects of silencing the GRKs. In isoproterenol-stimulated, control siRNA-transfected cells, ERK1/2 activation was robust at five min (typically 14-fold over basal), while the 15-min time point showed a lesser amount of ERK1/2 activation (4-fold over basal). Carvedilol stimulation in control siRNA-transfected cells led to lower ERK activation. GRK2 depletion by siRNA tended to increase ERK activation stimulated by isoproterenol or carvedilol. In stark contrast, GRK6-siRNA transfected cells stimulated with either isoproterenol or carvedilol showed significantly less ERK1/2 activation at the fifteen-minute point when compared with control-siRNA transfected cells. These data suggested that GRK6 is responsible for βarrestin-mediated ERK activation, whereas GRK2 opposes it (Table 2).

4.2 Molecular Mechanisms of GPCR Phosphorylation "Barcoding"

4.2.1 GRK2 and 6 Phosphorylation Dictate β-Arrestin2 Conformation

As mentioned above, inhibiting GRK5 or 6 expression abolished β-arrestin-mediated ERK activation, whereas lowering GRK2 or 3 led to an increase in this signaling. Consistent with this finding, β-arrestin-mediated ERK activation was enhanced by overexpression of GRK5 and 6, and reciprocally diminished by overexpression of GRK2 and 3. These findings further support the "barcode" theory, which posits that there are distinct functional capabilities of β-arrestins bound to receptors phosphorylated by different GRKs.

To test the hypothesis that phosphorylation of the β2AR, mediated by either GRK2 or GRK6, can elicit distinct conformations of β-arrestin, a bioluminescence resonance energy transfer (BRET)-based biosensor of β-arrestin2 was used [155, 156]. In this biosensor, the N-terminus of β-arrestin2 is fused to bioluminescent Renilla luciferase (RLuc) while the C-terminus is fused to yellow fluorescent protein (YFP). Isoproterenol stimulation of control-siRNA transfected cells results in an increase in the intramolecular BRET, indicating a conformational change in β-arrestin upon recruitment to the β2AR. In stark contrast, however, isoproterenol stimulation of β2AR after GRK2-siRNA treatment leads to a decrease in intramolecular BRET, suggesting a different conformation of β-arrestin in the GRK2-siRNA transfected cells compared to that in the CTL-siRNA transfected cells. Interestingly, GRK6-siRNA transfected cells showed no significant change in the BRET signal, suggesting that the β-arrestin conformation in the GRK6-siRNA transfected cells is different from that in either CTL- or GRK2-siRNA transfected cells. The differences in intramolecular BRET signals detected in the presence of CTL-, GRK2-, or GRK6-siRNA suggest that β-arrestin adopts different conformations under these conditions. Taken together, this study revealed that phosphorylation of β2AR by two different GRKs (GRK2 vs 6) results in distinct β-arrestin conformations.

4.2.2 Multiple Conformational Changes of β-Arrestin Induced by Different Phosphorylation Barcodes

It has been well established that phosphorylation of GPCRs by GRKs plays essential role in regulation of receptor function by promoting receptor interactions with β-arrestins. The binding to a phosphorylated receptor is usually a prerequisite for β-arrestin functions. In the study of the roles of different GRKs in V2R signaling, the authors found that agonist-dependent β-arrestin recruitment to the V2R was impaired significantly with GRK2 depletion compared with GRK5 or 6 siRNA-treated cells [15]. This result indicates that the V2R phosphorylated by GRK2 has a relatively higher binding affinity for β-arrestin, probably due to a unique conformation in β-arrestin induced by GRK2 phosphorylation. This unique β-arrestin conformation favors receptor uncoupling from the G protein. Simultaneously, there also exists the possibility that the

V2R phosphorylated by GRK5 and/or GRK6 might induce the proper conformation to promote ERK signaling via the β-arrestin2-mediated pathway. In agreement with this idea, it was previously reported that both β-arrestin1 and 2 could adopt activation-dependent conformations upon binding to V2Rpp, a phosphopeptide mimicking the phosphorylated C-terminus of V2R (V2Rpp sequence: ARGRpTPPpSLGPQDEpSCpTpTApSpSpSLAKDTSS) [157, 158]. These V2Rpp-activation-dependent conformations of β-arrestin1 and 2 are distinct from those adopted by free β-arrestins or β-arrestins in the presence of the non-phosphopeptide V2Rnp. Moreover, these active conformations could significantly enhance the binding affinity of clathrin for β-arrestins [157, 158].

The co-crystal structure of V2Rpp/β-arrestin1 complex revealed marked conformational differences in β-arrestin1 compared to its inactive conformation [159–164]. The binding of V2Rpp induced the rotation of the N-domain of β-arrestin1 with respect to its C-domain. Meanwhile, large conformational changes were observed in the "finger", "middle", and "lariat" loops previously implicated in β-arrestin–receptor interactions [13, 77, 78, 160, 164]. These results provided detailed structural information, at high resolution, of β-arrestin activated by a specific phosphorylation pattern of V2R, indicating a potentially general molecular mechanism for activation of β-arrestin.

To further characterize conformations of β-arrestins corresponding to different phosphorylation "barcodes" of GPCRs, unnatural amino acid incorporation and fluorine-19 nuclear magnetic resonance (^{19}F-NMR) spectroscopy were used to monitor the conformational changes in β-arrestin upon binding to a panel of synthetic phosphopeptides. These peptides mimic different phosphorylation "barcodes" corresponding to the C-terminus of β2AR phosphorylated by GRK2, GRK6, or PKA [165]. While all these phosphopeptides interact with a common phosphate binding site on the concave surface of β-arrestin1 and induce the movements of "finger" and "middle" loops, conformational changes induced by different phosphorylation patterns are distinct. Moreover, the phosphopeptides (GRK2App: DFVGHQGTVPpSDNIDpSQGRNCpSTNDpSLL and GRK2Bpp: NGNpTGEQpSGYHVEQEKENKLLCEDLPGTE), mimicking GRK2 phosphorylation of β2AR, promote the formation of the β-arrestin1/clathrin complex, whereas the phosphopeptide mimicking GRK6 phosphorylation (GRK6pp: RRSIKAYGNGYpSpSPSNGNTGEQSGYHVEQ) promotes the formation of the β-arrestin1/Src complex. In contrast, the phosphopeptide mimicking PKA phosphorylation (PKApp: DGRTGHGLRRpSpSKFCLKEHKALKTLGII) did not promote the formation of either β-arrestin1/Src and β-arrestin1/clathrin complexes. Taken together, these results provided further evidence for the "barcode" hypothesis and revealed that distinct receptor phosphorylation "barcodes" can translate into specific β-arrestin conformations and thus direct selective signaling (Fig. 6) [165]. The GRK6-mediated GPCR phosphorylation "barcode" selectively activates Src and GRK2-mediated receptor phosphorylation "barcode" specifically induces clathrin binding and facilitates receptor endocytosis.

4.2.3 "Barcode" Theory Explains Differential Functions of β-Arrestin

The studies summarized above provide accumulating evidence for the GPCR "barcode" theory and revealed detailed molecular mechanisms of receptor phosphorylation "barcoding" (Fig. 7) [166]. At the level of the receptor, different ligands stabilize different active receptor conformations. Subsequently, these unique conformations lead to the recruitment of unique GRK or subsets of GRKs to the ligand-activated receptors. As a consequence, differential phosphorylation patterns or "barcodes" are produced on the receptor. Receptor phosphorylation promotes the recruitment of β-arrestin to the receptor. At the level of β-arrestin, the distinct phosphorylation "barcodes" on the receptor induce distinct conformational changes in β-arrestin. The distinct β-arrestin conformations, in turn, promote binding of different signaling transducer molecules to the receptor–β-arrestin complexes, leading to the activation of distinct signaling networks. These distinct phosphorylation "barcodes" on the receptor ultimately lead to divergent physiological responses.

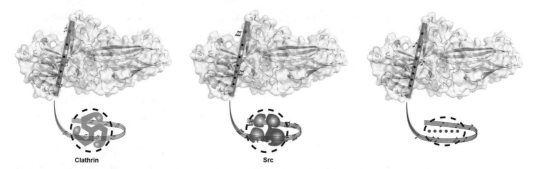

Clathrin   Src

Fig. 6 Phospho-pattern-selective mechanisms of β-arrestin conformations and specific functions. Experiments using unnatural amino acid incorporation and ^{19}F-NMR revealed that distinct receptor phosphorylation patterns ("barcode") can induce distinct conformation changes in β-arrestin. These distinct β-arrestin conformations promote the binding of different signaling proteins to the receptor–β-arrestin complexes. The GRK6-mediated GPCR phosphorylation "barcode" selectively activates Src, and the GRK2-mediated receptor phosphorylation "barcode" specifically induces clathrin binding

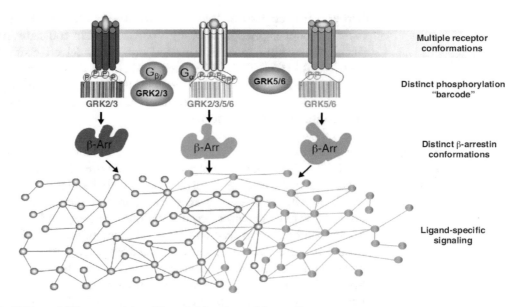

Fig. 7 "Barcode" theory explains differential functions of β-arrestins

5   The Ramifications of the GPCR "Barcode" Phenomenon for Biology and Medicine`

In the past several decades, the two-step regulatory process, receptor phosphorylation by GRKs followed by β-arrestin recruitment to the activated and phosphorylated receptor, forms the foundation to understanding how GPCRs function and how they are regulated. The GPCR "barcode" phenomenon extended this classic theory in GPCR regulation and expanded our understanding of GPCR function. It provides a fine-tuned molecular mechanism to explain how receptor function is precisely regulated and how complex signaling network is managed. This molecular mechanism offers a theoretical basis to explain many new discoveries in the field of GPCR biology and pharmacology. These observations were not previously well explained by the simple, two-step regulatory process of the GRK/β-arrestin system. As a result, the receptor "barcoding" provides a way to manage or manipulate GPCR signaling in a way that one favors for maximal pharmacological benefit. This signaling management or manipulation can be achieved through modification of the possible phosphorylation codes or by controlling specific GRKs or β-arrestin actions.

The "barcode" theory also provides a way to understand why the same receptor can exert different functions in different cells or tissue. By adopting a specific phosphorylation profile or "phosphorylation signature", a receptor could favor coupling to a particular pathway. In this way, the phosphorylation profile of a receptor could act as a "barcode" that encodes a particular signaling outcome. Hence, in each cell or tissue type a GPCR might adopt a different phosphorylation profile, or barcode, due the difference in the complement of the GRKs and β-arrestins. This would contribute to cell- or tissue-specific signaling related to the physiological function of the receptor.

As different ligands can induce distinct "phosphorylation signatures" on a given receptor, and these distinct "phosphorylation signatures" promote distinct conformational changes in β-arrestins, the β-arrestin signaling is therefore encoded via the phosphorylation "barcode". The "barcode" theory has great potential to be harnessed to develop novel therapeutics. Since specific ligands lead to specific phosphorylation "barcode" on a given receptor, the specific receptor "barcode" could be used to develop new assays for drug screening. For example, the phosphorylation "barcode" on the β2AR induced by β-arrestin-biased ligand carvedilol was found to be the sites phosphorylated by GRK6. These GRK6 sites therefore become a part of the unique profile for the β-arrestin-mediated β2AR signaling. Phospho-specific antibodies against these sites can be generated to enable screening assays for the β-arrestin-biased ligands for the β2AR. Such ligands may eliminate adverse effects by avoiding undesirable signaling, increase the efficacy by stimulating or avoiding specific negative or positive feedback loops in signaling pathways, and can also help to reveal previously unappreciated pharmacology with new benefits.

References

1. Rockman HA, Koch WJ, Lefkowitz RJ (2002) Seven-transmembrane-spanning receptors and heart function. Nature 415(6868):206–212
2. Pierce KL, Luttrell LM, Lefkowitz RJ (2001) New mechanisms in heptahelical receptor signaling to mitogen activated protein kinase cascades. Oncogene 20(13):1532–1539
3. Lefkowitz RJ (1998) G protein-coupled receptors. III New roles for receptor kinases and beta-arrestins in receptor signaling and desensitization. J Biol Chem 273(30):18677–18680
4. Lefkowitz RJ (1996) G protein-coupled receptors and receptor kinases: from molecular biology to potential therapeutic applications. Nat Biotechnol 14(3):283–286
5. Pierce KL, Premont RT, Lefkowitz RJ (2002) Seven-transmembrane receptors. Nat Rev Mol Cell Biol 3(9):639–650
6. Ma P, Zemmel R (2002) Value of novelty? Nat Rev Drug Discov 1(8):571–572
7. Neves SR, Ram PT, Iyengar R (2002) G protein pathways. Science 296(5573):1636–1639
8. Luttrell LM, Lefkowitz RJ (2002) The role of beta-arrestins in the termination and transduction of G-protein-coupled receptor signals. J Cell Sci 115(Pt 3):455–465
9. Shenoy SK, Lefkowitz RJ (2003) Multifaceted roles of beta-arrestins in the regulation of seven-membrane-spanning receptor trafficking and signalling. Biochem J 375(Pt 3):503–515
10. McDonald PH, Lefkowitz RJ (2001) Beta-Arrestins: new roles in regulating heptahelical receptors' functions. Cell Signal 13(10):683–689
11. Lefkowitz RJ, Shenoy SK (2005) Transduction of receptor signals by beta-arrestins. Science 308(5721):512–517
12. Lefkowitz RJ, Rajagopal K, Whalen EJ (2006) New roles for beta-arrestins in cell signaling: not just for seven-transmembrane receptors. Mol Cell 24(5):643–652
13. Gurevich VV, Gurevich EV (2006) The structural basis of arrestin-mediated regulation of G-protein-coupled receptors. Pharmacol Ther 110(3):465–502

14. Kim J, Ahn S, Ren XR, Whalen EJ, Reiter E, Wei H, Lefkowitz RJ (2005) Functional antagonism of different G protein-coupled receptor kinases for beta-arrestin-mediated angiotensin II receptor signaling. Proc Natl Acad Sci U S A 102(5):1442–1447

15. Ren XR, Reiter E, Ahn S, Kim J, Chen W, Lefkowitz RJ (2005) Different G protein-coupled receptor kinases govern G protein and beta-arrestin-mediated signaling of V2 vasopressin receptor. Proc Natl Acad Sci U S A 102(5):1448–1453

16. Shenoy SK, Drake MT, Nelson CD, Houtz DA, Xiao K, Madabushi S, Reiter E, Premont RT, Lichtarge O, Lefkowitz RJ (2006) beta-arrestin-dependent, G protein-independent ERK1/2 activation by the beta2 adrenergic receptor. J Biol Chem 281(2):1261–1273

17. Shichi H, Somers RL (1978) Light-dependent phosphorylation of rhodopsin. Purification and properties of rhodopsin kinase. J Biol Chem 253(19):7040–7046

18. Weiss ER, Raman D, Shirakawa S, Ducceschi MH, Bertram PT, Wong F, Kraft TW, Osawa S (1998) The cloning of GRK7, a candidate cone opsin kinase, from cone- and rod-dominant mammalian retinas. Mol Vis 4:27

19. Benovic JL, Strasser RH, Caron MG, Lefkowitz RJ (1986) Beta-adrenergic receptor kinase: identification of a novel protein kinase that phosphorylates the agonist-occupied form of the receptor. Proc Natl Acad Sci U S A 83(9):2797–2801

20. Benovic JL, Onorato JJ, Arriza JL, Stone WC, Lohse M, Jenkins NA, Gilbert DJ, Copeland NG, Caron MG, Lefkowitz RJ (1991) Cloning, expression, and chromosomal localization of beta-adrenergic receptor kinase 2. A new member of the receptor kinase family. J Biol Chem 266(23): 14939–14946

21. Sallese M, Lombardi MS, De Blasi A (1994) Two isoforms of G protein-coupled receptor kinase 4 identified by molecular cloning. Biochem Biophys Res Commun 199(2): 848–854

22. Premont RT, Koch WJ, Inglese J, Lefkowitz RJ (1994) Identification, purification, and characterization of GRK5, a member of the family of G protein-coupled receptor kinases. J Biol Chem 269(9):6832–6841

23. Kunapuli P, Benovic JL (1993) Cloning and expression of GRK5: a member of the G protein-coupled receptor kinase family. Proc Natl Acad Sci U S A 90(12):5588–5592

24. Benovic JL, Gomez J (1993) Molecular cloning and expression of GRK6. A new member of the G protein-coupled receptor kinase family. J Biol Chem 268(26):19521–19527

25. Benovic JL, Mayor F Jr, Staniszewski C, Lefkowitz RJ, Caron MG (1987) Purification and characterization of the beta-adrenergic receptor kinase. J Biol Chem 262(19):9026–9032

26. Chen CK, Burns ME, Spencer M, Niemi GA, Chen J, Hurley JB, Baylor DA, Simon MI (1999) Abnormal photoresponses and light-induced apoptosis in rods lacking rhodopsin kinase. Proc Natl Acad Sci U S A 96(7):3718–3722

27. Pitcher JA, Freedman NJ, Lefkowitz RJ (1998) G protein-coupled receptor kinases. Annu Rev Biochem 67:653–692

28. Premont RT, Inglese J, Lefkowitz RJ (1995) Protein kinases that phosphorylate activated G protein-coupled receptors. FASEB J 9(2):175–182

29. Willets JM, Challiss RA, Nahorski SR (2003) Non-visual GRKs: are we seeing the whole picture? Trends Pharmacol Sci 24(12): 626–633

30. Premont RT, Macrae AD, Aparicio SA, Kendall HE, Welch JE, Lefkowitz RJ (1999) The GRK4 subfamily of G protein-coupled receptor kinases. Alternative splicing, gene organization, and sequence conservation. J Biol Chem 274(41):29381–29389

31. Jiang X, Benovic JL, Wedegaertner PB (2007) Plasma membrane and nuclear localization of G protein coupled receptor kinase 6A. Mol Biol Cell 18(8):2960–2969

32. Thiyagarajan MM, Stracquatanio RP, Pronin AN, Evanko DS, Benovic JL, Wedegaertner PB (2004) A predicted amphipathic helix mediates plasma membrane localization of GRK5. J Biol Chem 279(17):17989–17995

33. Pitcher JA, Fredericks ZL, Stone WC, Premont RT, Stoffel RH, Koch WJ, Lefkowitz RJ (1996) Phosphatidylinositol 4,5-bisphosphate (PIP2)-enhanced G protein-coupled receptor kinase (GRK) activity. Location, structure, and regulation of the PIP2 binding site distinguishes the GRK subfamilies. J Biol Chem 271(40):24907–24913

34. Boguth CA, Singh P, Huang CC, Tesmer JJ (2010) Molecular basis for activation of G protein-coupled receptor kinases. EMBO J 29(19):3249–3259

35. Kohout TA, Lefkowitz RJ (2003) Regulation of G protein-coupled receptor kinases and arrestins during receptor desensitization. Mol Pharmacol 63(1):9–18

36. Jaber M, Koch WJ, Rockman H, Smith B, Bond RA, Sulik KK, Ross J Jr, Lefkowitz RJ, Caron MG, Giros B (1996) Essential role of beta-adrenergic receptor kinase 1 in cardiac development and function. Proc Natl Acad Sci U S A 93(23):12974–12979

37. Taneja M, Salim S, Saha K, Happe HK, Qutna N, Petty F, Bylund DB, Eikenburg DC (2011) Differential effects of inescapable stress on locus coeruleus GRK3, alpha2-adrenoceptor and CRF1 receptor levels in learned helpless and non-helpless rats: a potential link to stress resilience. Behav Brain Res 221(1):25–33

38. Bawa T, Altememi GF, Eikenburg DC, Standifer KM (2003) Desensitization of alpha 2A-adrenoceptor signalling by modest levels of adrenaline is facilitated by beta 2-adrenoceptor-dependent GRK3 up-regulation. Br J Pharmacol 138(5):921–931

39. Peppel K, Boekhoff I, McDonald P, Breer H, Caron MG, Lefkowitz RJ (1997) G protein-coupled receptor kinase 3 (GRK3) gene disruption leads to loss of odorant receptor desensitization. J Biol Chem 272(41): 25425–25428

40. Gainetdinov RR, Bohn LM, Walker JK, Laporte SA, Macrae AD, Caron MG, Lefkowitz RJ, Premont RT (1999) Muscarinic supersensitivity and impaired receptor desensitization in G protein-coupled receptor kinase 5-deficient mice. Neuron 24(4):1029–1036

41. Gainetdinov RR, Bohn LM, Sotnikova TD, Cyr M, Laakso A, Macrae AD, Torres GE, Kim KM, Lefkowitz RJ, Caron MG, Premont RT (2003) Dopaminergic supersensitivity in G protein-coupled receptor kinase 6-deficient mice. Neuron 38(2):291–303

42. Penela P, Ribas C, Mayor F Jr (2003) Mechanisms of regulation of the expression and function of G protein-coupled receptor kinases. Cell Signal 15(11):973–981

43. Chen CK, Zhang K, Church-Kopish J, Huang W, Zhang H, Chen YJ, Frederick JM, Baehr W (2001) Characterization of human GRK7 as a potential cone opsin kinase. Mol Vis 7:305–313

44. Somers RL, Klein DC (1984) Rhodopsin kinase activity in the mammalian pineal gland and other tissues. Science 226(4671):182–184

45. Yamamoto S, Sippel KC, Berson EL, Dryja TP (1997) Defects in the rhodopsin kinase gene in the Oguchi form of stationary night blindness. Nat Genet 15(2):175–178

46. Premont RT, Macrae AD, Stoffel RH, Chung N, Pitcher JA, Ambrose C, Inglese J, MacDonald ME, Lefkowitz RJ (1996) Characterization of the G protein-coupled receptor kinase GRK4. Identification of four splice variants. J Biol Chem 271(11): 6403–6410

47. Sallese M, Salvatore L, D'Urbano E, Sala G, Storto M, Launey T, Nicoletti F, Knopfel T, De Blasi A (2000) The G-protein-coupled receptor kinase GRK4 mediates homologous desensitization of metabotropic glutamate receptor 1. FASEB J 14(15):2569–2580

48. Felder RA, Sanada H, Xu J, Yu PY, Wang Z, Watanabe H, Asico LD, Wang W, Zheng S, Yamaguchi I, Williams SM, Gainer J, Brown NJ, Hazen-Martin D, Wong LJ, Robillard JE, Carey RM, Eisner GM, Jose PA (2002) G protein-coupled receptor kinase 4 gene variants in human essential hypertension. Proc Natl Acad Sci U S A 99(6):3872–3877

49. Villar VA, Jones JE, Armando I, Palmes-Saloma C, Yu P, Pascua AM, Keever L, Arnaldo FB, Wang Z, Luo Y, Felder RA, Jose PA (2009) G protein-coupled receptor kinase 4 (GRK4) regulates the phosphorylation and function of the dopamine D3 receptor. J Biol Chem 284(32):21425–21434

50. Brenninkmeijer CB, Price SA, Lopez Bernal A, Phaneuf S (1999) Expression of G-protein-coupled receptor kinases in pregnant term and non-pregnant human myometrium. J Endocrinol 162(3):401–408

51. Aguero J, Almenar L, D'Ocon P, Oliver E, Monto F, Moro J, Castello A, Rueda J, Martinez-Dolz L, Sanchez-Lazaro I, Montero JA (2008) Correlation between beta-adrenoceptors and G-protein-coupled receptor kinases in pretransplantation heart failure. Transplant Proc 40(9):3014–3016

52. Dzimiri N, Muiya P, Andres E, Al-Halees Z (2004) Differential functional expression of human myocardial G protein receptor kinases in left ventricular cardiac diseases. Eur J Pharmacol 489(3):167–177

53. Inglese J, Freedman NJ, Koch WJ, Lefkowitz RJ (1993) Structure and mechanism of the G protein-coupled receptor kinases. J Biol Chem 268(32):23735–23738

54. Monto F, Oliver E, Vicente D, Rueda J, Aguero J, Almenar L, Ivorra MD, Barettino D, D'Ocon P (2012) Different expression of adrenoceptors and GRKs in the human myocardium depends on heart failure etiology and correlates to clinical variables. Am J Physiol Heart Circ Physiol 303(3):H368–H376

55. Violin JD, Ren XR, Lefkowitz RJ (2006) G-protein-coupled receptor kinase specificity for beta-arrestin recruitment to the beta2-adrenergic receptor revealed by fluorescence resonance energy transfer. J Biol Chem 281(29):20577–20588

56. Bownds D, Dawes J, Miller J, Stahlman M (1972) Phosphorylation of frog photoreceptor membranes induced by light. Nat New Biol 237(73):125–127

57. Kuhn H, Dreyer WJ (1972) Light dependent phosphorylation of rhodopsin by ATP. FEBS Lett 20(1):1–6

58. Weller M, Virmaux N, Mandel P (1975) Light-stimulated phosphorylation of rhodopsin in the retina: the presence of a protein kinase that is specific for photobleached rhodopsin. Proc Natl Acad Sci U S A 72(1):381–385

59. Weller M, Virmaux N (1975) Proceedings: the role of rhodopsin phosphorylation in the control of permeability of rod segment discs to Ca2+. Exp Eye Res 20(2):185

60. Weller M, Virmaux N, Mandel P (1975) Role of light and rhodopsin phosphorylation in control of permeability of retinal rod outer segment disks to Ca2plus. Nature 256(5512):68–70

61. Weller M, Goridis C, Viramaux N, Mandel P (1975) Letter: a hypothetical model for the possible involvement of rhodopsin phosphorylation in light and dark adaptation in the retina. Exp Eye Res 21(4):405–408

62. Liebman PA, Pugh EN Jr (1980) ATP mediates rapid reversal of cyclic GMP phosphodiesterase activation in visual receptor membranes. Nature 287(5784):734–736

63. Stadel JM, Nambi P, Shorr RG, Sawyer DF, Caron MG, Lefkowitz RJ (1983) Catecholamine-induced desensitization of turkey erythrocyte adenylate cyclase is associated with phosphorylation of the beta-adrenergic receptor. Proc Natl Acad Sci U S A 80(11):3173–3177

64. Stadel JM, Nambi P, Shorr RG, Sawyer DF, Caron MG, Lefkowitz RJ (1983) Phosphorylation of the beta-adrenergic receptor accompanies catecholamine-induced desensitization of turkey erythrocyte adenylate cyclase. Trans Assoc Am Physicians 96:137–145

65. Sibley DR, Strasser RH, Caron MG, Lefkowitz RJ (1985) Homologous desensitization of adenylate cyclase is associated with phosphorylation of the beta-adrenergic receptor. J Biol Chem 260(7):3883–3886

66. Carman CV, Benovic JL (1998) G-protein-coupled receptors: turn-ons and turn-offs. Curr Opin Neurobiol 8(3):335–344

67. Stadel JM, Nambi P, Lavin TN, Heald SL, Caron MG, Lefkowitz RJ (1982) Catecholamine-induced desensitization of turkey erythrocyte adenylate cyclase. Structural alterations in the beta-adrenergic receptor revealed by photoaffinity labeling. J Biol Chem 257(16):9242–9245

68. Lorenz W, Inglese J, Palczewski K, Onorato JJ, Caron MG, Lefkowitz RJ (1991) The receptor kinase family: primary structure of rhodopsin kinase reveals similarities to the beta-adrenergic receptor kinase. Proc Natl Acad Sci U S A 88(19):8715–8719

69. Strasser RH, Benovic JL, Caron MG, Lefkowitz RJ (1986) Beta-agonist- and prostaglandin E1-induced translocation of the beta-adrenergic receptor kinase: evidence that the kinase may act on multiple adenylate cyclase-coupled receptors. Proc Natl Acad Sci U S A 83(17):6362–6366

70. Sibley DR, Strasser RH, Benovic JL, Daniel K, Lefkowitz RJ (1986) Phosphorylation/dephosphorylation of the beta-adrenergic receptor regulates its functional coupling to adenylate cyclase and subcellular distribution. Proc Natl Acad Sci U S A 83(24):9408–9412

71. Benovic JL, Mayor F Jr, Somers RL, Caron MG, Lefkowitz RJ (1986) Light-dependent phosphorylation of rhodopsin by beta-adrenergic receptor kinase. Nature 321(6073):869–872

72. Benovic JL, Kuhn H, Weyand I, Codina J, Caron MG, Lefkowitz RJ (1987) Functional desensitization of the isolated beta-adrenergic receptor by the beta-adrenergic receptor kinase: potential role of an analog of the retinal protein arrestin (48-kDa protein). Proc Natl Acad Sci U S A 84(24):8879–8882

73. Ramkumar V, Kwatra M, Benovic JL, Stiles GL, Stilesa GL (1993) Functional consequences of A1 adenosine-receptor phosphorylation by the beta-adrenergic receptor kinase. Biochim Biophys Acta 1179(1):89–97

74. Richardson RM, Kim C, Benovic JL, Hosey MM (1993) Phosphorylation and desensitization of human m2 muscarinic cholinergic receptors by two isoforms of the beta-adrenergic receptor kinase. J Biol Chem 268(18):13650–13656

75. Collins S, Bouvier M, Lohse MJ, Benovic JL, Caron MG, Lefkowitz RJ (1990) Mechanisms involved in adrenergic receptor desensitization. Biochem Soc Trans 18(4):541–544

76. Lohse MJ, Benovic JL, Codina J, Caron MG, Lefkowitz RJ (1990) beta-Arrestin: a protein that regulates beta-adrenergic receptor function. Science 248(4962):1547–1550

77. Gurevich VV, Dion SB, Onorato JJ, Ptasienski J, Kim CM, Sterne-Marr R, Hosey MM, Benovic JL (1995) Arrestin interactions with G protein-coupled receptors. Direct binding studies of wild type and mutant arrestins with rhodopsin, beta 2-adrenergic, and m2 muscarinic cholinergic receptors. J Biol Chem 270(2):720–731

78. Gurevich VV, Benovic JL (1993) Visual arrestin interaction with rhodopsin. Sequential multisite binding ensures strict selectivity toward light-activated phosphorylated rhodopsin. J Biol Chem 268(16):11628–11638

79. Ferguson SS, Downey WE 3rd, Colapietro AM, Barak LS, Menard L, Caron MG (1996) Role of beta-arrestin in mediating agonist-promoted G protein-coupled receptor internalization. Science 271(5247):363–366

80. DeWire SM, Ahn S, Lefkowitz RJ, Shenoy SK (2007) Beta-arrestins and cell signaling. Annu Rev Physiol 69:483–510

81. Shenoy SK, Lefkowitz RJ (2005) Seven-transmembrane receptor signaling through beta-arrestin. Sci STKE 2005(308):cm10

82. Moore CA, Milano SK, Benovic JL (2007) Regulation of receptor trafficking by GRKs and arrestins. Annu Rev Physiol 69:451–482

83. Laporte SA, Oakley RH, Holt JA, Barak LS, Caron MG (2000) The interaction of beta-arrestin with the AP-2 adaptor is required for the clustering of beta 2-adrenergic receptor into clathrin-coated pits. J Biol Chem 275(30):23120–23126

84. Krupnick JG, Goodman OB Jr, Keen JH, Benovic JL (1997) Arrestin/clathrin interaction. Localization of the clathrin binding domain of nonvisual arrestins to the carboxy terminus. J Biol Chem 272(23):15011–15016

85. Goodman OB Jr, Krupnick JG, Santini F, Gurevich VV, Penn RB, Gagnon AW, Keen JH, Benovic JL (1996) Beta-arrestin acts as a clathrin adaptor in endocytosis of the beta2-adrenergic receptor. Nature 383(6599):447–450

86. Krupnick JG, Santini F, Gagnon AW, Keen JH, Benovic JL (1997) Modulation of the arrestin-clathrin interaction in cells. Characterization of beta-arrestin dominant-negative mutants. J Biol Chem 272(51):32507–32512

87. Damke H, Baba T, Warnock DE, Schmid SL (1994) Induction of mutant dynamin specifically blocks endocytic coated vesicle formation. J Cell Biol 127(4):915–934

88. Oakley RH, Laporte SA, Holt JA, Caron MG, Barak LS (2000) Differential affinities of visual arrestin, beta arrestin1, and beta arrestin2 for G protein-coupled receptors delineate two major classes of receptors. J Biol Chem 275(22):17201–17210

89. Qian H, Pipolo L, Thomas WG (2001) Association of beta-Arrestin 1 with the type 1A angiotensin II receptor involves phosphorylation of the receptor carboxyl terminus and correlates with receptor internalization. Mol Endocrinol 15(10):1706–1719

90. Pals-Rylaarsdam R, Gurevich VV, Lee KB, Ptasienski JA, Benovic JL, Hosey MM (1997) Internalization of the m2 muscarinic acetylcholine receptor. Arrestin-independent and -dependent pathways. J Biol Chem 272(38):23682–23689

91. Vishnivetskiy SA, Paz CL, Schubert C, Hirsch JA, Sigler PB, Gurevich VV (1999) How does arrestin respond to the phosphorylated state of rhodopsin? J Biol Chem 274(17):11451–11454

92. Oakley RH, Laporte SA, Holt JA, Barak LS, Caron MG (1999) Association of beta-arrestin with G protein-coupled receptors during clathrin-mediated endocytosis dictates the profile of receptor resensitization. J Biol Chem 274(45):32248–32257

93. Reiter E, Lefkowitz RJ (2006) GRKs and beta-arrestins: roles in receptor silencing, trafficking and signaling. Trends Endocrinol Metab 17(4):159–165

94. Luttrell LM (2008) Reviews in molecular biology and biotechnology: transmembrane signaling by G protein-coupled receptors. Mol Biotechnol 39(3):239–264

95. Luttrell LM, Gesty-Palmer D (2010) Beyond desensitization: physiological relevance of arrestin-dependent signaling. Pharmacol Rev 62(2):305–330

96. Whalen EJ, Rajagopal S, Lefkowitz RJ (2011) Therapeutic potential of beta-arrestin- and G protein-biased agonists. Trends Mol Med 17(3):126–139

97. Lefkowitz RJ (2007) Seven transmembrane receptors: something old, something new. Acta Physiol (Oxford) 190(1):9–19

98. Rajagopal S, Rajagopal K, Lefkowitz RJ (2010) Teaching old receptors new tricks: biasing seven-transmembrane receptors. Nat Rev Drug Discov 9(5):373–386

99. Luttrell LM, Ferguson SS, Daaka Y, Miller WE, Maudsley S, Della Rocca GJ, Lin F, Kawakatsu H, Owada K, Luttrell DK, Caron MG, Lefkowitz RJ (1999) Beta-arrestin-dependent formation of beta2 adrenergic receptor-Src protein kinase complexes. Science 283(5402):655–661

100. Xiao K, McClatchy DB, Shukla AK, Zhao Y, Chen M, Shenoy SK, Yates JR 3rd, Lefkowitz RJ (2007) Functional specialization of beta-arrestin interactions revealed by proteomic analysis. Proc Natl Acad Sci U S A 104(29):12011–12016

101. Kim IM, Tilley DG, Chen J, Salazar NC, Whalen EJ, Violin JD, Rockman HA (2008) Beta-blockers alprenolol and carvedilol stimulate beta-arrestin-mediated EGFR transactivation. Proc Natl Acad Sci U S A 105(38):14555–14560

102. Wisler JW, DeWire SM, Whalen EJ, Violin JD, Drake MT, Ahn S, Shenoy SK, Lefkowitz RJ (2007) A unique mechanism of beta-blocker action: carvedilol stimulates beta-arrestin signaling. Proc Natl Acad Sci U S A 104(42):16657–16662

103. Zidar DA, Violin JD, Whalen EJ, Lefkowitz RJ (2009) Selective engagement of G protein coupled receptor kinases (GRKs) encodes distinct functions of biased ligands. Proc Natl Acad Sci U S A 106(24):9649–9654

104. Oppermann M, Freedman NJ, Alexander RW, Lefkowitz RJ (1996) Phosphorylation of the type 1A angiotensin II receptor by G protein-coupled receptor kinases and protein kinase C. J Biol Chem 271(22):13266–13272

105. Kohout TA, Nicholas SL, Perry SJ, Reinhart G, Junger S, Struthers RS (2004) Differential desensitization, receptor phosphorylation, beta-arrestin recruitment, and ERK1/2 activation by the two endogenous ligands for the CC chemokine receptor 7. J Biol Chem 279(22):23214–23222

106. Busillo JM, Armando S, Sengupta R, Meucci O, Bouvier M, Benovic JL (2010) Site-specific phosphorylation of CXCR4 is dynamically regulated by multiple kinases and results in differential modulation of CXCR4 signaling. J Biol Chem 285(10):7805–7817

107. Mueller W, Schutz D, Nagel F, Schulz S, Stumm R (2013) Hierarchical organization of multi-site phosphorylation at the CXCR4 C terminus. PLoS One 8(5):e64975

108. Raghuwanshi SK, Su Y, Singh V, Haynes K, Richmond A, Richardson RM (2012) The chemokine receptors CXCR1 and CXCR2 couple to distinct G protein-coupled receptor kinases to mediate and regulate leukocyte functions. J Immunol 189(6):2824–2832

109. Lipfert J, Odemis V, Engele J (2013) Grk2 is an essential regulator of CXCR7 signalling in astrocytes. Cell Mol Neurobiol 33(1): 111–118

110. Zhang X, Wang F, Chen X, Chen Y, Ma L (2008) Post-endocytic fates of delta-opioid receptor are regulated by GRK2-mediated receptor phosphorylation and distinct beta-arrestin isoforms. J Neurochem 106(2): 781–792

111. Arttamangkul S, Lau EK, Lu HW, Williams JT (2012) Desensitization and trafficking of mu-opioid receptors in locus ceruleus neurons: modulation by kinases. Mol Pharmacol 81(3):348–355

112. Bailey CP, Kelly E, Henderson G (2004) Protein kinase C activation enhances morphine-induced rapid desensitization of mu-opioid receptors in mature rat locus ceruleus neurons. Mol Pharmacol 66(6): 1592–1598

113. Bailey CP, Oldfield S, Llorente J, Caunt CJ, Teschemacher AG, Roberts L, McArdle CA, Smith FL, Dewey WL, Kelly E, Henderson G (2009) Involvement of PKC alpha and G-protein-coupled receptor kinase 2 in

agonist-selective desensitization of mu-opioid receptors in mature brain neurons. Br J Pharmacol 158(1):157–164

114. Hurle MA (2001) Changes in the expression of G protein-coupled receptor kinases and beta-arrestin 2 in rat brain during opioid tolerance and supersensitivity. J Neurochem 77(2):486–492

115. Johnson EA, Oldfield S, Braksator E, Gonzalez-Cuello A, Couch D, Hall KJ, Mundell SJ, Bailey CP, Kelly E, Henderson G (2006) Agonist-selective mechanisms of mu-opioid receptor desensitization in human embryonic kidney 293 cells. Mol Pharmacol 70(2):676–685

116. Kelly E, Bailey CP, Henderson G (2008) Agonist-selective mechanisms of GPCR desensitization. Br J Pharmacol 153(Suppl 1):S379–S388

117. Zhang J, Ferguson SS, Barak LS, Bodduluri SR, Laporte SA, Law PY, Caron MG (1998) Role for G protein-coupled receptor kinase in agonist-specific regulation of mu-opioid receptor responsiveness. Proc Natl Acad Sci U S A 95(12):7157–7162

118. Zhang J, Ferguson SS, Law PY, Barak LS, Caron MG (1999) Agonist-specific regulation of delta-opioid receptor trafficking by G protein-coupled receptor kinase and beta-arrestin. J Recept Signal Transduct Res 19(1-4):301–313

119. Nickolls SA, Humphreys S, Clark M, McMurray G (2013) Co-expression of GRK2 reveals a novel conformational state of the micro-opioid receptor. PLoS One 8(12), e83691

120. Cao J, Panetta R, Yue S, Steyaert A, Young-Bellido M, Ahmad S (2003) A naive Bayes model to predict coupling between seven transmembrane domain receptors and G-proteins. Bioinformatics 19(2):234–240

121. Holopainen I, Wojcik WJ (1993) A specific antisense oligodeoxynucleotide to mRNAs encoding receptors with seven transmembrane spanning regions decreases muscarinic m2 and gamma-aminobutyric acidB receptors in rat cerebellar granule cells. J Pharmacol Exp Ther 264(1):423–430

122. Watanabe H, Xu J, Bengra C, Jose PA, Felder RA (2002) Desensitization of human renal D1 dopamine receptors by G protein-coupled receptor kinase 4. Kidney Int 62(3):790–798

123. Ito K, Haga T, Lameh J, Sadee W (1999) Sequestration of dopamine D2 receptors depends on coexpression of G-protein-coupled receptor kinases 2 or 5. Eur J Biochem 260(1):112–119

124. Cho D, Zheng M, Min C, Ma L, Kurose H, Park JH, Kim KM (2010) Agonist-induced endocytosis and receptor phosphorylation

mediate resensitization of dopamine D(2) receptors. Mol Endocrinol 24(3):574–586

125. Cho DI, Zheng M, Min C, Kwon KJ, Shin CY, Choi HK, Kim KM (2013) ARF6 and GASP-1 are post-endocytic sorting proteins selectively involved in the intracellular trafficking of dopamine D(2) receptors mediated by GRK and PKC in transfected cells. Br J Pharmacol 168(6):1355–1374

126. Ohguro H, Palczewski K, Ericsson LH, Walsh KA, Johnson RS (1993) Sequential phosphorylation of rhodopsin at multiple sites. Biochemistry 32(21):5718–5724

127. Liu Q, Dewi DA, Liu W, Bee MS, Schonbrunn A (2008) Distinct phosphorylation sites in the SST2A somatostatin receptor control internalization, desensitization, and arrestin binding. Mol Pharmacol 73(2):292–304

128. Su Y, Ospina JK, Zhang J, Michelson AP, Schoen AM, Zhu AJ (2011) Sequential phosphorylation of smoothened transduces graded hedgehog signaling. Sci Signal 4(180):ra43

129. Tran TM, Friedman J, Qunaibi E, Baameur F, Moore RH, Clark RB (2004) Characterization of agonist stimulation of cAMP-dependent protein kinase and G protein-coupled receptor kinase phosphorylation of the beta2-adrenergic receptor using phosphoserine-specific antibodies. Mol Pharmacol 65(1):196–206

130. Tran TM, Jorgensen R, Clark RB (2007) Phosphorylation of the beta2-adrenergic receptor in plasma membranes by intrinsic GRK5. Biochemistry 46(50):14438–14449

131. Fredericks ZL, Pitcher JA, Lefkowitz RJ (1996) Identification of the G protein-coupled receptor kinase phosphorylation sites in the human beta2-adrenergic receptor. J Biol Chem 271(23):13796–13803

132. Hausdorff WP, Bouvier M, O'Dowd BF, Irons GP, Caron MG, Lefkowitz RJ (1989) Phosphorylation sites on two domains of the beta 2-adrenergic receptor are involved in distinct pathways of receptor desensitization. J Biol Chem 264(21):12657–12665

133. Krasel C, Zabel U, Lorenz K, Reiner S, Al-Sabah S, Lohse MJ (2008) Dual role of the beta2-adrenergic receptor C terminus for the binding of beta-arrestin and receptor internalization. J Biol Chem 283(46):31840–31848

134. Trester-Zedlitz M, Burlingame A, Kobilka B, von Zastrow M (2005) Mass spectrometric analysis of agonist effects on posttranslational modifications of the beta-2 adrenoceptor in mammalian cells. Biochemistry 44(16):6133–6143

135. Bouvier M, Hausdorff WP, De Blasi A, O'Dowd BF, Kobilka BK, Caron MG, Lefkowitz RJ (1988) Removal of phosphorylation sites from the beta 2-adrenergic receptor delays onset of agonist-promoted desensitization. Nature 333(6171):370–373

136. Tobin AB (2008) G-protein-coupled receptor phosphorylation: where, when and by whom. Br J Pharmacol 153(Suppl 1):S167–S176

137. Tobin AB, Butcher AJ, Kong KC (2008) Location, location, location...site-specific GPCR phosphorylation offers a mechanism for cell-type-specific signalling. Trends Pharmacol Sci 29(8):413–420

138. Charfi I, Nagi K, Mnie-Filali O, Thibault D, Balboni G, Schiller PW, Trudeau LE, Pineyro G (2014) Ligand- and cell-dependent determinants of internalization and cAMP modulation by delta opioid receptor (DOR) agonists. Cell Mol Life Sci 71(8):1529–1546

139. Kenakin T (1996) The classification of seven transmembrane receptors in recombinant expression systems. Pharmacol Rev 48(3):413–463

140. Stacey M, Lin HH, Gordon S, McKnight AJ (2000) LNB-TM7, a group of seven-transmembrane proteins related to family-B G-protein-coupled receptors. Trends Biochem Sci 25(6):284–289

141. Schulz R, Wehmeyer A, Schulz K (2002) Visualizing preference of G protein-coupled receptor kinase 3 for the process of kappa-opioid receptor sequestration. Mol Pharmacol 61(6):1444–1452

142. Curnow KM (1995) Expression cloning of type 2 angiotension II receptor reveals a unique class of seven-transmembrane receptors. J Endocrinol Invest 18(7):566–570

143. Just S, Illing S, Trester-Zedlitz M, Lau EK, Kotowski SJ, Miess E, Mann A, Doll C, Trinidad JC, Burlingame AL, von Zastrow M, Schulz S (2013) Differentiation of opioid drug effects by hierarchical multi-site phosphorylation. Mol Pharmacol 83(3):633–639

144. Mandyam CD, Thakker DR, Christensen JL, Standifer KM (2002) Orphanin FQ/nociceptin-mediated desensitization of opioid receptor-like 1 receptor and mu opioid receptors involves protein kinase C: a molecular mechanism for heterologous cross-talk. J Pharmacol Exp Ther 302(2):502–509

145. Thakker DR, Standifer KM (2002) Induction of G protein-coupled receptor kinases 2 and 3 contributes to the cross-talk between mu and ORL1 receptors following prolonged agonist exposure. Neuropharmacology 43(6):979–990

146. Kovoor A, Celver JP, Wu A, Chavkin C (1998) Agonist induced homologous desensitization of mu-opioid receptors mediated by G protein-coupled receptor kinases is dependent on agonist efficacy. Mol Pharmacol 54(4):704–711

147. Li J, Li JG, Chen C, Zhang F, Liu-Chen LY (2002) Molecular basis of differences in (-) (trans)-3,4-dichloro-N-methyl-N-[2-(1-pyrrolidiny)-cyclohexyl]benzeneacetamide-induced desensitization and phosphorylation between human and rat kappa-opioid receptors expressed in Chinese hamster ovary cells. Mol Pharmacol 61(1):73–84

148. Li JG, Benovic JL, Liu-Chen LY (2000) Mechanisms of agonist-induced down-regulation of the human kappa-opioid receptor: internalization is required for down-regulation. Mol Pharmacol 58(4):795–801

149. Li JG, Luo LY, Krupnick JG, Benovic JL, Liu-Chen LY (1999) U50,488H-induced internalization of the human kappa opioid receptor involves a beta-arrestin- and dynamin-dependent mechanism. Kappa receptor internalization is not required for mitogen-activated protein kinase activation. J Biol Chem 274(17):12087–12094

150. Nobles KN, Xiao K, Ahn S, Shukla AK, Lam CM, Rajagopal S, Strachan RT, Huang TY, Bressler EA, Hara MR, Shenoy SK, Gygi SP, Lefkowitz RJ (2011) Distinct phosphorylation sites on the beta(2)-adrenergic receptor establish a barcode that encodes differential functions of beta-arrestin. Sci Signal 4(185):ra51

151. Aramori I, Ferguson SS, Bieniasz PD, Zhang J, Cullen B, Cullen MG (1997) Molecular mechanism of desensitization of the chemokine receptor CCR-5: receptor signaling and internalization are dissociable from its role as an HIV-1 co-receptor. EMBO J 16(15):4606–4616

152. Mills A, Duggan MJ (1993) Orphan seven transmembrane domain receptors: reversing pharmacology. Trends Pharmacol Sci 14(11):394–396

153. Matsuoka S, Ballif BA, Smogorzewska A, McDonald ER 3rd, Hurov KE, Luo J, Bakalarski CE, Zhao Z, Solimini N, Lerenthal Y, Shiloh Y, Gygi SP, Elledge SJ (2007) ATM and ATR substrate analysis reveals extensive protein networks responsive to DNA damage. Science 316(5828):1160–1166

154. Mills A, Duggan MJ (1994) Orphan seven transmembrane domain receptors: reversing pharmacology. Trends Biotechnol 12(2):47–49

155. Charest PG, Terrillon S, Bouvier M (2005) Monitoring agonist-promoted conformational changes of beta-arrestin in living cells by intramolecular BRET. EMBO Rep 6(4):334–340

156. Shukla AK, Violin JD, Whalen EJ, Gesty-Palmer D, Shenoy SK, Lefkowitz RJ (2008) Distinct conformational changes in beta-arrestin report biased agonism at seven-transmembrane receptors. Proc Natl Acad Sci U S A 105(29):9988–9993

157. Nobles KN, Guan Z, Xiao K, Oas TG, Lefkowitz RJ (2007) The active conformation of beta-arrestin1: direct evidence for the phosphate sensor in the N-domain and conformational differences in the active states of beta-arrestins1 and -2. J Biol Chem 282(29):21370–21381

158. Xiao K, Shenoy SK, Nobles K, Lefkowitz RJ (2004) Activation-dependent conformational changes in {beta}-arrestin 2. J Biol Chem 279(53):55744–55753

159. Shukla AK, Manglik A, Kruse AC, Xiao K, Reis RI, Tseng WC, Staus DP, Hilger D, Uysal S, Huang LY, Paduch M, Tripathi-Shukla P, Koide A, Koide S, Weis WI, Kossiakoff AA, Kobilka BK, Lefkowitz RJ (2013) Structure of active beta-arrestin-1 bound to a G-protein-coupled receptor phosphopeptide. Nature 497(7447):137–141

160. Han M, Gurevich VV, Vishnivetskiy SA, Sigler PB, Schubert C (2001) Crystal structure of beta-arrestin at 1.9 A: possible mechanism of receptor binding and membrane translocation. Structure 9(9):869–880

161. Milano SK, Pace HC, Kim YM, Brenner C, Benovic JL (2002) Scaffolding functions of arrestin-2 revealed by crystal structure and mutagenesis. Biochemistry 41(10):3321–3328

162. Hirsch JA, Schubert C, Gurevich VV, Sigler PB (1999) The 2.8 A crystal structure of visual arrestin: a model for arrestin's regulation. Cell 97(2):257–269

163. Kim M, Vishnivetskiy SA, Van Eps N, Alexander NS, Cleghorn WM, Zhan X, Hanson SM, Morizumi T, Ernst OP, Meiler J, Gurevich VV, Hubbell WL (2012) Conformation of receptor-bound visual arrestin. Proc Natl Acad Sci U S A 109(45):18407–18412

164. Gurevich EV, Gurevich VV (2006) Arrestins: ubiquitous regulators of cellular signaling pathways. Genome Biol 7(9):236

165. Yang F, Yu X, Liu C, Qu CX, Gong Z, Liu HD, Li FH, Wang HM, He DF, Yi F, Song C, Tian CL, Xiao KH, Wang JY, Sun JP (2015) Phospho-selective mechanisms of arrestin conformations and functions revealed by unnatural amino acid incorporation and (19)F-NMR. Nat Commun 6:8202

166. Wisler JW, Xiao K, Thomsen AR, Lefkowitz RJ (2014) Recent developments in biased agonism. Curr Opin Cell Biol 27:18–24

167. Feng YH, Ding Y, Ren S, Zhou L, Xu C, Karnik SS (2005) Unconventional homolo-

gous internalization of the angiotensin II type-1 receptor induced by G-protein-independent signals. Hypertension 46(2):419–425

168. Heitzler D, Durand G, Gallay N, Rizk A, Ahn S, Kim J, Violin JD, Dupuy L, Gauthier C, Piketty V, Crepieux P, Poupon A, Clement F, Fages F, Lefkowitz RJ, Reiter E (2012) Competing G protein-coupled receptor kinases balance G protein and beta-arrestin signaling. Mol Syst Biol 8:590

169. Diviani D, Lattion AL, Cotecchia S (1997) Characterization of the phosphorylation sites involved in G protein-coupled receptor kinase- and protein kinase C-mediated desensitization of the alpha1B-adrenergic receptor. J Biol Chem 272(45):28712–28719

170. Desai AN, Salim S, Standifer KM, Eikenburg DC (2006) Involvement of G protein-coupled receptor kinase (GRK) 3 and GRK2 in down-regulation of the alpha2B-adrenoceptor. J Pharmacol Exp Ther 317(3):1027–1035

171. Desai AN, Standifer KM, Eikenburg DC (2005) Cellular G protein-coupled receptor kinase levels regulate sensitivity of the {alpha}2b-adrenergic receptor to undergo agonist-induced down-regulation. J Pharmacol Exp Ther 312(2):767–773

172. Fu Q, Xu B, Parikh D, Cervantes D, Xiang YK (2015) Insulin induces IRS2-dependent and GRK2-mediated beta2AR internalization to attenuate betaAR signaling in cardiomyocytes. Cell Signal 27(3):707–715

173. Tutunea-Fatan E, Caetano FA, Gros R, Ferguson SS (2015) GRK2 targeted knockdown results in spontaneous hypertension, and altered vascular GPCR signaling. J Biol Chem 290(8):5141–5155

174. Dehvari N, Hutchinson DS, Nevzorova J, Dallner OS, Sato M, Kocan M, Merlin J, Evans BA, Summers RJ, Bengtsson T (2012) beta(2)-Adrenoceptors increase translocation of GLUT4 via GPCR kinase sites in the receptor C-terminal tail. Br J Pharmacol 165(5):1442–1456

175. Zhu W, Petrashevskaya N, Ren S, Zhao A, Chakir K, Gao E, Chuprun JK, Wang Y, Talan M, Dorn GW 2nd, Lakatta EG, Koch WJ, Feldman AM, Xiao RP (2012) Gi-biased beta2AR signaling links GRK2 upregulation to heart failure. Circ Res 110(2):265–274

176. Zhu W, Tilley DG, Myers VD, Coleman RC, Feldman AM (2013) Arginine vasopressin enhances cell survival via a G protein-coupled receptor kinase 2/beta-arrestin1/extracellular-regulated kinase 1/2-dependent pathway in H9c2 cells. Mol Pharmacol 84(2):227–235

177. Orsini MJ, Parent JL, Mundell SJ, Marchese A, Benovic JL (1999) Trafficking of the HIV coreceptor CXCR4. Role of arrestins and identification of residues in the c-terminal tail that mediate receptor internalization. J Biol Chem 274(43):31076–31086

178. Clift IC, Bamidele AO, Rodriguez-Ramirez C, Kremer KN, Hedin KE (2014) beta-Arrestin1 and distinct CXCR4 structures are required for stromal derived factor-1 to downregulate CXCR4 cell-surface levels in neuroblastoma. Mol Pharmacol 85(4):542–552

179. Tong X, Zhang L, Zhang L, Hu M, Leng J, Yu B, Zhou B, Hu Y, Zhang Q (2009) The mechanism of chemokine receptor 9 internalization triggered by interleukin 2 and interleukin 4. Cell Mol Immunol 6(3):181–189

180. Tiberi M, Nash SR, Bertrand L, Lefkowitz RJ, Caron MG (1996) Differential regulation of dopamine D1A receptor responsiveness by various G protein-coupled receptor kinases. J Biol Chem 271(7):3771–3778

181. Namkung Y, Dipace C, Javitch JA, Sibley DR (2009) G protein-coupled receptor kinase-mediated phosphorylation regulates post-endocytic trafficking of the D2 dopamine receptor. J Biol Chem 284(22):15038–15051

182. Kim KM, Gainetdinov RR, Laporte SA, Caron MG, Barak LS (2005) G protein-coupled receptor kinase regulates dopamine D3 receptor signaling by modulating the stability of a receptor-filamin-beta-arrestin complex. A case of autoreceptor regulation. J Biol Chem 280(13):12774–12780

183. Kara E, Crepieux P, Gauthier C, Martinat N, Piketty V, Guillou F, Reiter E (2006) A phosphorylation cluster of five serine and threonine residues in the C-terminus of the follicle-stimulating hormone receptor is important for desensitization but not for beta-arrestin-mediated ERK activation. Mol Endocrinol 20(11):3014–3026

184. Willets JM, Taylor AH, Shaw H, Konje JC, Challiss RA (2008) Selective regulation of H1 histamine receptor signaling by G protein-coupled receptor kinase 2 in uterine smooth muscle cells. Mol Endocrinol 22(8):1893–1907

185. Rodriguez-Pena MS, Timmerman H, Leurs R (2000) Modulation of histamine H(2) receptor signalling by G-protein-coupled receptor kinase 2 and 3. Br J Pharmacol 131(8):1707–1715

186. Fernandez N, Gottardo FL, Alonso MN, Monczor F, Shayo C, Davio C (2011) Roles of phosphorylation-dependent and -independent mechanisms in the regulation of histamine H2 receptor by G protein-coupled

receptor kinase 2. J Biol Chem 286(33):28697–28706

187. Zheng H, Worrall C, Shen H, Issad T, Seregard S, Girnita A, Girnita L (2012) Selective recruitment of G protein-coupled receptor kinases (GRKs) controls signaling of the insulin-like growth factor 1 receptor. Proc Natl Acad Sci U S A 109(18):7055–7060

188. Wei Z, Hurtt R, Gu T, Bodzin AS, Koch WJ, Doria C (2013) GRK2 negatively regulates IGF-1R signaling pathway and cyclins' expression in HepG2 cells. J Cell Physiol 228(9):1897–1901

189. Aziziyeh AI, Li TT, Pape C, Pampillo M, Chidiac P, Possmayer F, Babwah AV, Bhattacharya M (2009) Dual regulation of lysophosphatidic acid (LPA1) receptor signalling by Ral and GRK. Cell Signal 21(7):1207–1217

190. Iacovelli L, Capobianco L, D'Ancona GM, Picascia A, De Blasi A (2002) Regulation of lysophosphatidic acid receptor-stimulated response by G-protein-coupled receptor kinase-2 and beta-arrestin1 in FRTL-5 rat thyroid cells. J Endocrinol 174(1):103–110

191. Moughal NA, Waters C, Sambi B, Pyne S, Pyne NJ (2004) Nerve growth factor signaling involves interaction between the Trk A receptor and lysophosphatidate receptor 1 systems: nuclear translocation of the lysophosphatidate receptor 1 and Trk A receptors in pheochromocytoma 12 cells. Cell Signal 16(1):127–136

192. Moughal NA, Waters CM, Valentine WJ, Connell M, Richardson JC, Tigyi G, Pyne S, Pyne NJ (2006) Protean agonism of the lysophosphatidic acid receptor-1 with Ki16425 reduces nerve growth factor-induced neurite outgrowth in pheochromocytoma 12 cells. J Neurochem 98(6):1920–1929

193. Obara Y, Okano Y, Ono S, Yamauchi A, Hoshino T, Kurose H, Nakahata N (2008) Betagamma subunits of G(i/o) suppress EGF-induced ERK5 phosphorylation, whereas ERK1/2 phosphorylation is enhanced. Cell Signal 20(7):1275–1283

194. Li J, Xiang B, Su W, Zhang X, Huang Y, Ma L (2003) Agonist-induced formation of opioid receptor-G protein-coupled receptor kinase (GRK)-G beta gamma complex on membrane is required for GRK2 function in vivo. J Biol Chem 278(32):30219–30226

195. Hong MH, Xu C, Wang YJ, Ji JL, Tao YM, Xu XJ, Chen J, Xie X, Chi ZQ, Liu JG (2009) Role of Src in ligand-specific regulation of delta-opioid receptor desensitization and internalization. J Neurochem 108(1):102–114

196. Marie N, Aguila B, Hasbi A, Davis A, Jauzac P, Allouche S (2008) Different kinases desensitize the human delta-opioid receptor (hDOP-R) in the neuroblastoma cell line SK-N-BE upon peptidic and alkaloid agonists. Cell Signal 20(6):1209–1220

197. Willets J, Kelly E (2001) Desensitization of endogenously expressed delta-opioid receptors: no evidence for involvement of G protein-coupled receptor kinase 2. Eur J Pharmacol 431(2):133–141

198. McLaughlin JP, Xu M, Mackie K, Chavkin C (2003) Phosphorylation of a carboxyl-terminal serine within the kappa-opioid receptor produces desensitization and internalization. J Biol Chem 278(36):34631–34640

199. Dang VC, Chieng B, Azriel Y, Christie MJ (2011) Cellular morphine tolerance produced by betaarrestin-2-dependent impairment of mu-opioid receptor resensitization. J Neurosci 31(19):7122–7130

200. Dang VC, Napier IA, Christie MJ (2009) Two distinct mechanisms mediate acute mu-opioid receptor desensitization in native neurons. J Neurosci 29(10):3322–3327

201. He L, Whistler JL (2011) Chronic ethanol consumption in rats produces opioid antinociceptive tolerance through inhibition of mu opioid receptor endocytosis. PLoS One 6(5), e19372

202. Saland LC, Chavez JB, Lee DC, Garcia RR, Caldwell KK (2008) Chronic ethanol exposure increases the association of hippocampal mu-opioid receptors with G-protein receptor kinase 2. Alcohol 42(6):493–497

203. Lowe JD, Sanderson HS, Cooke AE, Ostovar M, Tsisanova E, Withey SL, Chavkin C, Husbands SM, Kelly E, Henderson G, Bailey CP (2015) Role of G protein-coupled receptor kinases 2 and 3 in mu-Opioid receptor desensitization and internalization. Mol Pharmacol 88(2):347–356

204. Huang J, Nalli AD, Mahavadi S, Kumar DP, Murthy KS (2014) Inhibition of Galphai activity by Gbetagamma is mediated by PI 3-kinase-gamma- and cSrc-dependent tyrosine phosphorylation of Galphai and recruitment of RGS12. Am J Physiol Gastrointest Liver Physiol 306(9):G802–G810

205. Kenski DM, Zhang C, von Zastrow M, Shokat KM (2005) Chemical genetic engineering of G protein-coupled receptor kinase 2. J Biol Chem 280(41):35051–35061

206. Ozaita A, Escriba PV, Ventayol P, Murga C, Mayor F Jr, Garcia-Sevilla JA (1998) Regulation of G protein-coupled receptor kinase 2 in brains of opiate-treated rats and human opiate addicts. J Neurochem 70(3):1249–1257

207. Malecz N, Bambino T, Bencsik M, Nissenson RA (1998) Identification of phosphorylation

sites in the G protein-coupled receptor for parathyroid hormone. Receptor phosphorylation is not required for agonist-induced internalization. Mol Endocrinol 12(12):1846–1856

208. Luo J, Busillo JM, Benovic JL (2008) M3 muscarinic acetylcholine receptor-mediated signaling is regulated by distinct mechanisms. Mol Pharmacol 74(2):338–347

209. Holroyd EW, Szekeres PG, Whittaker RD, Kelly E, Edwardson JM (1999) Effect of G protein-coupled receptor kinase 2 on the sensitivity of M4 muscarinic acetylcholine receptors to agonist-induced internalization and desensitization in NG108-15 cells. J Neurochem 73(3):1236–1245

210. Chen Z, Gaudreau R, Le Gouill C, Rola-Pleszczynski M, Stankova J (2004) Agonist-induced internalization of leukotriene B(4) receptor 1 requires G-protein-coupled receptor kinase 2 but not arrestins. Mol Pharmacol 66(3):377–386

211. Sanchez-Mas J, Guillo LA, Zanna P, Jimenez-Cervantes C, Garcia-Borron JC (2005) Role of G protein-coupled receptor kinases in the homologous desensitization of the human and mouse melanocortin 1 receptors. Mol Endocrinol 19(4):1035–1048

212. Freedman NJ, Ament AS, Oppermann M, Stoffel RH, Exum ST, Lefkowitz RJ (1997) Phosphorylation and desensitization of human endothelin A and B receptors. Evidence for G protein-coupled receptor kinase specificity. J Biol Chem 272(28):17734–17743

213. Tseng CC, Zhang XY (2000) Role of G protein-coupled receptor kinases in glucose-dependent insulinotropic polypeptide receptor signaling. Endocrinology 141(3):947–952

214. Vinge LE, von Lueder TG, Aasum E, Qvigstad E, Gravning JA, How OJ, Edvardsen T, Bjornerheim R, Ahmed MS, Mikkelsen BW, Oie E, Attramadal T, Skomedal T, Smiseth OA, Koch WJ, Larsen TS, Attramadal H (2008) Cardiac-restricted expression of the carboxyl-terminal fragment of GRK3 Uncovers Distinct Functions of GRK3 in regulation of cardiac contractility and growth: GRK3 controls cardiac alpha1-adrenergic receptor responsiveness. J Biol Chem 283(16):10601–10610

215. Lowe JD, Celver JP, Gurevich VV, Chavkin C (2002) mu-Opioid receptors desensitize less rapidly than delta-opioid receptors due to less efficient activation of arrestin. J Biol Chem 277(18):15729–15735

216. Gluck L, Loktev A, Mouledous L, Mollereau C, Law PY, Schulz S (2014) Loss of morphine reward and dependence in mice lacking G protein-coupled receptor kinase 5. Biol Psychiatry 76(10):767–774

217. Zhang NR, Planer W, Siuda ER, Zhao HC, Stickler L, Chang SD, Baird MA, Cao YQ, Bruchas MR (2012) Serine 363 is required for nociceptin/orphanin FQ opioid receptor (NOPR) desensitization, internalization, and arrestin signaling. J Biol Chem 287(50):42019–42030

218. Dautzenberg FM, Braun S, Hauger RL (2001) GRK3 mediates desensitization of CRF1 receptors: a potential mechanism regulating stress adaptation. Am J Physiol Regul Integr Comp Physiol 280(4):R935–R946

219. Fraga S, Jose PA, Soares-da-Silva P (2004) Involvement of G protein-coupled receptor kinase 4 and 6 in rapid desensitization of dopamine D1 receptor in rat IEC-6 intestinal epithelial cells. Am J Physiol Regul Integr Comp Physiol 287(4):R772–R779

220. Rankin ML, Marinec PS, Cabrera DM, Wang Z, Jose PA, Sibley DR (2006) The D1 dopamine receptor is constitutively phosphorylated by G protein-coupled receptor kinase 4. Mol Pharmacol 69(3):759–769

221. Kanaide M, Uezono Y, Matsumoto M, Hojo M, Ando Y, Sudo Y, Sumikawa K, Taniyama K (2007) Desensitization of GABA(B) receptor signaling by formation of protein complexes of GABA(B2) subunit with GRK4 or GRK5. J Cell Physiol 210(1):237–245

222. Iacovelli L, Salvatore L, Capobianco L, Picascia A, Barletta E, Storto M, Mariggio S, Sallese M, Porcellini A, Nicoletti F, De Blasi A (2003) Role of G protein-coupled receptor kinase 4 and beta-arrestin 1 in agonist-stimulated metabotropic glutamate receptor 1 internalization and activation of mitogen-activated protein kinases. J Biol Chem 278(14):12433–12442

223. Oppermann M, Diverse-Pierluissi M, Drazner MH, Dyer SL, Freedman NJ, Peppel KC, Lefkowitz RJ (1996) Monoclonal antibodies reveal receptor specificity among G-protein-coupled receptor kinases. Proc Natl Acad Sci U S A 93(15):7649–7654

224. Hu LA, Chen W, Premont RT, Cong M, Lefkowitz RJ (2002) G protein-coupled receptor kinase 5 regulates beta 1-adrenergic receptor association with PSD-95. J Biol Chem 277(2):1607–1613

225. Appleyard SM, Celver J, Pineda V, Kovoor A, Wayman GA, Chavkin C (1999) Agonist-dependent desensitization of the kappa opioid receptor by G protein receptor kinase and beta-arrestin. J Biol Chem 274(34):23802–23807

226. Simon V, Robin MT, Legrand C, Cohen-Tannoudji J (2003) Endogenous G protein-coupled receptor kinase 6 triggers homologous beta-adrenergic receptor desensitization in primary uterine smooth muscle cells. Endocrinology 144(7):3058–3066

227. Aiyar N, Disa J, Dang K, Pronin AN, Benovic JL, Nambi P (2000) Involvement of G protein-coupled receptor kinase-6 in desensitization of CGRP receptors. Eur J Pharmacol 403(1-2):1–7

228. Fraga S, Luo Y, Jose P, Zandi-Nejad K, Mount DB, Soares-da-Silva P (2006) Dopamine D1-like receptor-mediated inhibition of Cl/HCO3- exchanger activity in rat intestinal epithelial IEC-6 cells is regulated by G protein-coupled receptor kinase 6 (GRK 6). Cell Physiol Biochem 18(6):347–360

229. Willets JM, Mistry R, Nahorski SR, Challiss RA (2003) Specificity of g protein-coupled receptor kinase 6-mediated phosphorylation and regulation of single-cell m3 muscarinic acetylcholine receptor signaling. Mol Pharmacol 64(5):1059–1068

230. Willets JM, Brighton PJ, Mistry R, Morris GE, Konje JC, Challiss RA (2009) Regulation of oxytocin receptor responsiveness by G protein-coupled receptor kinase 6 in human myometrial smooth muscle. Mol Endocrinol 23(8):1272–1280

Part III

GRKs in Cell Signaling

Chapter 6

Cell-Type Specific GRK2 Interactomes: Pathophysiological Implications

Federico Mayor Jr., Rocío Vila-Bedmar, Laura Nogués, Marta Cruces-Sande, Elisa Lucas, Verónica Rivas, Clara Reglero, Petronila Penela, and Cristina Murga

Abstract

G protein-coupled receptor kinase 2 (GRK2) is emerging as a key hub in cell signaling cascades. In addition to modulating activated G protein-coupled receptors, GRK2 can phosphorylate and/or functionally interact with a complex network of cellular proteins in a cell-type and physiological context-dependent way. A combination of such canonical and noncanonical interactions underlies the participation of this kinase in the control of cell migration, proliferation or metabolism and in integrated processes at the tissue or whole organism levels, such as angiogenesis, cardiovascular function, or insulin resistance, among others. Its role as a signaling node and the fact that altered levels of GRK2 are detected in a variety of pathological conditions put forward this protein as a potentially relevant diagnostic and therapeutic target.

Key words GRK2, Arrestin, GPCR, Migration, Proliferation, Hypertension, Insulin resistance, Obesity, Angiogenesis, Cardiovascular diseases

1 Introduction

G protein-coupled receptor kinases (GRKs) were initially identified as negative regulators of G protein-coupled receptors (GPCR). Once activated, GPCR become selectively phosphorylated by GRKs [1], which promotes the association of β-arrestins, leading to uncoupling from G proteins. The fact that arrestins can act as scaffold proteins for endocytic adaptors and several signaling mediators lead to the new paradigm that the GRK/arrestin axis is also involved in GPCR internalization and triggers the modulation of additional signaling cascades by these receptors [2]. Further adding to this complexity, research by different laboratories has established that GRKs, and, in particular, the ubiquitous and essential GRK2 isoform, in addition to promoting arrestin recruitment to GPCRs, engage in specific signalosomes with varied cellular functions [3–5].

Vsevolod V. Gurevich et al. (eds.), *G Protein-Coupled Receptor Kinases*, Methods in Pharmacology and Toxicology, DOI 10.1007/978-1-4939-3798-1_6, © Springer Science+Business Media New York 2016

Moreover, GRK2 can also impact cell signaling networks by directly interacting and/or phosphorylating non-GPCR components of transduction cascades [1, 4, 6].

In this context, key challenges ahead are:

(a) to dissect the relevant spatiotemporal GRK2 "interactomes" and to identify specific partners engaged in different cell types and contexts depending on environmental cues and on the relative levels of expression of GRK2 as well as on the intracellular concentrations of its potential interacting proteins, leading to distinct cellular responses.

(b) to decipher how the diverse GRK2 interactions (both canonical/GPCR-related and noncanonical, scaffold or kinase-activity dependent) are functionally integrated within a given cell type, and how the physiological integration of such cell-type specific GRK2 "interactomes" is achieved and potentially disturbed in specific pathological conditions at the organism level.

Notably, GRK2 expression and activity is tightly regulated by several mechanisms/stimuli, and these parameters are altered in humans in relevant and prevalent pathologies such as hypertension, heart failure, metabolic syndrome, inflammation and in certain tumors, suggesting that changes in GRK2 function may be involved in the triggering or development of relevant pathological situations, and that this protein could be a useful biomarker or therapeutic target. In this review we summarize recent work describing that combinations of GRK2 interactions with different cellular partners underlie its participation in basic cellular processes, such as cell migration or cell proliferation and that integration of cell type- and tissue-specific GRK2 functions may play a key role in relevant physiological and pathological situations such as angiogenesis, tumor progression, insulin resistance, and cardiovascular disease.

2   Canonical and Noncanonical Roles of GRK2

GRK2 was initially identified as a serine–threonine kinase able to phosphorylate agonist-engaged GPCRs, thus promoting the association of arrestins, leading to both desensitization of GPCR-dependent G protein signaling and to the initiation of arrestin-dependent responses [1, 2]. In addition to the decrease in responsiveness of GPCR to specific agonists, it is important to note that GRK2 functionality may modulate GPCR signaling in more subtle ways. For instance, changes in GRK2 levels or activity may control the balance/bias between G protein-dependent vs. GRK/β-arrestin-dependent cascades and/or affect the response to biased agonists. On the other hand, although the β-arrestin recruitment markedly depends on the extent of bulk receptor phosphorylation, β-arrestin-mediated functions do not. For instance, upon phosphorylation of certain GPCR by GRK6, β-arrestin/receptor complexes preferentially initiate MAPK signaling, while GRK2 phosphorylation instructs β-arrestins to perform internalization. Therefore, the relative expression and activity of the different GRK isoforms in a given cell type and physiological context may lead to distinct patterns of GPCR phosphorylation and thus to the differential recruitment of β-arrestin in diverse conformations, able to preferentially interact with defined signaling partners [4, 7, 8].

In addition to its canonical function as a GPCR kinase, GRK2 phosphorylates a variety of non-GPCR membrane receptors (as receptor tyrosine kinases) and other downstream effectors of signal transduction cascades (phosducins, Smads, HDAC6, ezrin, IRS1, or p38 MAPK, among others), which can contribute to receptor signaling either in a positive or negative way [1, 4–6]. Interestingly, GRK2- and GRK3-mediated phosphorylation of GPCRs is strictly dependent on ligand activation, while other GRKs have the capacity to target inactive receptors and to promote basal desensitization [9]. Such differential dependence provides a functional specialization for GRK2 versus the other isoforms on their activity in the context of GPCR signaling, but raises the question of how GRK2 activity toward non-receptor substrates is modulated. In this regard, allosteric activation of GRK2 by means of posttranslational modifications (as tyrosine phosphorylation of the N-terminal Y13 residue or C-terminal S670 phosphorylation) and interaction with allosteric factors (lipids or protein partners) [3] may provide a mechanistic basis for non-GPCR phosphorylation in a ligand/receptor complex-independent fashion.

In recent years, work from different laboratories has demonstrated that GRK2 dynamically interacts with other partners (for instance Gαq, PI3K/Akt, GIT1, MEK, IRS1, EPAC, Pin1, or Mdm2) acting as a scaffold protein [1, 4–6]. Therefore, it is tempting to suggest that combinations of sequential or parallel functional interactions of GRK2 with these potential partners would be triggered in response to specific stimuli and could underlie the role of this protein in cellular processes and physiological functions (Fig. 1). Moreover, on the basis of this complex interactome, GRK2 has the potential to regulate some signaling circuits without the involvement of an upstream active receptor. The fact that global GRK2 knockout mice are embryonically lethal [10] further supports the notion that GRK2 is a key node involved in the control of organ development and/or growth and viability.

126   Federico Mayor Jr. et al.

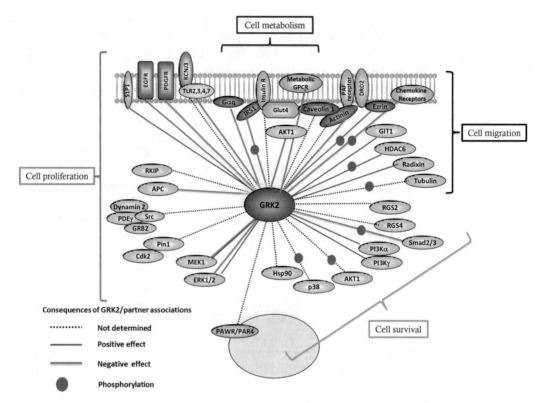

Fig. 1 Combinations of sequential or parallel functional interactions of GRK2 with a variety of GPCR and other signal transduction partners underlie the role of this protein in cellular processes such as cell proliferation, migration, survival, or metabolism

3   GRK2 Modulates Pathways Related to Cell Proliferation and Survival

GRK2 may control cell proliferation by modulating MAPK activation at several mechanistic levels including (1) direct GPCR desensitization and down-modulation of G protein-dependent MAPK pathways; (2) engagement of β-arrestins to GPCRs in conformations noncompetent to stimulate MAPK cascades, thus competing with the formation of MAPK activating β-arrestin-complexes triggered by phosphorylation of certain GPCR by the GRK5/6 subfamily; and (3) the ability to phosphorylate or dynamically interact (in a kinase activity-independent way) with important modulators/effectors engaged along the MAPK pathway, such as GIT-1, Raf, RhoA, Epac, PDEγ, RKIP, or Pin1 [11–15] upon stimulation of the epidermal growth factor (EGF) receptor or of several mitogenic GPCRs.

As a result of such complex intertwinement of GRK2 with the MAPK pathway, the impact of changes in the GRK2 expression on cell proliferation and mitogenic signaling is not straightforward and depends on both the cell type and the mitogenic stimuli involved. GRK2 appears to play a positive role as mediator of

MAPK activation and/or growth signaling by the bioactive lipid sphingosine-1-phosphate (S1P) and integrins [13] in epithelial cells and fibroblasts, by the chemokine receptor CXCR7 in astrocytes [16], by EGF in several cell types, including HEK-293 cells [15], vascular smooth muscles cells [14], or epithelial cells [17]. GRK2 kinase activity is required for IGF-1-triggered proliferation and mitogenic signaling in osteoblasts [18]. GRK2 has also been found to potentiate the Smoothened receptor signaling and cooperate with Smoothened to transform the fibroblastic cell line C3H10T1/2 [19–21]. On the other hand, GRK2 attenuates serum- or PDGF-induced proliferation of thyroid cancer cell lines [22] and smooth muscle cells [23], as well as IGF-1-dependent signaling and cell growth in human hepatocellular carcinoma (HCC) HepG2 cells [24] or HEK-293 cells [25, 26], consistent with the ability of GRK2 to desensitize the receptors of such mitogenic factors in these cellular types. Therefore, the physiological outcome of altered GRK2 expression would depend on the cell-type-specific multimolecular signaling complexes assembled by growth factors, and may involve both kinase activity-dependent and independent functions of this protein [4].

In addition, the intrinsic dynamic of the cell cycle, namely the length of the different cell cycle phases, is a cell context-specific factor that contributes to the rate of cell proliferation triggered by mitogenic factors. We and others have recently reported that GRK2 is necessary to ensure a proper and timely progression of cell cycle, particularly during G1–S and G2–M transitions in response to extrinsic and intrinsic cues, respectively (reviewed in ref. 4). GRK2 levels fluctuate along the cell cycle, being down-regulated during the G2–M transition. Phosphorylation of the GRK2 S670 residue by the cell-cycle kinase CDK2-Cyclin A and the subsequent binding of Pin1 underlie this transient GRK2 degradation, which in turn is required for normal cell cycle progression [27]. Consistently, cells with reduced GRK2 levels by expression of a silencing construct display a more efficient progression through G2/M, while the presence of extra levels of GRK2 mutants unable to be phosphorylated and degraded results in G2/M arrest [27]. Interestingly, the proliferation rate of cells expressing GRK2 silencing constructs can be either reduced (Nogués et al., submitted) or unaltered [24, 28] suggesting that a specific threshold level of GRK2 protein is required for the proper progression of other phases of the cell cycle. The ability of GRK2 to interact with Patched and to relieve the Patched-induced cytosolic retention of cyclin B in response to Hedgehog ligand appears to underlie the stimulatory effect of GRK2 in cell division [29].

GRK2 is also able to interact with some key players in the processes of cellular stress response and growth arrest such as p38, Smad2/3, PI3K, Akt, HDAC6, or Hsp90 (reviewed in ref. 4, 30), what might positively impact cell survival and the resistance to cell death. p38 MAPK, a critical player in apoptosis or survival in a cell-type specific context and a mediator of p53 activation in response to different stresses [31], is phosphorylated by GRK2, which prevents its binding to the p38's upstream activator MKK6 [32]. Interestingly, the default GRK2 protein decay in G2 is prevented in the presence of DNA damaging agents that trigger cell cycle arrest such as doxorubicin. Moreover, such preservation of GKR2 inversely correlated with the activation of p53 triggered by G2/M checkpoints mechanisms, helping to restrict the apoptotic fate of arrested cells [27]. Accordingly, we hypothesized that GRK2 might allow cells to cope with genotoxic stress by potentiating protective cell cycle arrest and survival response pathways. In this regard, GRK2 also interacts with both PI3K and Akt proteins, although the functional outcome of such interactions is not straightforward, as positive and negative effects have been described in cell type-specific contexts. In non-epithelial cells, a GRK2-mediated inhibition of Akt phosphorylation and canonical activation has been shown [33]. A role for GRK2 in the cellular response to environmental stresses is also suggested by the fact that GRK2 is a novel scaffolding and catalytic modulator of histone deacetylase HDAC6 [17]. Under cellular stress, the assembly of stress granules (SG) contributes to reprogram the expression of key mediators and regulators at the post-transcriptional level in order to counterbalance damage, while misfolded proteins are sequestered into protein aggregates (aggresomes) for cell protection. HDAC6 is required for SG assembly [34] and for protein trafficking to the aggresome and their clearance [35].

4   GRK2 Is an Important Modulator of Cell Motility

Compelling evidences indicate a relevant role of GRK2 in cellular motility (reviewed in ref. 5). Initial reports ascribed the effects of GRK2 on chemotaxis to its ability to trigger desensitization of particular chemokine receptors, thus controlling the intensity and duration of chemokine-triggered signaling [1, 36, 37]. Consistent with this notion, decreased GRK2 levels increases chemotactic responses to different agonists in immune cell types, whereas its enhanced expression attenuates chemotaxis, consistent with its canonical negative role in GPCR signaling. However, GRK2 downregulation can lead to decreased migration of immune cell types towards certain stimuli [38], and GRK2 has been recently shown to be an important positive player in epithelial cell migration [30, 39]. These results indicate that the global effect of GRK2 on chemotaxis would depend on the integrated modulation of different steps of the chemotactic process (receptor sensing, cell polarization, membrane protrusion, adhesion/de-adhesion cycles) in given cell types and in response to specific stimuli [5].

We have hypothesized that the "canonical" role of GRK2—triggering desensitization/internalization of chemotactic GPCRs in immune cells—would influence how these receptors sense the strength and steepness of chemotactic gradients (less GRK2, steeper; more GRK2, weaker gradients), thus facilitating the formation of robust directional sensing responses, the specification of stable pseudopodia and cell polarization [5]. Such function of the kinase would be more relevant in immune cells, particularly when cells migrate between opposed chemoattractant gradients. In contrast, in intrinsically polarized epithelial cells and fibroblasts, the stimuli-dependent interaction of GRK2 with other cellular partners would result in a positive role of this protein in the migration process [30, 39, 40]. The positive contribution of GRKs to epithelial cell migration seems to involve several molecular mechanisms that would amplify the intensity and duration of pro-migratory signaling downstream of chemotactic receptors.

First, GRK2 could promote reorganization of the actin cytoskeleton via ERM proteins. The ERM proteins ezrin and radixin contribute to local F-actin polymerization-dependent membrane protrusion. GRK2 phosphorylates ezrin at a single Thr567 residue in a PIP_2-and Gβγ-dependent manner, which is important for maintaining ezrin in an active conformation with both its plasma membrane and F-actin binding domains accessible [41]. Similarly, GRK2 phosphorylates radixin at the analogous Thr564 residue [42].

In addition, GRK2 can potentiate pathways linked to polarity persistence by increasing MAPK activation and focal adhesion turnover via GIT1-scaffolding functions [5, 13]. GIT1 plays an important role in cell motility as an adaptor protein promoting MAPK and Rac/PAK activation both at focal adhesions and at the cell leading edge [43, 44]. In response to either fibronectin or S1P, GRK2 translocates to the plasma membrane of epithelial cells and dynamically interacts with GIT1, in a process modulated by the sequential phosphorylation of GRK2 by c-Src and MAPK. Such transient GRK2/GIT1 interaction at the leading edge enhances both Rac1 activation leading to F-actin cortical remodeling and MAPK activation in a β-arrestin-independent manner, thereby resulting in increased migration [13].

On the other hand, GRK2 has been reported to control microtubule (MT) dynamics through the activation of the cytosolic histone deacetylase type II protein HDAC6 [5, 17], responsible for the de-acetylation of tubulin and other substrates involved in motility such as cortactin [45]. The protruding and retracting cell regions display different MT dynamics, polarization and posttranslational modifications during cell migration. In particular, MTs become acetylated in the stable subset present in the lamella region, while highly dynamic MTs facing the lamellipodium are de-acetylated [17, 46]. GRK2 directly interacts with and phosphorylates HDAC6 at residues serine 1060/1062 and 1068, and this phosphorylation event enhances HDAC6-mediated α-tubulin (but not cortactin) deacetylation and is necessary for the positive effect of HDAC6 in the migration of epithelial cells and fibroblasts challenged by fibronectin or EGF [17, 47]. The functional interactions of GRK2 with both GIT-1 and HDAC6 could also be relevant to increasing focal adhesion turnover, thus modulating cell adhesion and tension and increasing cell motility [5].

One emerging question is how such different GRK2 interactions are orchestrated during cell migration. We have suggested that changes in the subcellular localization and phosphorylation status of GRK2 would allow the dynamic and stimuli-specific switching of partners relevant to cell migration, allowing its sequential and coordinated participation in several steps of the motility process [5, 47]. Migratory stimuli would promote GRK2 recruitment to activated GPCR in the leading edge membrane, and transient Src-mediated tyrosine phosphorylation of GRK2 at such locations, enhancing its interaction with GIT1 and facilitating localized activation of the Rac/Pak/Mek/Erk pathway. Subsequent phosphorylation of GRK2 at S670 by MAPK disrupts interactions with GIT-1 and GPCR, simultaneously switching on the ability of GRK2 to phosphorylate HDAC6 co-localized at the lamellipodium, resulting in dynamic, local HDAC6-mediated de-acetylation of MTs. The concerted action of de-acetylated MTs and GIT1 signalosomes at the leading edge would contribute to cortical polarity and membrane protrusion and thus lead to enhanced cell motility [5, 13, 17, 40].

It is important to note that several of the GRK2-interacting signaling modules in epithelial cell migration play well-known roles in invasive motility, including integrins, GPCRs (S1P, chemokine or PAR receptors), the EGFR family, RhoA, Rac1, or ERMs. HDAC6 is overexpressed in a high proportion of breast tumors and contributes to cell motility and to invadopodia formation and maturation, through the regulation of acetylation–deacetylation of a growing number of proteins [48–50]. It is thus tempting to speculate that GRK2 levels may contribute to tumor cell invasiveness. In order to assess such potential role of GRK2 and to define the underlying molecular mechanisms, it would be important to combine 2D, 3D, and in vivo experimental models, to take into account the different stimuli that can converge in modulating GRK2 function.

5   GRK2 Plays a Role in the Tumoral Angiogenic Switch

Tumor microvasculature is usually highly angiogenic and leaky, leading to deficient blood supply and hypoxia [51]. In such microenvironment, transformed cells often became more aggressive, displaying increased proliferation, invasiveness, and drug resistance. The reciprocal interactions among tumor-associated vasculature, tumor-infiltrated immune cells and transformed cells emerge are the key factor for cancer progression. We have shown that downregulation of GRK2 in endothelial cells (EC) is a relevant event in the tumoral angiogenic switch that impairs endothelial TGF-β signaling and EC interaction with mural cells, what results in the formation of immature and fragile vessels [28]. Moreover, decreased EC GRK2 dosage is observed in the presence of cocultured breast transformed cells and occurs in human breast cancer vessels. Remarkably, reduced GRK2 in the endothelium accelerates tumor growth in mice, increases the size of intra-tumor vessels, reduces pericyte coverage, and enhances macrophage infiltration, thereby strengthening many of the hallmarks of the tumor microvasculature [28].

Angiogenesis involves early steps during which ECs polarize, migrate, establish cell–cell contacts, and form vessel lumens, followed by a stabilization period characterized by pericyte apposition to form mature vessels [52, 53]. The study of the effects of altering GRK2 dosage in cell and animal models indicates that this kinase acts as a hub in signaling pathways involved in vascular stabilization and remodeling. Upon GRK2 downregulation, primary microvascular ECs display an increase in motility and enhanced downstream signaling in response to key angiogenic stimuli (VEGF, S1P, serum). In parallel, these cells lose the capability to organize into tubular structures, and the balanced secretion of pro-inflammatory and pro-angiogenic factors is disrupted [28, 54].

Moreover, endothelial GRK2 dosage modulates TGFβ1-mediated pathways. Cellular responses triggered by TGFβ1 in ECs are complex, contributing positive or negatively to endothelial activation, due to the coexistence of two receptors that drive opposite effects, ALK1 and ALK5, and their functional cross-modulation [55–57]. Decreased GRK2 levels alter the balance in TGFβ1 signaling through ALK5 and ALK1 receptors towards enhanced ALK5 signaling and impair the actions of the ALK1-specific BMP9 ligand, a member of TGFβ family that functions as a vascular quiescence factor [28, 54]. GRK2 would inhibit the ALK5 pathway in endothelial cells at the level of Smad2/3, consistent with the previously reported effect in other cell types [58, 59], while the positive effect of the kinase in the ALK1 signaling branch does not involve a negative-crosstalk from ALK5 to ALK1 at the Smad level, which suggests the occurrence of additional mechanisms of GRK2 modulation in the ALK1–Smad1,7 interface. Interestingly, a lower GRK2 abundance in EC alters the secretome of these cells, leading to altered levels of PDGF-BB, critical for pericyte recruitment, as well as of several chemokines as CCL2 or CCL5, relevant for the attraction and activation of mononuclear cells, suggesting that reduced EC GRK2 expression might help to recruit monocytes to tumors [28, 54]. Consistent with this array of cell-autonomous endothelial defects, neovascularization is impaired in both global and endothelium-specific GRK2 knockout mice, which develop vessels with altered morphometrics and reduced mural coating [28]. Moreover, decreased EC GRK2 dosage accelerates tumor growth in mice, by impairing the pericytes ensheathing of vessels, thereby promoting hypoxia and macrophage infiltration along with enhanced macrophage infiltration [28].

These results raise new questions regarding the mechanisms by which transformed cells trigger the decrease in GRK2 observed in human breast cancer vessels and as to how GRK2 can modulate the interactions between different cell types that occur in the tumor microenvironment [54].

6   GRK2 as an Oncomodulator?

The overall available data indicating that GRK2 can modulate several of the hallmarks of cancer (proliferation, survival, migration, angiogenesis) suggest that this protein may act as an onco-modifier, contributing to tumoral transformation in a cell-specific manner. Moreover, the connection of GRK2 with the TGFβ signaling axis described in the previous section provides a means by which upregulation of GRK2 may restrict the tumoral suppressor role of TGFβ. Indeed, this factor elicits paradoxical effects on cell proliferation and migration in a cellular context-dependent manner [60]. In response to TGFβ-bound ALK5, GRK2 can associate with and phosphorylate Smad2/3 in their regulatory linker domain, preventing activation and nuclear translocation of the Smad complex, thereby leading to the inhibition of pro-arresting and pro-apoptotic TGF-β effects [58, 59]. Such regulation might favor a potential TGFβ switch from a tumor suppressor to a tumor promoter, akin to that induced by oncogenic H-Ras-dependent, Jnk-mediated phosphorylation of Smad3 [61]. On the other hand, a role for GRK2 in the regulation of centrosome dynamics has recently been demonstrated, with potential implications in cell transformation [62]. GRK2 mediates the EGF-induced separation of centrosomes during G2 progression, and "excessive" EGF signaling promotes centrosome amplification that could lead to the formation of multipolar spindles and result in aneuploidy, a hallmark of tumor cells. Therefore, cells with abnormal GRK2 levels may be more prone to genomic instability.

Consistent with these findings, GRK2 levels are altered in granulose cell tumors, thyroid and prostate cancer (reviewed in refs. 4, 6) or upregulated in malignant mammary cell lines with aberrant activation of the PI3K/Akt pathway [63]. In support of the notion that upregulation of GRK2 in breast tumoral cells is not a bystander effect of the transformation process but instead an active player in aberrant proliferation and survival, depletion of GRK2 significantly attenuated the cell viability and colony-formation ability of the basal breast tumor cell line MDA-MB231 [64]. Moreover, GRK2 silencing in these cells led to a cell arrest in the G0/G1 phase, which is consistent with our data suggesting that the G1/G0 and G2/M cell cycle phases have a different requirement for GRK2 levels. Ongoing research in our laboratory has shown that increased expression of GRK2 also plays a relevant role in luminal breast cancer (Nogues et al., submitted). Enhanced GRK2 functionality fosters proliferation, survival, anchorage-independent growth, and tumor growth in vivo, by mechanisms involving a reinforced GRK2-HDAC6 signaling module, putting forward GRK2 as an essential oncomodulator of breast tumor progression. Together with our previous data in tumoral endothelial cells ([28], see Sect. 5), these results suggest that concurrent and opposite changes of GRK2 in the epithelial (upregulation) and stromal (downregulation) components of breast tumors might act synergistically to promote tumor growth, stressing that a better knowledge of cell type-specific modulation and roles of GRK2 is key to understand its integrated role in pathophysiological processes.

7   GRK2 and Insulin Resistance-Related Conditions

Insulin resistance (IR) characterized by a reduced responsiveness to the effects of insulin is a common feature of obesity and a susceptibility factor for several pathological conditions, including glucose intolerance, hypertension, dyslipidemias, nonalcoholic fatty liver disease (NAFLD), cardiovascular disease, and type 2 diabetes (T2D), that is becoming a global public health problem [65]. Thus, a better knowledge of how different intracellular pathways integrate to finely tune the response to insulin, body weight gain, and metabolic rate is needed that helps identify novel therapeutic strategies beyond diet, physical exercise, or drugs.

Interestingly, accumulating evidence indicates that GRK2 plays an important integrative role in the homeostasis of cellular metabolism, energy production and expenditure [66–68]. Consistent with this notion, GRK2 levels are elevated during IR in a cell line of human adipocytes, in white adipose tissue (WAT) and muscle in either TNFα, aging or high-fat diet (HFD)-induced murine models, also in peripheral blood cells from metabolic syndrome patients [69] and in cells chronically stimulated with insulin [70] or in the hearts of mice fed with a long-term high-fat diet (Lucas et al., in preparation). On the other hand, peptide inhibitors of GRK2 have been reported to ameliorate glucose homeostasis in several murine models [71], and mice hemizygous for GRK2 maintain glucose tolerance and insulin signaling in the major insulin-responsive tissues during TNFα, aging or HFD-induced IR models [69]. These data indicate that high GRK2 levels markedly impair insulin sensitivity in vivo and that a moderate decrease in GRK2 levels/activity could be a valid therapeutic strategy for T2D.

Importantly, we have recently shown that lowering GRK2 levels can not only prevent but also revert ongoing IR and obesity, by using a tamoxifen (Tx)-inducible GRK2 deletion strategy during a HFD feeding [72]. A reduction of GRK2 levels reverts key aspects of an already established diabetic-linked phenotype: impedes further body weight gain in the face of high fat feeding, normalizes glucose intolerance and leads to preserved insulin sensitivity in skeletal muscle and in liver, thus maintaining glucose homeostasis. Moreover, Tx-induced GRK2 knockout mice display reduced fat mass and smaller adipocyte size, are resistant to the development of liver steatosis and show reduced expression of pro-inflammatory markers in the liver [72].

These results put forward the GRK2 as a novel potential therapeutic target for IR and obesity and raise important questions as to the role of GRK2 in specific tissues/cell types, the integration of these effects in the organism and the molecular mechanisms involved.

7.1 GRK2 Interactome in the Modulation of Metabolism and Energy Expenditure

There are a number of molecular mechanisms by which GRK2 may impact insulin signaling, glucose homeostasis, adiposity, and energy expenditure. Regarding canonical GPCR-modulating functions, GRK2 regulates key GPCR related to metabolic rate, such as β-adrenergic receptors (βARs). βARs are necessary for diet-induced thermogenesis and play a critical role in the control of energy homeostasis, glucose metabolism, and in the body's response to diet-induced obesity. Moreover, sympathetic downregulation is a hallmark of animal models of obesity. GRK2 has a well-established role in downregulating adrenergic receptor signaling, and decreased GRK2 levels enhance βAR signaling in WAT and BAT [67]. It also should be noted that some key determinants of insulin secretion belong to the GPCR family, such as the GLP-1 receptors or the recently identified receptors for fatty acids and metabolites. GLP-1 released from intestinal cells in response to nutrients promotes glucose-stimulated insulin secretion (GSIS) by the pancreas and protects β cells from apoptosis. In fact, GLP-1R agonists are currently used for glycemic control in T2D patients [73]. GRK2 has been reported to translocate to the activated GLP-1R [74] but its possible role in GLP-1 signaling regulation remains to be established. Also, several GPCRs for intermediate metabolites such as FA, lactate, and ketone bodies detect changes in the levels of different energy substrates, and use this information to regulate the metabolic activity of cells and tissues [75]. Most of these receptors show a causal involvement in the pathophysiology of metabolic diseases such as T2D, dyslipidemia, and obesity, in addition to cardiovascular diseases [76]. The receptor for long chain FA GPR120 regulates the action of insulin, appetite control and adipogenesis. GPR120 also binds omega-3 fatty acids mediating potent anti-inflammatory and insulin-sensitizing effects [77]. This receptor is phosphorylated by GRKs and PKC [78]. Similarly, GPR40 agonists increase insulin-stimulated glucose uptake, improve glucose tolerance and some have reached human clinical T2D trials [79]. The potential physiological role of GRK2 and other GRKs in the modulation of these receptors in pathophysiological contexts remains to be established.

As for noncanonical mechanisms, GRK2 has been reported to act as an inhibitor of insulin-mediated glucose transport in 3T3L1 adipocytes by interfering with $G_{q/11}$ function [80], and it inhibits basal and insulin-stimulated glycogen synthesis [81]. Our group has shown that in adipocytes and myoblasts, increased GRK2 levels inhibit, and GRK2 silencing enhances, insulin-dependent signaling by controlling GRK2/IRS1 complexes and IRS1 levels [69]. An inhibitory phosphorylation on IRS1 serines by GRK2 has also been reported [82]. In addition, it has been described that GRK2 can localize to the mitochondrial outer membrane by means of a cellular stress-induced MAPK-mediated phosphorylation of GRK2 and its subsequent interaction with Hsp90. The consequences of such mitochondrial translocation of GRK2 are controversial, because both detrimental (increased cytochrome C release and apoptosis) and protective (increased biogenesis and ATP production) effects have been reported [83, 84].

7.2 Tissue-Specific Actions and Integration

At least four potentially interrelated tissue-specific processes have been found to be involved in the integrated physiological effects of GRK2 reduction in HFD-fed mice. First, insulin signaling is maintained in the face of HFD in peripheral insulin-targeted tissues. Second, enhanced lipolysis is detected in GRK2-deficient WAT and BAT. Also, increased expression of thermogenic markers and FA oxidation are found in BAT that may help burn the excess fat spilled over by WAT lipolysis. Finally, reduced steatosis and inflammation and altered patterns of M1/M2 macrophages are detected in the liver [72].

Based on our data, we believe that such pleiotropic effects of GRK2 are due to its unique ability to directly modulate in different tissues both the insulin receptor cascade and key GPCRs related to the control of adiposity and metabolic rate, such as β ARs. We next describe the effects of GRK2 and its cell-specific interactomes in different tissues.

WAT and BAT. WAT is a primary regulator of metabolism in food-deprived states: through its regulation of lipolysis, it influences the availability of different substrates, and also secretes adipokines (such as adiponectin, leptin, and resistin) controlling whole-body energy and fuel metabolism. WAT from GRK2 hemizygous mice presents a reduced expression of perilipins A and B (essential lipid-droplet associated proteins), as well as key de novo lipogenic enzymes, such as fatty acid synthase (FAS), acetyl-CoA carboxylase (ACC), and the FA transporter aP2 [67], which may indicate a decrease in lipogenesis and is consistent with the decreased size of white adipocytes in aged or HFD-fed mice [69]. GRK2 also appears to play an important role in BAT function and architecture, as well as in brown adipocyte differentiation [67]. In this regard, the decreased weight observed in 9-month-old GRK2+/– mice seems to be due, at least in part, to an increased function of BAT in these animals [67],since a more pronounced increase upon cold exposure of the expression of UCP1 as well as of beta-oxidation markers (CPT1 and COXIV) was observed in the BAT of GRK2+/– animals. Furthermore, phosphorylation of proteins such as AMPK and ACC regulating lipid metabolism and brown fat function was also increased. Importantly, Tx-induced GRK2 loss enhances the β-adrenergic-dependent lipolytic capacity of WAT by increasing the response to adrenergic agonists and also the expression levels of HSL. The enhanced BAT function observed in GRK2+/– mice would make this tissue more able to consume the extra FFA released by WAT and thus prevent lipotoxicity in these animals [67, 72].

7.2.1   Liver

The liver's metabolic buffering system controls macronutrient and micronutrient homeostasis, allowing other tissues to perform normally under physiological stresses, thus playing a significant role in how the body responds to changing fuel needs and nutritional challenges. Hepatic IR and steatosis triggered by HFD or other conditions is an essential element in the pathogenesis of nonalcoholic fatty liver disease (NAFLD). NAFLD is the liver manifestation of the metabolic syndrome and is independently associated with obesity, IR, cardiovascular disease and T2D, and has been associated with metabolic inflexibility [85]. Interestingly, GRK2 levels are increased in the liver of mice fed HFD [69]. Along the same lines, Sprague-Dawley rats fed HFD for two weeks presented increased hepatic plasma membrane GRK2 [86]. Moreover, insulin-mediated Akt phosphorylation was preserved in the liver of GRK2+/– mice in the face of different IR-inducing conditions [69]. In vitro experiments in mouse liver FL83B cells demonstrated that GRK2 negatively regulates basal and insulin-stimulated glycogen synthesis downstream of the insulin receptor. Mechanistically, GRK2 seems to affect phosphorylation of Ser307 on IRS1, reducing insulin receptor-IRS1 interaction and, thus, insulin receptor-mediated phosphorylation of Tyr612 on IRS1 [81]. Accordingly, an increase of IRS1 phosphorylation at Tyr612 was found in HepG2 cells with reduced GRK2 protein levels after IGF-1 treatment [24]. Whether GRK2 is directly or indirectly causing the phosphorylation of Ser307 on IRS1, as detected in other cell types [82], remains a subject for future investigation, but undoubtedly IRS1 and components of the insulin receptor cascade represent some of the most relevant directly interacting partners to explain the regulation of hepatic functions by GRK2.

Notably, reduced GRK2 level protects against HFD-induced hepatic insulin resistance and lipid accumulation, an effect that was associated with reduced expression of the genes encoding fatty acid synthase (FAS) and PPARγ, which are increased in fatty liver. Moreover, the accumulation of M1-like macrophages and pro-inflammatory markers observed in control HFD-fed mice was not present in livers from HFD-fed tamoxifen-induced GRK2−/− animals, which were characterized by lower activation of inflammatory pathways such as that of JNK, scattered distribution of macrophages, and elevated M2 to M1 ratio [72]. Although the actual mechanisms and molecules involved are currently unknown, they may involve a direct effect on the polarization or migration of these cells. These data warrant further investigation of the role of GRK2 in the control of hepatic steatosis and metabolism and in the development of NAFLD.

7.2.2   Skeletal Muscle   Skeletal muscle is the critical tissue for glycemic control. It represents the quantitatively major site of insulin-stimulated glucose clearance in the postprandial state, accounting for approximately 80% of glucose disposal under insulin-stimulated conditions [87] and also represents the largest glycogen storage organ. Thus, IR and metabolic dysfunction in the skeletal muscle play a major role in the development of the metabolic syndrome and T2D. GRK2 levels are elevated in the muscle in either TNFα, aging or HFD-fed murine models, whereas GRK2+/− mice retain enhanced insulin signaling in this tissue [69], and tamoxifen-induced GRK2 deletion enhances insulin signaling to Akt in HFD-fed animals [72]. This is consistent with the suggested negative role for GRK2 in the regulation of insulin signaling in skeletal muscle both in cultured myocytes and in vivo, most probably by mechanisms independent of kinase activity and involving the formation of dynamic GRK2/IRS1 complexes [69]. It is worth noting that the skeletal muscle fibers in GRK2+/− mice are hypertrophied as compared to those of WT littermates [88], but whether this fact contributes to the improved glucose homeostasis observed in hemizygous GRK2 mice is still unknown. In addition, in C2C12 myoblasts, GRK2 levels and functionality have been reported to affect muscle cell differentiation networks by mechanisms involving timely modulation of the p38MAPK and Akt pathways. The impaired differentiation promoted by increased GRK2 levels were recapitulated by a p38MAPK mutant mimicking the inhibitory phosphorylation of p38MAPK by GRK2 [88]. These data suggest that noncanonical kinase functions of GRK2, and, in particular, p38MAPK phosphorylation, represent the most relevant GRK2 interactome to explain its effects on muscle differentiation.

8   New Players in the GRK2 Interactome in Cardiovascular Disease

GRK2 is known to be a key regulator of the cardiovascular function and dysfunction, and its levels are increased in hypertension, cardiac ischemia, and in early stages of maladaptive myocardial remodeling

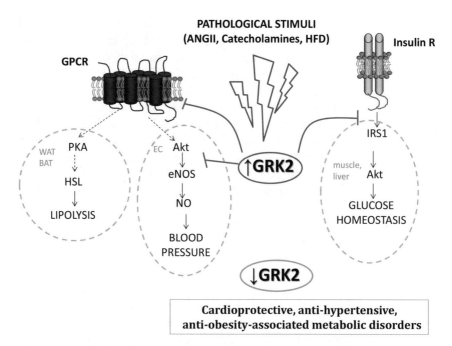

Fig. 2 GRK2 as an integrative node in cardiovascular and metabolic diseases. Several pathogenic stimuli (high circulating levels of catecholamines or angiotensin, high-fat diet feeding) converge in promoting increased GRK2 abundance in several relevant tissues/cell types (adipose, muscle, liver, heart, endothelial cells (EC), …). This increase in the GRK2 levels would simultaneously alter GPCR and insulin receptor-dependent signaling cascades or other signaling pathways, thus contributing to disease progression. On the contrary, downregulation of GRK2 functionality has a protective role

and heart failure in patients and in animal experimental models (reviewed in refs. 82, 89, 90). Emerging evidence indicates that the integrated regulation of GPCR, in addition to noncanonical pathways, underlies the role of GRK2 in such physiological and pathological contexts (Fig. 2).

8.1 GRK2 and the Molecular Mechanisms of Hypertension

The impact of increased GRK2 levels in hypertension has been largely ascribed to its effects on the modulation of a variety of vasoconstrictor and vasodilator GPCRs. We have recently compared vascular responses using global adult (9 months old) GRK2 hemizygous mice and found that these GRK2+/− animals are resistant to the development of vascular remodeling, mechanical alterations, endothelial dysfunction, increased vasoconstrictor responses, and hypertension-induced by AngII. The underlying mechanisms involve differential GPCR modulation and the preservation of the impaired Akt/eNOS pathway and eNOS levels leading to enhanced NO availability [91]. Earlier studies demonstrated that Akt physically interacts with GRK2 and this interaction inhibits Akt activity and NO production [33]. In addition, lower GRK2 abundance might potentiate the activation of endothelial muscarinic GPCR triggering alternative

NO synthesis modulatory pathways. The mechanisms leading to preservation of total eNOS levels in GRK2+/− mice deserve further investigation.

It should be noted that different mediators involved in the development of hypertension and vascular damage during obesity/diabetes appear to converge in upregulating the GRK2 expression in the vasculature. Increased GRK2 expression observed in vessels from diabetic mice [92–95] is abolished by AngII type I receptor blockade [93] suggesting that AngII is per se able to increase the GRK2 expression, as also shown by our group [91]. Moreover, high glucose/high insulin enhances GRK2 abundance in cultured endothelial cells by an unknown mechanism, what results in the inhibition of the insulin/Akt/eNOS pathway [96]. In diabetes, the increased levels of GRK2 seem to prevent the translocation of β-arrestin2 to the membrane where it acts as a scaffold molecule for Akt and the insulin receptor [97], thereby contributing to impaired Akt/eNOS/NO production in response to insulin and other agonists [92, 94–96]. The fact that GRK2 inhibition or partial GRK2 deletion improved the endothelial dysfunction observed in obese/diabetic [93, 95, 98] or hypertensive [91] animal models strongly supports the notion that GRK2 is an important signaling hub in vascular function.

8.2 GRK2 as an Integrative Sensor and Signaling Node in Cardiac Tissue

The overall importance of GRK2 in the heart has been demonstrated through several studies with genetically engineered mice (see references above) and in zebrafish [90, 99]. The global loss of GRK2 leads to embryonic lethality with cardiac malformations and dysplasia [10]. However, cardiac-specific GRK2 knockout mice developed normally and exhibited no adult cardiac phenotype at baseline other than a modestly enhanced contractile function [100], which demonstrated that GRK2 has a broader extra-cardiac role in embryogenesis. For instance, GRK2 KO mice embryos display marked vascular malformations involving impaired recruitment of mural cells [28]. On the other hand, in the conditional cardiac GRK2 ablation mouse model, in which cardiac myocyte GRK2 expression was normal during embryonic development, but was ablated after birth, improved function and prevention of heart failure (HF) development was observed after myocardial infarction. Moreover, when the downregulation of GRK2 is induced in the cardiomyocytes after HF development by tamoxifen administration (αMHC-MerCreMer × GRK2 fl/fl), there is an active reverse remodeling and improved cardiac function [101]. On the contrary, cardiac-specific GRK2-overexpressing mice display the loss of β-AR-mediated inotropic reserve, as well as desensitized AngII receptors (AT1R) in their hearts [102]. To study the contribution of GRK2 to different cellular processes in the cardiovascular disease, animal models that overexpress a carboxy-terminal peptide of GRK2 (βARKct) have been extensively used. βARKct overexpression seems to act by inhibiting endogenous GRK2 activation by competing with Gβγ binding. Transgenic βARKct mice have increased function at baseline and in response to the β-AR agonist isoproterenol [102]. In fact, overexpression of βARKct rescued several mouse models of HF, such as after pressure overload induced by transverse aortic constriction [103] or after acute myocardial ischemia/reperfusion injury [104]. Furthermore, the cross breeding of βARKct mice with different animal models of chronic HF induced by genetic manipulation also rescued overt cardiac failure in these animals [105, 106]. A recent report indicates that paroxetine-mediated GRK2 inhibition reverses cardiac dysfunction and remodeling after myocardial infarction [107].

The molecular mechanisms underlying both the deleterious and beneficial effects in cardiovascular function of the reported changes in GRK2 levels are not fully understood. GRK2 is known to attenuate cardiac contractile responses to β-AR stimulation and to modulate Ang II receptor-mediated contraction [102, 108], and heterozygous GRK2 knockout mice show increased cardiac function and responses to adrenergic input [109]. It was proposed that increased GRK2 levels resulted from enhanced neurohumoral activation would further alter β-adrenergic signaling, leading to HF. However, the fact that GRK2 inhibition acts in a synergistic manner with established β-blocker treatments in HF models suggests that the functional impact of altered GRK2 levels involves cellular partners additional to the β-adrenergic axis. Recent findings [68, 82, 110] suggest that GRK2 upregulation may inhibit cardiac insulin signaling, a critical cardioprotective pathway, thus putting forward GRK2 as a new molecular link among insulin resistance/obesity and cardiovascular comorbidities.

It has been shown that increased GRK2 levels upon chronic β-AR stimulation can lead to IRS1 phosphorylation and insulin resistance in cardiomyocytes [82]. On the other hand, activation of insulin receptor induces GRK2-mediated phosphorylation of the β2AR, which attenuates adrenergic stimulation [111]. The insulin-induced phosphorylation of the β-AR seems to be dependent on IRS1 and IRS2 and involve PKA and GRK2 activity. Thus GRK2 would link the cardiac remodeling and IR to impaired contractility and cardiac dysfunction, features that are present in obese individuals and may contribute to heart failure. In this context, we have recently uncovered that cardiac GRK2 levels increase in situations where IR develops, such as in ob/ob mice or after HFD, whereas 9-month-old GRK2+/− mice display preserved cardiac insulin sensitivity and the gene expression reprogramming that would confer cardioprotection [110].

We have observed that GLUT4 translocation and glucose uptake as well as insulin-dependent Akt and p70S6K activation were impaired in WT but not in 9-month-old GRK2+/− animals [110]. Interestingly, although GRK2+/− mice displayed a slightly larger cardiac area and cardiomyocyte diameter, they did not exhibit pathological cardiac hypertrophy, consistent with a physiological hypertrophy situation. In this line, decreased GRK2 levels correlate with higher expression of key genes implicated in physiological hypertrophy and cardioprotection. Notably, such difference in cardiac gene expression profiles between WT and GRK2+/− genotypes was detected at 9 but not at 4 months of age, suggesting that they are the consequence of GRK2 dosage together with age-related factors, such as the systemic prediabetic state with higher insulin and glucose levels in plasma present in WT compared to GRK2+/− animals [69]. In support of this notion, cardiac GRK2 expression is increased in adult ob/ob mice and upon HFD feeding for 12 weeks, leading to higher amounts of GRK2/IRS1 complexes and impaired cardiac insulin sensitivity observed in these situations [110].

Overall, our data indicate that age- and HFD-induced insulin resistance in the heart can be prevented by maintaining the GRK2 levels below a certain threshold. In this regard, it is worth keeping in mind that the incidence of pathological conditions such as T2D, metabolic syndrome and cardiovascular diseases is significantly higher in the adult/elderly population as compared to young individuals. It should be stressed, however, that most studies in the field use young animals (2–3 months old) that would not adequately mimic the "physiological environment" present in older animals (such as mild insulin resistance) when these pathologies begin to develop. Thus, the use of adequate experimental models is necessary, if the differential molecular mechanisms underlying these conditions are to be accurately identified.

The available evidence suggests that, in addition to the previously reported upregulation of cardiac GRK2 levels by increased catecholamine levels, systemic insulin resistance-inducing conditions such as high dietary fat, also cause enhanced GRK2 expression in the heart. GRK2 levels would thus act as an integrative sensor of a variety of pathological inputs, triggering dysfunctionality both in the adrenergic and insulin signaling cascades and allowing progression towards maladaptive remodeling. Sustained β-AR desensitization could fuel a detrimental cycle where the adrenal glands would try to compensate the lower β-adrenergic output by increasing catecholamine secretion. This in turn further upregulates GRK2 levels in the cardiac tissue [112], thus triggering an impairment of cardiac insulin signaling and cardiac metabolism. Altered GRK2 levels may also affect the function of other relevant GPCRs in HF, such as the adiponectin receptor [113]. Together, these events would eventually bring about maladaptive changes in global gene expression patterns. On the contrary, exercise, which is critical for the prevention and treatment of obesity, is able to decrease myocardial GRK2 levels [114] in accordance with the cardioprotective role of lowering GRK2 levels for the obese heart.

Overall, our data put forward GRK2 as a new molecular link among aging, insulin resistance/obesity, and cardiovascular comorbidities. Since circulating GRK2 levels have been shown to mirror cardiac expression [115], and increased GRK2 expression is present in peripheral blood cells from metabolic syndrome and from heart failure patients, in particular those with diabetes mellitus [116], it will be interesting to explore the potential use of GRK2 as a prognostic cardiovascular risk marker in such conditions [117].

9   Conclusions and Future Perspectives

As summarized in this review, available data indicate that GRK2 is a critical signaling node with important roles in cellular functions and in the whole body homeostasis. Depending on the stimuli, the cell type and the physiological or pathological context, diverse canonical and noncanonical functions of GRK2 are coordinately engaged, thus contributing to integrated cellular responses orchestrated by different stimuli and guided by various extracellular cues. Moreover, several factors altered in prevalent pathologies appear to converge in modulating the GRK2 expression and or phosphorylation/functionality status, putting forward this kinase as an integrative homeostatic sensor, which would in turn simultaneously target GPCR, RTK, and other noncanonical networks, leading to coordinated adaptive (or maladaptive) responses (Fig. 3). The

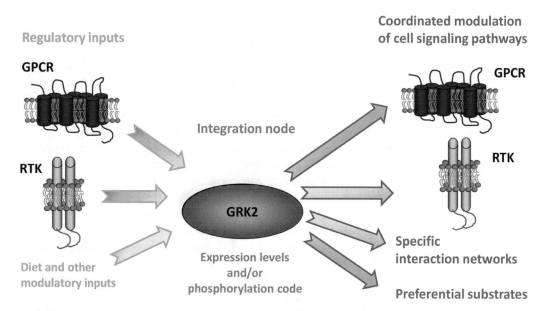

Fig. 3 The GRK2 signaling hub. Factors altered in prevalent pathologies acting through GPCR, growth factor receptors or via other mechanisms converge in modulating the GRK2 expression and/or phosphorylation status. These parameters modulate the functionality of GRK2 towards its target GPCR and RTK in a given cell, and determine its preferential/sequential interactions with specific substrates and partners. The integrated modulation of signaling cascades achieved through these combination of canonical and noncanonical GRK2 functions allow for coordinated adaptive (or maladaptive) physiological responses

mechanisms controlling changes in GRK2 levels and functionality in specific cell types, how GPCR activation influences noncanonical functions of GRK2 (or vice versa), and how concurrent changes in GRK2 functionality taking place in different cell types/tissues impact the whole body homeostasis in pathological conditions remain exciting areas of research for the future.

Acknowledgments

Our laboratory is supported by Grants SAF2014-55511-R (to F.M. and C.M.) from Ministerio de Economía y Competitividad (MINECO), Spain; PI14/00435 from Instituto de Salud Carlos III to P.P., S2010/BMD-2332 (INDISNET) from Comunidad de Madrid, Spain (to F.M.); The Cardiovascular Network (RD12/0042/0012), from Ministerio Sanidad y Consumo-Instituto Carlos III, Spain (to F.M.), an European Foundation for the Study of Diabetes (EFSD) Novo Nordisk Partnership for Diabetes Research in Europe Grant (to F.M.); Fundación Ramón Areces (to C.M. and P.P.). We also acknowledge the support of a Contrato para la Formación Postdoctoral from MINECO to R.V.B., and institutional support from Fundación Ramón Areces.

References

1. Gurevich EV, Tesmer JJ, Mushegian A, Gurevich VV (2012) G protein-coupled receptor kinases: more than just kinases and not only for GPCRs. Pharmacol Ther 133(1):40–69. doi:10.1016/j.pharmthera.2011.08.001

2. Shenoy SK, Lefkowitz RJ (2011) beta-Arrestin-mediated receptor trafficking and signal transduction. Trends Pharmacol Sci 32(9):521–533. doi:10.1016/j.tips.2011.05.002

3. Ribas C, Penela P, Murga C, Salcedo A, Garcia-Hoz C, Jurado-Pueyo M, Aymerich I, Mayor F Jr (2007) The G protein-coupled receptor kinase (GRK) interactome: role of GRKs in GPCR regulation and signaling. Biochim Biophys Acta 1768(4):913–922. doi:10.1016/j.bbamem.2006.09.019

4. Penela P, Murga C, Ribas C, Lafarga V, Mayor F Jr (2010) The complex G protein-coupled receptor kinase 2 (GRK2) interactome unveils new physiopathological targets. Br J Pharmacol 160(4):821–832. doi:10.1111/j.1476-5381.2010.00727.x

5. Penela P, Nogues L, Mayor F Jr (2014) Role of G protein-coupled receptor kinases in cell migration. Curr Opin Cell Biol 27:10–17. doi:10.1016/j.ceb.2013.10.005

6. Evron T, Daigle TL, Caron MG (2012) GRK2: multiple roles beyond G protein-coupled receptor desensitization. Trends Pharmacol Sci 33(3):154–164. doi:10.1016/j.tips.2011.12.003

7. Lymperopoulos A, Rengo G, Koch WJ (2012) GRK2 inhibition in heart failure: something old, something new. Curr Pharm Des 18(2):186–191. doi:10.2174/138161212799040510

8. Liggett SB (2011) Phosphorylation barcoding as a mechanism of directing GPCR signaling. Sci Signal 4(185):pe36. doi:10.1126/scisignal.2002331

9. Li L, Homan KT, Vishnivetskiy SA, Manglik A, Tesmer JJ, Gurevich VV, Gurevich EV (2015) G protein-coupled receptor kinases of the GRK4 protein subfamily phosphorylate inactive G Protein-coupled Receptors (GPCRs). J Biol Chem 290(17):10775–10790. doi:10.1074/jbc.M115.644773

10. Jaber M, Koch WJ, Rockman H, Smith B, Bond RA, Sulik KK, Ross J Jr, Lefkowitz RJ, Caron MG, Giros B (1996) Essential role of beta-adrenergic receptor kinase 1 in cardiac development and function. Proc Natl Acad Sci U S A 93(23):12974–12979

11. Deiss K, Kisker C, Lohse MJ, Lorenz K (2012) Raf kinase inhibitor protein (RKIP) dimer formation controls its target switch from Raf1 to G protein-coupled receptor kinase (GRK) 2. J Biol Chem 287(28):23407–23417. doi:10.1074/jbc.M112.363812

12. Eijkelkamp N, Wang H, Garza-Carbajal A, Willemen HL, Zwartkruis FJ, Wood JN, Dantzer R, Kelley KW, Heijnen CJ, Kavelaars A (2010) Low nociceptor GRK2 prolongs prostaglandin E2 hyperalgesia via biased cAMP signaling to Epac/Rap1, protein kinase Cepsilon, and MEK/ERK. J Neurosci 30(38):12806–12815. doi:10.1523/JNEUROSCI.3142-10.2010

13. Penela P, Ribas C, Aymerich I, Eijkelkamp N, Barreiro O, Heijnen CJ, Kavelaars A, Sanchez-Madrid F, Mayor F Jr (2008) G protein-coupled receptor kinase 2 positively regulates epithelial cell migration. EMBO J 27(8):1206–1218. doi:10.1038/emboj.2008.55

14. Robinson JD, Pitcher JA (2013) G protein-coupled receptor kinase 2 (GRK2) is a Rho-activated scaffold protein for the ERK MAP kinase cascade. Cell Signal 25(12):2831–2839. doi:10.1016/j.cellsig.2013.08.031

15. Wan KF, Sambi BS, Tate R, Waters C, Pyne NJ (2003) The inhibitory gamma subunit of the type 6 retinal cGMP phosphodiesterase functions to link c-Src and G-protein-coupled receptor kinase 2 in a signaling unit that regulates p42/p44 mitogen-activated protein kinase by epidermal growth factor. J Biol Chem 278(20):18658–18663. doi:10.1074/jbc.M212103200

16. Lipfert J, Odemis V, Engele J (2013) Grk2 is an essential regulator of CXCR7 signalling in astrocytes. Cell Mol Neurobiol 33(1):111–118. doi:10.1007/s10571-012-9876-5

17. Lafarga V, Aymerich I, Tapia O, Mayor F Jr, Penela P (2012) A novel GRK2/HDAC6 interaction modulates cell spreading and motility. EMBO J 31(4):856–869. doi:10.1038/emboj.2011.466

18. Bliziotes M, Gunness M, Zhang X, Nissenson R, Wiren K (2000) Reduced G-protein-coupled-receptor kinase 2 activity results in impairment of osteoblast function. Bone 27(3):367–373

19. Chen W, Ren XR, Nelson CD, Barak LS, Chen JK, Beachy PA, de Sauvage F, Lefkowitz RJ (2004) Activity-dependent internalization of smoothened mediated by beta-arrestin 2 and GRK2. Science 306(5705):2257–2260. doi:10.1126/science.1104135

20. Meloni AR, Fralish GB, Kelly P, Salahpour A, Chen JK, Wechsler-Reya RJ, Lefkowitz RJ, Caron MG (2006) Smoothened signal transduction is promoted by G protein-coupled receptor kinase 2. Mol Cell Biol 26(20):7550–7560. doi:10.1128/MCB.00546-06

21. Molnar C, Holguin H, Mayor F Jr, Ruiz-Gomez A, de Celis JF (2007) The G protein-coupled receptor regulatory kinase GPRK2 participates in Hedgehog signaling in Drosophila. Proc Natl Acad Sci U S A 104(19):7963–7968. doi:10.1073/pnas.0702374104

22. Metaye T, Levillain P, Kraimps JL, Perdrisot R (2008) Immunohistochemical detection, regulation and antiproliferative function of G-protein-coupled receptor kinase 2 in thyroid carcinomas. J Endocrinol 198(1):101–110. doi:10.1677/JOE-07-0562

23. Peppel K, Jacobson A, Huang X, Murray JP, Oppermann M, Freedman NJ (2000) Overexpression of G protein-coupled receptor kinase-2 in smooth muscle cells attenuates mitogenic signaling via G protein-coupled and platelet-derived growth factor receptors. Circulation 102(7):793–799

24. Wei Z, Hurtt R, Gu T, Bodzin AS, Koch WJ, Doria C (2013) GRK2 negatively regulates IGF-1R signaling pathway and cyclins' expression in HepG2 cells. J Cell Physiol 228(9):1897–1901. doi:10.1002/jcp.24353

25. Zheng H, Worrall C, Shen H, Issad T, Seregard S, Girnita A, Girnita L (2012) Selective recruitment of G protein-coupled receptor kinases (GRKs) controls signaling of the insulin-like growth factor 1 receptor. Proc Natl Acad Sci U S A 109(18):7055–7060. doi:10.1073/pnas.1118359109

26. Fu X, Koller S, Abd Alla J, Quitterer U (2013) Inhibition of G-protein-coupled receptor kinase 2 (GRK2) triggers the growth-promoting mitogen-activated protein kinase (MAPK) pathway. J Biol Chem 288(11):7738–7755. doi:10.1074/jbc.M112.428078

27. Penela P, Rivas V, Salcedo A, Mayor F Jr (2010) G protein-coupled receptor kinase 2 (GRK2) modulation and cell cycle progression. Proc Natl Acad Sci U S A 107(3):1118–1123. doi:10.1073/pnas.0905778107

28. Rivas V, Carmona R, Munoz-Chapuli R, Mendiola M, Nogues L, Reglero C, Miguel-Martin M, Garcia-Escudero R, Dorn GW 2nd, Hardisson D, Mayor F Jr, Penela P (2013) Developmental and tumoral vascularization is regulated by G protein-coupled receptor kinase 2. J Clin Invest 123(11):4714–4730. doi:10.1172/JCI67333

29. Jiang X, Yang P, Ma L (2009) Kinase activity-independent regulation of cyclin pathway by GRK2 is essential for zebrafish early development. Proc Natl Acad Sci U S A 106(25):10183–10188. doi:10.1073/pnas.0812105106

30. Lafarga V, Mayor F Jr, Penela P (2012) The interplay between G protein-coupled receptor kinase 2 (GRK2) and histone deacetylase 6 (HDAC6) at the crossroads of epithelial cell motility. Cell Adhes Migr 6(6):495–501. doi:10.4161/cam.21585

31. Bulavin DV, Fornace AJ Jr (2004) p38 MAP kinase's emerging role as a tumor suppressor. Adv Cancer Res 92:95–118. doi:10.1016/S0065-230X(04)92005-2

32. Peregrin S, Jurado-Pueyo M, Campos PM, Sanz-Moreno V, Ruiz-Gomez A, Crespo P, Mayor F Jr, Murga C (2006) Phosphorylation of p38 by GRK2 at the docking groove unveils a novel mechanism for inactivating p38MAPK. Curr Biol 16(20):2042–2047. doi:10.1016/j.cub.2006.08.083

33. Liu S, Premont RT, Kontos CD, Zhu S, Rockey DC (2005) A crucial role for GRK2 in regulation of endothelial cell nitric oxide synthase function in portal hypertension. Nat Med 11(9):952–958. doi:10.1038/nm1289

34. Boyault C, Zhang Y, Fritah S, Caron C, Gilquin B, Kwon SH, Garrido C, Yao TP, Vourc'h C, Matthias P, Khochbin S (2007) HDAC6 controls major cell response pathways to cytotoxic accumulation of protein aggregates. Genes Dev 21(17):2172–2181. doi:10.1101/gad.436407

35. Kawaguchi Y, Kovacs JJ, McLaurin A, Vance JM, Ito A, Yao TP (2003) The deacetylase HDAC6 regulates aggresome formation and cell viability in response to misfolded protein stress. Cell 115(6):727–738

36. Cotton M, Claing A (2009) G protein-coupled receptors stimulation and the control of cell migration. Cell Signal 21(7):1045–1053. doi:10.1016/j.cellsig.2009.02.008

37. Vroon A, Heijnen CJ, Kavelaars A (2006) GRKs and arrestins: regulators of migration and inflammation. J Leukoc Biol 80(6):1214–1221. doi:10.1189/jlb.0606373

38. Arnon TI, Xu Y, Lo C, Pham T, An J, Coughlin S, Dorn GW, Cyster JG (2011) GRK2-dependent S1PR1 desensitization is required for lymphocytes to overcome their attraction to blood. Science 333(6051):1898–1903. doi:10.1126/science.1208248

39. Penela P, Murga C, Ribas C, Salcedo A, Jurado-Pueyo M, Rivas V, Aymerich I, Mayor F Jr (2008) G protein-coupled receptor kinase 2 (GRK2) in migration and inflammation. Arch Physiol Biochem 114(3):195–200. doi:10.1080/13813450802181039

40. Penela P, Ribas C, Aymerich I, Mayor F Jr (2009) New roles of G protein-coupled receptor kinase 2 (GRK2) in cell migration. Cell Adhes Migr 3(1):19–23

41. Cant SH, Pitcher JA (2005) G protein-coupled receptor kinase 2-mediated phosphorylation of ezrin is required for G protein-coupled receptor-dependent reorganization of the actin cytoskeleton. Mol Biol Cell 16(7):3088–3099. doi:10.1091/mbc.E04-10-0877

42. Kahsai AW, Zhu S, Fenteany G (2010) G protein-coupled receptor kinase 2 activates radixin, regulating membrane protrusion and motility in epithelial cells. Biochim Biophys Acta 1803(2):300–310. doi:10.1016/j.bbamcr.2009.11.002

43. Hoefen RJ, Berk BC (2006) The multifunctional GIT family of proteins. J Cell Sci 119(Pt 8):1469–1475. doi:10.1242/jcs.02925

44. Yin G, Zheng Q, Yan C, Berk BC (2005) GIT1 is a scaffold for ERK1/2 activation in focal adhesions. J Biol Chem 280(30):27705–27712. doi:10.1074/jbc.M502271200

45. Kaluza D, Kroll J, Gesierich S, Yao TP, Boon RA, Hergenreider E, Tjwa M, Rossig L, Seto E, Augustin HG, Zeiher AM, Dimmeler S, Urbich C (2011) Class IIb HDAC6 regulates endothelial cell migration and angiogenesis by deacetylation of cortactin. EMBO J 30(20):4142–4156. doi:10.1038/emboj.2011.298

46. Etienne-Manneville S (2010) From signaling pathways to microtubule dynamics: the key players. Curr Opin Cell Biol 22(1):104–111. doi:10.1016/j.ceb.2009.11.008

47. Penela P, Lafarga V, Tapia O, Rivas V, Nogues L, Lucas E, Vila-Bedmar R, Murga C, Mayor F, Jr. (2012) Roles of GRK2 in cell signaling beyond GPCR desensitization: GRK2-HDAC6 interaction modulates cell spreading and motility. Sci Signal 5 (224):pt3. doi:10.1126/scisignal.2003098

48. Duong V, Bret C, Altucci L, Mai A, Duraffourd C, Loubersac J, Harmand PO, Bonnet S, Valente S, Maudelonde T, Cavailles V, Boulle N (2008) Specific activity of class II histone deacetylases in human breast cancer cells. Mol Cancer Res 6(12):1908–1919. doi:10.1158/1541-7786.MCR-08-0299

49. Lee YS, Lim KH, Guo X, Kawaguchi Y, Gao Y, Barrientos T, Ordentlich P, Wang XF, Counter CM, Yao TP (2008) The cytoplasmic deacetylase HDAC6 is required for efficient oncogenic tumorigenesis. Cancer Res 68(18):7561–7569. doi:10.1158/0008-5472.CAN-08-0188

50. Zhang M, Xiang S, Joo HY, Wang L, Williams KA, Liu W, Hu C, Tong D, Haakenson J, Wang C, Zhang S, Pavlovicz RE, Jones A, Schmidt KH, Tang J, Dong H, Shan B, Fang B, Radhakrishnan R, Glazer PM, Matthias P, Koomen J, Seto E, Bepler G, Nicosia SV,

Chen J, Li C, Gu L, Li GM, Bai W, Wang H, Zhang X (2014) HDAC6 deacetylates and ubiquitinates MSH2 to maintain proper levels of MutSalpha. Mol Cell 55(1):31–46. doi:10.1016/j.molcel.2014.04.028

51. Potente M, Gerhardt H, Carmeliet P (2011) Basic and therapeutic aspects of angiogenesis. Cell 146(6):873–887. doi:10.1016/j.cell.2011.08.039

52. Carmeliet P, Jain RK (2011) Molecular mechanisms and clinical applications of angiogenesis. Nature 473(7347):298–307. doi:10.1038/nature10144

53. Gerhardt H, Betsholtz C (2003) Endothelial-pericyte interactions in angiogenesis. Cell Tissue Res 314(1):15–23. doi:10.1007/s00441-003-0745-x

54. Rivas V, Nogues L, Reglero C, Mayor F Jr, Penela P (2014) Role of G protein-coupled receptor kinase 2 in tumoral angiogenesis. Mol Cell Oncol 1(4):e969166. doi:10.4161/23723548.2014.969166

55. van Meeteren LA, Goumans MJ, ten Dijke P (2011) TGF-beta receptor signaling pathways in angiogenesis; emerging targets for anti-angiogenesis therapy. Curr Pharm Biotechnol 12(12):2108–2120

56. Goumans MJ, Valdimarsdottir G, Itoh S, Lebrin F, Larsson J, Mummery C, Karlsson S, ten Dijke P (2003) Activin receptor-like kinase (ALK)1 is an antagonistic mediator of lateral TGFbeta/ALK5 signaling. Mol Cell 12(4):817–828

57. Orlova VV, Liu Z, Goumans MJ, ten Dijke P (2011) Controlling angiogenesis by two unique TGF-beta type I receptor signaling pathways. Histol Histopathol 26(9):1219–1230

58. Ho J, Cocolakis E, Dumas VM, Posner BI, Laporte SA, Lebrun JJ (2005) The G protein-coupled receptor kinase-2 is a TGFbeta-inducible antagonist of TGFbeta signal transduction. EMBO J 24(18):3247–3258. doi:10.1038/sj.emboj.7600794

59. Ho J, Chen H, Lebrun JJ (2007) Novel dominant negative Smad antagonists to TGFbeta signaling. Cell Signal 19(7):1565–1574. doi:10.1016/j.cellsig.2007.02.001

60. Siegel PM, Massague J (2003) Cytostatic and apoptotic actions of TGF-beta in homeostasis and cancer. Nat Rev Cancer 3(11):807–821. doi:10.1038/nrc1208

61. Liu IM, Schilling SH, Knouse KA, Choy L, Derynck R, Wang XF (2009) TGFbeta-stimulated Smad1/5 phosphorylation requires the ALK5 L45 loop and mediates the pro-migratory TGFbeta switch. EMBO J 28(2):88–98. doi:10.1038/emboj.2008.266

62. So CH, Michal A, Komolov KE, Luo J, Benovic JL (2013) G protein-coupled receptor kinase 2 (GRK2) is localized to centrosomes and mediates epidermal growth factor-promoted centrosomal separation. Mol Biol Cell 24(18):2795–2806. doi:10.1091/mbc.E13-01-0013

63. Salcedo A, Mayor F Jr, Penela P (2006) Mdm2 is involved in the ubiquitination and degradation of G-protein-coupled receptor kinase 2. EMBO J 25(20):4752–4762. doi:10.1038/sj.emboj.7601351

64. Zhang C, Chen X, Li Y, SWA H, Wu J, Shi X, Liu X, Kim S (2014) si-RNA-mediated silencing of ADRBK1 gene attenuates breast cancer cell proliferation. Cancer Biother Radiopharm 29(8):303–309. doi:10.1089/cbr.2014.1653

65. Eckel RH, Kahn SE, Ferrannini E, Goldfine AB, Nathan DM, Schwartz MW, Smith RJ, Smith SR (2011) Obesity and type 2 diabetes: what can be unified and what needs to be individualized? J Clin Endocrinol Metab 96(6):1654–1663. doi:10.1210/jc.2011-0585

66. Ciccarelli M, Cipolletta E, Iaccarino G (2012) GRK2 at the control shaft of cellular metabolism. Curr Pharm Des 18(2):121–127

67. Vila-Bedmar R, Garcia-Guerra L, Nieto-Vazquez I, Mayor F Jr, Lorenzo M, Murga C, Fernandez-Veledo S (2012) GRK2 contribution to the regulation of energy expenditure and brown fat function. FASEB Journal 26(8):3503–3514. doi:10.1096/fj.11-202267

68. Woodall MC, Ciccarelli M, Woodall BP, Koch WJ (2014) G protein-coupled receptor kinase 2: a link between myocardial contractile function and cardiac metabolism. Circ Res 114(10):1661–1670. doi:10.1161/CIRCRESAHA.114.300513

69. Garcia-Guerra L, Nieto-Vazquez I, Vila-Bedmar R, Jurado-Pueyo M, Zalba G, Diez J, Murga C, Fernandez-Veledo S, Mayor F Jr, Lorenzo M (2010) G protein-coupled receptor kinase 2 plays a relevant role in insulin resistance and obesity. Diabetes 59(10):2407–2417. doi:10.2337/db10-0771

70. Cipolletta E, Campanile A, Santulli G, Sanzari E, Leosco D, Campiglia P, Trimarco B, Iaccarino G (2009) The G protein coupled receptor kinase 2 plays an essential role in beta-adrenergic receptor-induced insulin resistance. Cardiovasc Res 84(3):407–415. doi:10.1093/cvr/cvp252

71. Anis Y, Leshem O, Reuveni H, Wexler I, Ben Sasson R, Yahalom B, Laster M, Raz I, Ben Sasson S, Shafrir E, Ziv E (2004) Antidiabetic effect of novel modulating peptides of G-protein-coupled kinase in experimental models of diabetes. Diabetologia 47(7):1232–1244. doi:10.1007/s00125-004-1444-1

72. Vila-Bedmar R, Cruces-Sande M, Lucas E, Willemen HLD, Heijnen CJ, Kavelaars A, Mayor F, Jr., Murga C (2015) Reversal of diet-induced obesity and insulin resistance by inducible genetic ablation of GRK2. Sci Signal 8 (386): (in press)

73. Owens DR, Monnier L, Bolli GB (2013) Differential effects of GLP-1 receptor agonists on components of dysglycaemia in individuals with type 2 diabetes mellitus. Diabetes Metabol 39(6):485–496. doi:10.1016/j. diabet.2013.09.004

74. Jorgensen R, Norklit Roed S, Heding A, Elling CE (2011) Beta-arrestin2 as a competitor for GRK2 interaction with the GLP-1 receptor upon receptor activation. Pharmacology 88(3-4):174–181. doi:10.1159/000330742

75. Offermanns S (2014) Free fatty acid (FFA) and hydroxy carboxylic acid (HCA) receptors. Annu Rev Pharmacol Toxicol 54:407–434. doi:10.1146/annurev-pharmtox-011613-135945

76. Tonack S, Tang C, Offermanns S (2013) Endogenous metabolites as ligands for G protein-coupled receptors modulating risk factors for metabolic and cardiovascular disease. Am J Physiol Heart Circ Physiol 304(4):H501–H513. doi:10.1152/ajpheart.00641.2012

77. Oh DY, Talukdar S, Bae EJ, Imamura T, Morinaga H, Fan W, Li P, Lu WJ, Watkins SM, Olefsky JM (2010) GPR120 is an omega-3 fatty acid receptor mediating potent anti-inflammatory and insulin-sensitizing effects. Cell 142(5):687–698. doi:10.1016/j. cell.2010.07.041

78. Burns RN, Singh M, Senatorov IS, Moniri NH (2014) Mechanisms of homologous and heterologous phosphorylation of FFA receptor 4 (GPR120): GRK6 and PKC mediate phosphorylation of Thr(3)(4)(7), Ser(3)(5)(0), and Ser(3)(5)(7) in the C-terminal tail. Biochem Pharmacol 87(4):650–659. doi:10.1016/j.bcp.2013.12.016

79. Burant CF (2013) Activation of GPR40 as a therapeutic target for the treatment of type 2 diabetes. Diabetes Care 36(Suppl 2):S175–S179. doi:10.2337/dcS13-2037

80. Usui I, Imamura T, Babendure JL, Satoh H, Lu JC, Hupfeld CJ, Olefsky JM (2005) G protein-coupled receptor kinase 2 mediates endothelin-1-induced insulin resistance via the inhibition of both Galphaq/11 and insulin receptor substrate-1 pathways in 3T3-L1 adipocytes. Mol Endocrinol 19(11):2760–2768. doi:10.1210/me.2004-0429

81. Shahid G, Hussain T (2007) GRK2 negatively regulates glycogen synthesis in mouse liver FL83B cells. J Biol Chem 282(28):20612–20620. doi:10.1074/jbc.M700744200

82. Ciccarelli M, Chuprun JK, Rengo G, Gao E, Wei Z, Peroutka RJ, Gold JI, Gumpert A, Chen M, Otis NJ, Dorn GW 2nd, Trimarco B, Iaccarino G, Koch WJ (2011) G protein-coupled receptor kinase 2 activity impairs cardiac glucose uptake and promotes insulin resistance after myocardial ischemia. Circulation 123(18):1953–1962. doi:10.1161/CIRCULATIONAHA.110.988642

83. Fusco A, Santulli G, Sorriento D, Cipolletta E, Garbi C, Dorn GW 2nd, Trimarco B, Feliciello A, Iaccarino G (2012) Mitochondrial localization unveils a novel role for GRK2 in organelle biogenesis. Cell Signal 24(2):468–475. doi:10.1016/j.cellsig.2011.09.026

84. Huang ZM, Gao E, Chuprun JK, Koch WJ (2014) GRK2 in the heart: a GPCR kinase and beyond. Antioxid Redox Signal 21(14):2032–2043. doi:10.1089/ars.2014.5876

85. Galgani JE, Moro C, Ravussin E (2008) Metabolic flexibility and insulin resistance. Am J Physiol Endocrinol Metab 295(5):E1009–E1017. doi:10.1152/ajpendo.90558.2008

86. Charbonneau A, Unson CG, Lavoie JM (2007) High-fat diet-induced hepatic steatosis reduces glucagon receptor content in rat hepatocytes: potential interaction with acute exercise. J Physiol 579(Pt 1):255–267. doi:10.1113/jphysiol.2006.121954

87. DeFronzo RA, Tripathy D (2009) Skeletal muscle insulin resistance is the primary defect in type 2 diabetes. Diabetes Care 32(Suppl 2):S157–S163. doi:10.2337/dc09-S302

88. Garcia-Guerra L, Vila-Bedmar R, Carrasco-Rando M, Cruces-Sande M, Martin M, Ruiz-Gomez A, Ruiz-Gomez M, Lorenzo M, Fernandez-Veledo S, Mayor F Jr, Murga C, Nieto-Vazquez I (2014) Skeletal muscle myogenesis is regulated by G protein-coupled receptor kinase 2. J Mol Cell Biol 6(4):299–311. doi:10.1093/jmcb/mju025

89. Penela P, Murga C, Ribas C, Tutor AS, Peregrin S, Mayor F Jr (2006) Mechanisms of regulation of G protein-coupled receptor kinases (GRKs) and cardiovascular disease. Cardiovasc Res 69(1):46–56. doi:10.1016/j.cardiores.2005.09.011

90. Sato PY, Chuprun JK, Schwartz M, Koch WJ (2015) The evolving impact of g protein-coupled receptor kinases in cardiac health and disease. Physiol Rev 95(2):377–404. doi:10.1152/physrev.00015.2014

91. Avendano MS, Lucas E, Jurado-Pueyo M, Martinez-Revelles S, Vila-Bedmar R, Mayor F Jr, Salaices M, Briones AM, Murga C (2014) Increased nitric oxide bioavailability in adult GRK2 hemizygous mice protects against angiotensin II-induced hypertension.

Hypertension 63(2):369–375. doi:10.1161/ HYPERTENSIONAHA.113.01991

92. Taguchi K, Kobayashi T, Matsumoto T, Kamata K (2011) Dysfunction of endothelium-dependent relaxation to insulin via PKC-mediated GRK2/Akt activation in aortas of ob/ob mice. Am J Physiol Heart Circ Physiol 301(2):H571–H583. doi:10.1152/ajpheart.01189.2010, ajpheart.01189.2010 [pii]

93. Taguchi K, Kobayashi T, Takenouchi Y, Matsumoto T, Kamata K (2011) Angiotensin II causes endothelial dysfunction via the GRK2/Akt/eNOS pathway in aortas from a murine type 2 diabetic model. Pharmacol Res 64(5):535–546. doi:10.1016/j. phrs.2011.05.001

94. Taguchi K, Matsumoto T, Kamata K, Kobayashi T (2012) G protein-coupled receptor kinase 2, with beta-arrestin 2, impairs insulin-induced Akt/endothelial nitric oxide synthase signaling in ob/ob mouse aorta. Diabetes 61(8):1978–1985. doi:10.2337/ db11-1729

95. Taguchi K, Matsumoto T, Kamata K, Kobayashi T (2012) Inhibitor of G protein-coupled receptor kinase 2 normalizes vascular endothelial function in type 2 diabetic mice by improving beta-arrestin 2 translocation and ameliorating Akt/eNOS signal dysfunction. Endocrinology 153(7):2985–2996. doi:10.1210/en.2012-1101

96. Taguchi K, Sakata K, Ohashi W, Imaizumi T, Imamura J, Hattori Y (2014) Tonic inhibition by G protein-coupled receptor kinase 2 of Akt/endothelial nitric oxide synthase signaling in human vascular endothelial cells under conditions of hyperglycemia with high insulin levels. J Pharmacol Exp Ther 349(2): 199–208. doi:jpet.113.211854 [pii]

97. Luan B, Zhao J, Wu H, Duan B, Shu G, Wang X, Li D, Jia W, Kang J, Pei G (2009) Deficiency of a beta-arrestin-2 signal complex contributes to insulin resistance. Nature 457(7233):1146–1149. doi:10.1038/ nature07617

98. Taguchi K, Matsumoto T, Kamata K, Kobayashi T (2013) Suppressed G-protein-coupled receptor kinase 2 activity protects female diabetic-mouse aorta against endothelial dysfunction. Acta Physiol (Oxford) 207(1):142–155. doi:10.1111/j.1748-1716. 2012.02473.x

99. Philipp M, Berger IM, Just S, Caron MG (2014) Overlapping and opposing functions of G protein-coupled receptor kinase 2 (GRK2) and GRK5 during heart development. J Biol Chem 289(38):26119–26130. doi:10.1074/jbc.M114.551952

100. Matkovich SJ, Diwan A, Klanke JL, Hammer DJ, Marreez Y, Odley AM, Brunskill EW, Koch WJ, Schwartz RJ, Dorn GW 2nd (2006) Cardiac-specific ablation of G-protein receptor kinase 2 redefines its roles in heart development and beta-adrenergic signaling. Circ Res 99(9):996–1003. doi:10.1161/01. RES.0000247932.71270.2c

101. Raake PW, Vinge LE, Gao E, Boucher M, Rengo G, Chen X, DeGeorge BR Jr, Matkovich S, Houser SR, Most P, Eckhart AD, Dorn GW 2nd, Koch WJ (2008) G protein-coupled receptor kinase 2 ablation in cardiac myocytes before or after myocardial infarction prevents heart failure. Circ Res 103(4):413–422. doi:10.1161/ CIRCRESAHA.107.168336

102. Koch WJ, Rockman HA, Samama P, Hamilton RA, Bond RA, Milano CA, Lefkowitz RJ (1995) Cardiac function in mice overexpressing the beta-adrenergic receptor kinase or a beta ARK inhibitor. Science 268(5215):1350–1353

103. Tachibana H, Naga Prasad SV, Lefkowitz RJ, Koch WJ, Rockman HA (2005) Level of beta-adrenergic receptor kinase 1 inhibition determines degree of cardiac dysfunction after chronic pressure overload-induced heart failure. Circulation 111(5):591–597. doi:10.1161/01.CIR.0000142291.70954.DF

104. Brinks H, Boucher M, Gao E, Chuprun JK, Pesant S, Raake PW, Huang ZM, Wang X, Qiu G, Gumpert A, Harris DM, Eckhart AD, Most P, Koch WJ (2010) Level of G protein-coupled receptor kinase-2 determines myocardial ischemia/reperfusion injury via pro- and anti-apoptotic mechanisms. Circ Res 107(9):1140–1149. doi:10.1161/ CIRCRESAHA.110.221010

105. Rockman HA, Chien KR, Choi DJ, Iaccarino G, Hunter JJ, Ross J Jr, Lefkowitz RJ, Koch WJ (1998) Expression of a beta-adrenergic receptor kinase 1 inhibitor prevents the development of myocardial failure in gene-targeted mice. Proc Natl Acad Sci U S A 95(12): 7000–7005

106. Harding VB, Jones LR, Lefkowitz RJ, Koch WJ, Rockman HA (2001) Cardiac beta ARK1 inhibition prolongs survival and augments beta blocker therapy in a mouse model of severe heart failure. Proc Natl Acad Sci U S A 98(10):5809–5814. doi:10.1073/pnas.091102398

107. Schumacher SM, Gao E, Zhu W, Chen X, Chuprun JK, Feldman AM, Tesmer JJ, Koch WJ (2015) Paroxetine-mediated GRK2 inhibition reverses cardiac dysfunction and remodeling after myocardial infarction. Sci Transl Med 7(277):277ra231. doi:10.1126/ scitranslmed.aaa0154

108. Rockman HA, Choi DJ, Rahman NU, Akhter SA, Lefkowitz RJ, Koch WJ (1996) Receptor-specific in vivo desensitization by the G protein-coupled receptor kinase-5 in transgenic mice. Proc Natl Acad Sci U S A 93(18):9954–9959

109. Rockman HA, Choi DJ, Akhter SA, Jaber M, Giros B, Lefkowitz RJ, Caron MG, Koch WJ (1998) Control of myocardial contractile function by the level of beta-adrenergic receptor kinase 1 in gene-targeted mice. J Biol Chem 273(29):18180–18184

110. Lucas E, Jurado-Pueyo M, Fortuno MA, Fernandez-Veledo S, Vila-Bedmar R, Jimenez-Borreguero LJ, Lazcano JJ, Gao E, Gomez-Ambrosi J, Fruhbeck G, Koch WJ, Diez J, Mayor F Jr, Murga C (2014) Downregulation of G protein-coupled receptor kinase 2 levels enhances cardiac insulin sensitivity and switches on cardioprotective gene expression patterns. Biochim Biophys Acta 1842:2448–2456. doi:10.1016/j.bbadis.2014.09.004

111. Fu Q, Xu B, Liu Y, Parikh D, Li J, Li Y, Zhang Y, Riehle C, Zhu Y, Rawlings T, Shi Q, Clark RB, Chen X, Abel ED, Xiang YK (2014) Insulin inhibits cardiac contractility by inducing a Gi-biased beta2 adrenergic signaling in hearts. Diabetes. doi:10.2337/db13-1763

112. Lymperopoulos A, Rengo G, Koch WJ (2007) Adrenal adrenoceptors in heart failure: fine-tuning cardiac stimulation. Trends Mol Med 13(12):503–511. doi:10.1016/j.molmed.2007.10.005

113. Wang Y, Gao E, Lau WB, Wang Y, Liu G, Li JJ, Wang X, Yuan Y, Koch WJ, Ma XL (2015) G-protein-coupled receptor kinase 2-mediated desensitization of adiponectin receptor 1 in failing heart. Circulation 131(16):1392–1404. doi:10.1161/CIRCULATIONAHA.114.015248

114. MacDonnell SM, Kubo H, Crabbe DL, Renna BF, Reger PO, Mohara J, Smithwick LA, Koch WJ, Houser SR, Libonati JR (2005) Improved myocardial beta-adrenergic responsiveness and signaling with exercise training in hypertension. Circulation 111(25):3420–3428. doi:10.1161/CIRCULATIONAHA.104.505784

115. Hata JA, Williams ML, Schroder JN, Lima B, Keys JR, Blaxall BC, Petrofski JA, Jakoi A, Milano CA, Koch WJ (2006) Lymphocyte levels of GRK2 (betaARK1) mirror changes in the LVAD-supported failing human heart: lower GRK2 associated with improved beta-adrenergic signaling after mechanical unloading. J Card Fail 12(5):360–368. doi:10.1016/j.cardfail.2006.02.011

116. Rengo G, Pagano G, Paolillo S, de Lucia C, Femminella GD, Liccardo D, Cannavo A, Formisano R, Petraglia L, Komici K, Rengo F, Trimarco B, Ferrara N, Leosco D, Perrone-Filardi P (2015) Impact of diabetes mellitus on lymphocyte GRK2 protein levels in patients with heart failure. Eur J Clin Investig 45(2):187–195. doi:10.1111/eci.12395

117. Lucas E, Jurado-Pueyo M, Vila-Bedmar R, Díez J, Mayor F Jr, Murga C (2015) Linking cardiac insulin resistance and heart failure: GRK2 as an integrative node. Cardiovasc Regen Med 2:e586. doi:10.14800/crm.586

Chapter 7

Differential Regulation of IGF-1 and Insulin Signaling by GRKs

Leonard Girnita, Ada Girnita, and Caitrin Crudden

Abstract

Textbooks depict box-to-box signaling schematics downstream of G-protein-coupled receptors (GPCRs) and receptor tyrosine kinases (RTKs), yet it is now widely accepted that cellular signaling is much more web-like than linear, and the nodes of crosstalk between pathways and receptors increase in complexity and intricacy with each additional study. A complex network involving bidirectional crosstalk between GPCRs and RTKs is emerging, and this phenomenon is commonly termed "transactivation." In this process, RTKs or components of RTK pathways are utilized by GPCRs or, conversely, components of classical GPCRs such as G proteins, GRKs, and β-arrestins are recruited downstream of activated RTKs. This chapter aims to summarize the emerging evidence of RTKs utilizing GPCR components, thus blurring the boundaries we have given them. In particular, we will follow how all of the functional components of the GPCR system have been described for the insulin receptor (IR) and the insulin-like growth factor type 1 receptor (IGF-1R) and hence the rationale behind the development of a functional RTK/GPCR hybrid model. Given the IGF-1R's important role in the development and maintenance of a malignant phenotype, GPCR components, such as the GRK/β-arrestin system, may yield important future targets in anti-IGF-1R therapeutics.

Key words Receptor tyrosine kinase, RTK, Insulin-like growth factor type 1 receptor, IGF-1R, Insulin receptor, IR, Cancer, GRK, Beta-arrestin

---

1 Introduction

Shakespeare's famous line *"That which we call a rose, by any other name, would smell as sweet,"* aimed to remind us that it does not matter what names or categories we choose to give to things, it does not change what they truly are or how things truly exist. In that respect, the naming of RTKs solely on their tyrosine kinase activity masks the fact that they can also work completely independent of their kinase domain and outside of the "group" characteristics we have given them. Indeed, it is now clear that RTKs can utilize all components of the GPCR machinery, giving rise to new perspectives on functional classifications. In this chapter, we describe

Vsevolod V. Gurevich et al. (eds.), *G Protein-Coupled Receptor Kinases*, Methods in Pharmacology and Toxicology, DOI 10.1007/978-1-4939-3798-1_7, © Springer Science+Business Media New York 2016

152 Leonard Girnita et al.

the IR/IGF-1R signaling from the GPCR-paradigm perspective, focusing specifically on the roles played in this process by GRKs and β-arrestins.

1.1 RTK Classical Paradigm

Second to the GPCRs, the RTKs represent another major cell surface receptor family, containing around 60 members, subdivided into at least 13 families [1, 2]. RTKs are structurally defined by the presence of a tyrosine kinase domain. In most cases this is joined to the extracellular ligand binding domain via a single transmembrane anchor [3]. RTKs are traditionally defined by their ligands and hence the ligand binding domains vary between receptors to encode specificity. In addition, there are also significant differences in terms of cytoplasmic kinase regions, juxtamembrane domain and carboxyl (C)-terminal tail among members of the same family and these differences are often even more important between different RTK classes.

The canonical signaling activation model describes the majority of RTKs as an "OFF/ON" system. The "switch-ON" mechanism is a two-step process: binding of their respective ligand induces the formation of receptor dimers which initiate conformational changes within intracellular domains, and secondly, trans-autophosphorylation of tyrosine residues within the kinase domain stabilizes this "ON" state [4, 5]. Dimerization can take place between two identical receptors (homodimerization), between different members of the same receptor family (heterodimerization), or in some cases, between a receptor and an accessory protein [6, 7]. Autophosphorylation of adjacent receptors results in an exponential increase in kinase activity and subsequent activation of intracellular signaling pathways [8]. The main two signaling cascades emanating from RTKs are MAPK/ERK and PI3K/Akt, which culminate in biological effects on cell survival, cell cycle progression, proliferation, and metabolism [9].

Over the last few decades, RTKs have received particular attention, not only as essential regulators of normal cellular processes but also as key factors involved in the development and progression of human cancers. In 1983, two groups published their observations of sequence homology between an oncogene and an RTK, namely the simian sarcoma virus oncogene *v-sis* and the platelet-derived growth factor (PDGF) [10, 11]. A year later came the first description of a mutated RTK in cancer [12], and the list of growth factors, RTKs, or molecules within their signaling cascade which contribute to transformation and malignancy began to grow. Clinical data supported the fact that RTKs were intimately linked to tumorigenesis through various mechanisms: gene amplification, overexpression, mutation, or autocrine growth factor loops [13]. As such, RTK therapeutic exploration has been a large research focus, and many strategies targeting RTKs have been developed and successfully translated into clinic, e.g. trastuzumab (Herceptin), an anti-HER2 antibody used in the treatment of breast cancers [14], PDGFR inhibitors for gastrointestinal cancers [15], and c-KIT targeting in cancers containing these oncogenic mutations [16].

1.2 IGF-1R and IR

Among RTKs, the IGF system of ligands, receptors, and binding proteins is undoubtedly a major player in normal cellular growth and differentiation, as well as in aberrant growth or metabolic dysregulation such as in cancer or diabetes. The IGF system is organized on three distinct levels: (1) the input layer of ligands, receptors, and regulatory proteins of ligand–receptor interaction; (2) the second layer, transmission, is orchestrated by adaptors and enzymes of the signaling cascades, directing the information toward the (3) output layer of effectors through transcription factors, ultimately controlling the biological responses (Fig. 1). The input layer is represented by three ligands: insulin, IGF-1, and IGF-2, and although some cross activation can occur at supraphysiological concentrations [17], the receptors bind to their respective ligands with by far the greatest affinity. IGF ligand availability is controlled by insulin-like growth factor binding proteins (IGFBPs) of which at least 7 are described [18]. The cell membrane receptor members are the IR, the IGF-1R, and the IGF-2R. Both the IR and the IGF-1R consist of two α and two β subunits linked together by disulfide bonds. Overall there is high sequence homology (≈70%) between the IGF-1R and the IR [19], each domain to different degrees: TK domain ≈84%, juxtamembrane domain ≈61%, C-terminal domain ≈44% [9]. Recent work has extended the family with additional members, including the antimicrobial peptide LL-37 [20], the orphan insulin-related receptor (IRR) [21], and the insulin-IGF-1R hybrid receptor [22].

Whilst two-step ligand-induced dimerization and kinase activation is the RTK rule, the IR and the IGF-1R are the major exceptions. The IGF-1R and the IR both exist within the cell membrane as preformed dimers. Much like GPCRs, these receptors are already expressed as fully assembled functional units, and ligand binding triggers the second step only: conformational changes within the receptor that trans-activates the kinases located on the β-subunits. In an unphosphorylated state, the kinase activity is kept very low by the inhibitory conformation of an activation loop (A-loop) within the kinase region that interferes with ATP-binding [23]. Once agonist activated, receptor-kinase-dependent autophosphorylation of tyrosine residues within this A-loop; 1131, 1135, and 1136 in the IGF-1R and 1161, 1165, and 1166 in the IR, exponentially increase the receptor kinase efficiency. This activation in turn phosphorylates other residues within the β subunit that creates docking sites for the signal transduction molecules of the second layer, including insulin receptor substrates (IRSs) and the src homology 2 (SH2)-domain containing transforming protein 1 (Shc) [9]. These molecules set up the transmission of two main

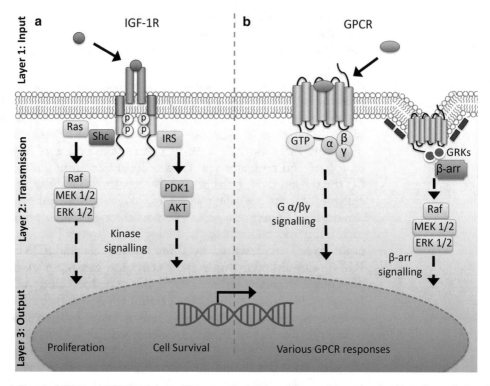

Fig. 1 Classical RTK and GPCR pathways. The canonical IGF system can be categorized into three distinct layers. The input layer (1) is made up of ligands (insulin, IGF-1, IGF-2), IGFBPs, and surface receptors. Upon stimulation, entry into layer (2) (the signaling cascade) is initiated by two main adaptor proteins: Shc and the IRSs (1–4). Through stepwise enzymatic activation the signal cascade is set up, following two main routes: the mitogen-activated protein kinase (MAPK) route and the phosphoinositide 3-kinase (PI3K) route. The signaling cascade arms culminate in the activation of transcription factors in layer (3), which control site-specific transcription and generate the resulting biological effects. (**a**, **b**) GPCR functional classification is based on: (1) ligand-induced receptor activation leading to the activation of heterotrimeric G proteins. (2) Subsequent GRK-dependent phosphorylation of C-terminal serine and/or threonine residues allowing β-arrestin binding to these specific phosphorylated residues with (3) β-arrestin recruitment. (4) Subsequent signaling desensitization, (5) activation of a β-arrestin-dependent second signaling wave, and (6) receptor endocytosis with the β-arrestin/GRK isoform determining receptor degradation or recycling

signaling cascades: RAS/RAF/ERK and PI3K/Akt. The IRS family consists of 4 proteins, and IRS1 and IRS2 are well known to play important roles in IGF's metabolic effects. IRS binding reaches maximum 1–2 min after phosphorylation of the tyrosine residues. The C-terminal domain of IRS contains multiple phosphorylation sites, which bind with high affinity to SH2 domain-containing proteins, guided by the specific phosphorylation tyrosine motif [9]. IRS interaction with a p85 subunit of PI3K leads to its activation and induces phospholipid activation of the downstream signaling pathway. The second major pathway begins with the binding of Shc, reaching maximal phosphorylation 5–10 min after IGF-1 stimulation. Shc family consists of four members (A, B, C, and D), which contain a PTB domain and an SH2 domain at the N-terminal and C-terminal regions respectively. Either Shc or IRS can mediate the activation of the MAPK cascade via Grb2 interaction. Grb2 acts as an adaptor protein, bringing son of sevenless (sos), a guanine nucleotide exchange protein that promotes the release of GDP and binding of GTP to the membrane bound Ras protein. Ras then sets up a phosphorylation cascade through Raf and the MAPKs pathway. Both signals culminate in nuclear translocation of transcription factors such as STAT3, CREB, and ElK1 orchestrating the output later through various biological activities such as cell growth, proliferation, survival, and metabolism (Fig. 1).

Despite their similarities in structure and signaling, the IGF-1R and the IR have distinct biological roles. The IR is a key regulator of metabolic processes such as glucose transport and biosysnthesis of fat and glycogen, whereas the IGF-1R functions primarily in cell growth, proliferation, and differentiation. Mice with the IGF-1R gene knocked out (−/−) die at birth of respiratory failure and display a generalized growth deficiency (≈50% of normal size) [24]. Mice lacking IR are born almost phenotypically normal (≈10% growth retardation), but develop early postnatal diabetes and die from ketoacidosis [25]. Interestingly, combined abolition of both IGF-1R and IR results in a more severe growth phenotype (≈30% normal size) highlighting the redundancy of the two systems [26].

In addition to its physiological role in normal cell growth, the IGF-1R turned out to be an important player in cancer development. The fundamental evidence for this was the demonstration that IGF-1R knock-out mouse embryonic cells are refractory to transformation by several oncogenes, viruses, or overexpression of other RTKs [27]. Cells from wild-type littermates, as well as these knockout cells (R-) with the IGF-1R reinserted were readily transformed. Subsequently, IGF-1R has been demonstrated to regulate multiple cellular functions that are intrinsically essential for the malignant phenotype, e.g. proliferation, survival, anchorage-independent growth, tumor neovascularization, migration, and invasion [28, 29].

Accumulating new data suggest that insulin also plays a key role in tumorigenesis, both in the fact that it can act in a redundant manner when the IGF-1R is inhibited, and in the formation of hybrid receptors. In a transgenic mouse model of pancreatic β-cell neuroendocrine tumor, upregulating IGF-1R accelerates tumorigenesis, however, antibody inhibition of IGF-1R alone had only modest effects on tumor growth. Notably, only combined IGF-1R and IR blockage significantly hindered tumor growth [30]. In addition to their structural similarity, it has been shown in multiple studies that the IGF-1R and the IR can heterodimerize to form IGF-1R/IR hybrid receptors [22, 31, 32]. The role of hybrid receptors is not clear, but some studies suggest that they may be expressed by cancer cells to make use of additional ligands for signaling activation [33]. There are studies that show that one of the two IR isoforms (IR-A) is especially overexpressed in cancer. IR-A is the fetal isoform and importantly can bind IGF-2 as well as insulin [34]. Epidemiology also supports their interaction, as several types of cancer (including liver, breast, colorectal, urinary tract, and female reproductive organs) are increased in diabetic patients, both in terms of incidence and mortality [35].

Lending support to the cell transformation studies, a wide range of experimental data clearly demonstrate that inhibition of IGF-1R would be beneficial for cancer treatment [36–39]. In vivo and in vitro studies targeting IGF-1R, including antibodies, small molecule inhibitors, and antisense technology, have shown that IGF-1R is functionally essential for tumor cell growth and proliferation [40, 41]. However, unlike other RTKs, no clear mechanism of aberrant IGF-1R can be recognized: IGF-1 or IGF-1R overexpression is not a general rule [42], nor does the receptor show intrinsic abnormalities [43]. Altogether, this suggests that other regulatory pathways and as yet unappreciated changes are likely to be involved. One recently recognized characteristic is the GPCR-like capabilities of the IR and the IGF-1R.

2   IR/IGF-1R Utilize GPCR Components

2.1   G-Protein Signaling Activation

The term G-protein-coupled receptor was selected to highlight the main functional characteristic of the cell surface receptors that couple to and activate heterotrimeric G protein signaling and this term was used mainly for the seven-transmembrane receptors (7TMRs). Yet, the 7TMRs are not the only receptor family initiating G protein signaling and a major advancement in RTK biology is their recognition as activators of G-protein-mediated signaling [9, 44]. At least two mechanisms were described for the G-protein signaling activation downstream of RTKs: direct recruitment and activation of heterotrimeric G protein or transactivation of a 7TMR by an RTK or its ligands [45]. In the case of the IR family, over two decades ago, Luttrell et al. reported that IR was sensitive to pertussis toxin [46], a toxin that uncouples the G protein subunit $G\alpha i$ from an activated receptor. IR subjected to pertussis toxin showed decreased insulin-induced inhibition of adenylyl cyclase in isolated hepatocytes [47], which lead to altered insulin-mediated biological outcomes [48]. In addition, Imamura et al. found that insulin stimulation lead to tyrosine phosphorylation of $G\alpha_{q/11}$ and antibodies against this form inhibited insulin-stimulated translocation of the GLUT4 glucose transporter. Overexpression of a constitutively active form of $G\alpha_{q/11}$, in the absence of insulin, stimulated glucose uptake and GLUT4 translocation to 70% of an insulin-stimulated effect [49]. Given their high degree of similarity, it may be not surprising that the pertussis toxin sensitivity was also described to occur at the IGF-1R. Lefkowitz's laboratory reported that IGF-1R activation of the MAPK pathway was sensitive to both pertussis toxin and sequestration of the G protein βγ subunits [50]. In rat fibroblasts, stimulation of MAPK via the IGF-1R was also demonstrated to be sensitive to cellular expression of a specific Gβγ-binding peptide [50]. This study clearly demonstrated that in addition to kinase signaling, the IGF-1R employs a GPCR-like mechanism for activation of mitogenic signaling. Strengthening this finding, subsequent studies went on to demonstrate the association of Gαi and Gβ with the IGF-1R in rat neuronal cells and mouse fibroblasts [51, 52]. Importantly, Gαi inhibition (pertussis toxin) or Gβγ sequestration selectively inhibited IGF-1-induced proliferation with no effect on EGFR or insulin action [52].

The IGF-1R and the IR are not the only RTKs employing G proteins for downstream signaling activation. In an excellent review, Waters et al. [53] described the state of results by which many RTKs, such as PDGFR, EGFR, and VEGFR, can use proximal heterotrimeric G proteins to exert their biological activities. In addition, signaling downstream of several RTKs (e.g. TRK A, the receptor for the neuronal growth factor neurotrophin (NGF)), is pertussis toxin-sensitive, suggesting the involvement of G proteins [53, 54]. The authors postulate the existence of what they term "RTK-GPCR signaling platforms" which come about due to close receptor proximity and allow sharing of signaling components [55]. Most, if not all, RTKs either directly associate with the heterotrimeric G proteins or "hijack" them from neighboring GPCRs (Table 1). Yet, in addition to G-protein signaling activation, as a distinctive functional hallmark, GPCRs employ the GRK/arrestin system to control the intensity and duration of the signals as well as receptor trafficking. Thus, a key question arises in how the IR/IGF-1R and other RTKs fit within this paradigm?

2.2 IGF-1R/IR Engage the β-Arrestin/GRK System

2.2.1 β-Arrestin and IGF-1R Trafficking

The IGF-1R is probably the first acknowledged case of an RTK engaging β-arrestins [56]. Following the discovery of Gβγ-mediated MAPK activation by a ligand-occupied IGF-1R [50], it has been recognized that both β-arrestin isoforms are recruited by the IGF-1R in a ligand-dependent manner [56]. In line with this, β-arrestins were found to orchestrate receptor endocytosis and a dominant negative β-arrestin1 mutant was shown to impair IGF-1R internalization [56]. Classically, IGF-1R internalization was known to be ubiquitin-dependent, through both clathrin and caveolin routes [57–60]. Following endocytosis, the receptor either follows a degradation or recycling route, and the balance between the two can be manipulated in different instances [60]. The mechanism was further elucidated by a distinct line of research investigating IGF-1R trafficking [42], identifying MDM2 as a ubiquitin ligase for the IGF-1R [60]. Subsequent studies revealed that both β-arrestins isoforms mediate MDM2/IGF-1R interaction as

Table 1
RTKs utilize GPCR components

	G-protein activation	GRK recruitment	β-Arrestin recruitment/signaling	β-Arrestin-mediated receptor degradation
IGF-1R	Sensitive to G-protein toxin [50] Ligand-dependent phosphorylation of G-protein subunit [51]	GRK2 and GRK6 phosphorylation (also possibly GRK3 and GRK5) [66]	β-Arrestin binding [52] IGF-1R MAPK signaling through β-arrestin [63]	Ubiquitination and downregulation of IGF-1R dependent on β-arrestin [61]
IR	Sensitive to G-protein toxin [46] Ligand-dependent phosphorylation of G-protein subunit [49]	GRK2 inhibits the G-protein signaling [81] (kinase independent)		
PDGFR	Sensitive to G-protein toxin [102]	GRK2 phosphorylates PDGF for desensitization [85]		PDGFβ-R internalization via GRK2/β-arrestin [83] possibly indirect through S1P (GPCR)
EGFR	Sensitivity to G-protein toxin [103] Ligand promotes G subunit associated with receptor [104]	GRK2 serine phosphorylation [85] (but does not desensitize)		
VEGFR	G-protein utilization for MAPK activation [105]			β-Arrestin2 controls VE-cadherin endocytosis after VEGF stimulation [106] (indirect)
TRK A	Sensitive to G-protein toxin—possibly indirect through GPCR LPA [54]	GRK2 promotes β-arrestin binding [54]	Overexpression of β-arrestin increased NGF-dependent ERK activation [83]	
FGFR	FGF-2 migration sensitive to G-protein toxin [107], proliferation not [108]			

Summary of receptor tyrosine kinase members and the experimental evidence of their use of GPCR pathway components. RTKs stated are the insulin-like growth factor type 1 receptor (IGF-1R), insulin receptor (IR), platelet derived growth factor receptor (PDGFR), epidermal growth factor receptor (EGFR), vascular endothelial growth factor receptor (VEGFR), nerve growth factor receptor (TRK A), and fibroblast growth factor receptor (FGFR)

MDM2 and β-arrestins co-immunoprecipitated with the IGF-1R. Both in vitro and in vivo, β-arrestins enhanced MDM2-mediated ligand-dependent IGF-1R ubiquitination [61] and degradation, yet the β-arrestin isoform 1 appeared to be more strongly associated with receptor downregulation than isoform 2. Altogether, β-arrestin 1 was demonstrated to act as an essential component in the ubiquitination and endocytosis of the IGF-1R [61].

2.2.2 β-Arrestin and IGF-1R Signaling

Whilst initially categorized as GPCR's desensitization route, β-arrestin is now understood to be a multi-task protein. Integral to retaining receptor sensitivity, β-arrestin uncouples G proteins from an activated receptor and internalizes the receptor via clathrin-mediated endocytosis, for degradation or recycling. In addition, β-arrestin activates a second wave of signaling, independent of G proteins by acting as a scaffold to the MAPK components [62]. At least three lines of evidence indicate that the IGF-1R/β-arrestin interaction follows this model. Firstly, IGF-1R's mitogenic signaling is sensitive to β-arrestin1 inhibition, demonstrated through microinjection of a β-arrestin1-specific antibody [52]. Secondly, it was shown that IGF-1R stimulation leads to the ubiquitination of β-arrestin1, which regulates vesicular trafficking and activation of ERK1/2. This β-arrestin1-dependent ERK activity occurred even when the classical tyrosine kinase signaling was impaired. Through siRNA suppression of β-arrestin1, this ERK signaling was shown to contribute to cell cycle progression, and thus is an integral part of IGF-1R's mitogenic signaling [63]. The corollary of these studies is that in addition to kinase-mediated signaling, the IGF-1R activates MAPK through G proteins and β-arrestin1 (Fig. 2). Yet, a key question to be answered is whether the latter are mutually exclusive thus supporting the desensitizing paradigm. For an RTK, due to the intrinsic kinase activity, separating different branches of MAPK activation is more complicated than for a prototypical GPCR. Nevertheless, the third line of evidence supports a β-arrestin-desenzitization model for the IGF-1R. Experimental models promoting a IGF-1R/β-arrestin association, without kinase activation, revealed the tendency for unbalanced IGF-1-induced MAPK signaling with a decreased early (G-protein) and enhanced late (β-arrestin) component, supporting a desensitizing role for the β-arrestin [63–65]. Moreover, identification of the GRKs, as mediators of β-arrestin recruitment to an activated IGF-1R, further supports a GPCR-like mechanism (see below and [9, 44, 66]).

There are different ways by which β-arrestin mediates signaling downstream of the IGF-1R. Signaling mediation can be through β-arrestin's control of IGF-1R endocytosis. It has been shown that IGF-1-mediated Shc phosophorylation and p42/44 activation rely on endocytosis of the IGF-1R [56], as demonstrated by using low temperature and dansylcadaverine (chemical inhibitor of endocytosis) [67]. In addition, β-arrestin regulates IGF-1R

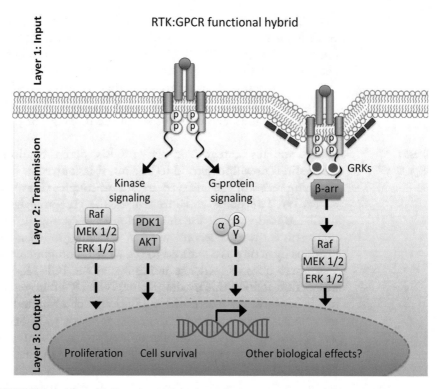

Fig. 2 RTK/GPCR hybrid model. Experimental evidence has shown that in addition to the prototypical kinase signaling, the IGF-1R (in a ligand-dependent fashion) (1) leads to the activation of heterotrimeric G proteins, (2) subsequent GRK-dependent phosphorylation of C-terminal serine residues which leads to (3) β-arrestin recruitment, (4) subsequent signaling desensitization, (5) activation of a β-arrestin-dependent second signaling wave followed by (6) receptor degradation or recycling. Altogether it is concluded that by all functional definitions the IGF-1R can act as a GPCR

endocytosis by controlling its ubiquitination [61]. While not yet studied directly in the case of the IGF-1R, it is well documented in the GPCR field, as well as for IR (see below), that β-arrestin acts as a scaffold for the components of the MAPK pathway [68]. By acting as a physical scaffold β-arrestin can create functional signaling modules that control MAPK signal specificity [69, 70]. In the case of the IGF-1R, β-arrestin is also required for an anti-apoptotic response through Akt activation and this action is independent of G proteins and ERK activity [71].

2.2.3 β-Arrestin and IR Trafficking and Signaling

The IR, like most receptors, undergoes degradation upon persistent ligand stimulation. The IR shares 85 % sequence homology with the IGF-1R, yet their C-terminal (β-arrestin binding domain) tails are less conserved (44 %) explaining why the two receptors respond differently to β-arrestin perturbations [1]. The IR has been shown to bind β-arrestin1 in a ligand-dependent manner [52] with similar kinetics to IGF-1R, however, IR trafficking is not modified by β-arrestin alterations. Nevertheless, in the case of IR, β-arrestins recruitment has a major impact on IR biological activities by controlling the signaling pathways downstream of an activated receptor. Upon insulin stimulation, the major IR substrate (IRS-1) is ubiquitinated [72, 73] by the same E3 ligase as IGF-1R, MDM2. Usui et al. demonstrated that MDM2 associates with IRS-1 in a ligand-dependent manner and is targeting IRS-1 for proteasomal degradation. This process was demonstrated to be dependent on β-arrestin1, yet in the opposite way to IGF-1R. Overexpressing β-arrestin1 prevented insulin-induced IRS-1 ubiquitination, and β-arrestin1 downregulation enhanced IRS-1 degradation. One possible scenario is that IRS-1 and IGF-1R compete for the same ligase, while β-arrestin1 directs MDM2 toward either substrate. Another possibility is that IGF-1R and IR preferentially utilize different arrestin isoform and the competition is at this level. This scenario is supported by the studies investigating the effects of β-arrestin1-mediated signaling downstream of IR. β-arrestin1 inhibition, which impaired IGF-1 signaling, had no effect on insulin mediated metabolic (GLUT4 translocation, glucose uptake) or mitogenic effects (ERK phosphorylation, DNA synthesis, or ERK-mediated transcriptional activity) [52, 74]. On the other hand, a crucial role has been reported for β-arrestin2 in controlling IR metabolic effects [75]. Insulin resistance, a hallmark of type 2 diabetes, includes a defective IR that is less responsive to insulin stimulation. Diabetic mouse models show decreased expression of β-arrestin2. In addition, knockdown of β-arrestin2 exacerbates insulin resistance, whereas administration of β-arrestin2 restores insulin sensitivity by scaffolding Akt and Src to the IR [75]. Increasing the complexity of the system, competition between IGF-1R and IR for β-arrestins was demonstrated by heterologous desensitization of IGF-1R (and adrenergic receptor) following prolonged IR stimulation. Insulin treatment for 12 h reduced IGF-1R mitogenic signaling ability, by inducing ≈50% decrease in cellular β-arrestin levels [74]. In contrast to utilizing it for signaling activation, IR activation leads to β-arrestin ubiquitination and proteasome-mediated degradation, impairing both IGF-1R and GPCR signaling.

Through numerous studies, the IR's use of β-arrestin is being built. It is clear that although both the IR and the IGF-1R utilize β-arrestin, their exact mechanisms differ. At multiple points, use of the same substrate infers points of competition and crosstalk between the closely related receptors.

2.2.4 GRKs and IGF-1R/IR Signaling

In the case of the IGF-1R, β-arrestins play a dual regulatory role; receptor downregulation (with subsequent kinase and possible G-protein signaling attenuation), and a new wave of β-arrestin-dependent signaling activation. This model fully resembles the β-arrestin paradigm for the larger GPCR family; while internalizing the GPCR and ending G-protein signaling, β-arrestins activate the

MAPK pathway [62, 76, 77]. The next logical question is whether the mechanism of GRK-dependent serine phosphorylation to create β-arrestins binding sites [62, 78, 79] is conserved in the case of IGF-1R.

Investigating this scenario we uncovered that an activated IGF-1R allows recruitment of GRK proteins, specifically with balancing effects between GRK2 and GRK6 [66]. The GRK isoform employed, as well as phosphorylated serine residue, confer specificity for the β-arrestin action by controlling the duration and strength of its interaction with the IGF-1R [49]. GRK2 and GRK6 coimmunoprecipitate with the IGF-1R and increase IGF-1R serine phosphorylation, promoting β-arrestin1 association. By suppressing GRK expression with siRNA, we found that GRK5/6 inhibition mitigates IGF-1-mediated ERK and AKT activation, whereas GRK2 inhibition has opposing effects on ERK signaling. Conversely, β-arrestin-mediated ERK activation is enhanced by overexpression of GRK6 and diminished by GRK2. The same balancing effects of GRK2 and GRK6 were observed for IGF-1R downregulation: GRK2 decreases whereas GRK6 enhances ligand-induced degradation. Mutation analysis identified serine 1248 and 1291 as the major serine phosphorylation sites and potential β-arrestin binding sites of the IGF-1R. Targeted mutation of S1248 recapitulates GRK2 modulation, promoting a transient receptor/arrestin interaction whereas S1291 mutation resembles GRK6 effects and a stable IGF-1R/arrestin association with enhanced receptor degradation and signaling activation. The corollary of this study is that GRK2 or GRK5/6-dependent phosphorylation of IGF-1R C-terminal serine residues 1248 or 1291, respectively, allows β-arrestin1 recruitment, with the residue that is phosphorylated controlling the duration and strength of the β-arrestin/IGF-1R association.

2.2.5 GRKs and IR Signaling

Building on the findings that an activated IR can phosphorylate the heterotrimeric protein component Gαq/11 with downstream glucose transport stimulation [49, 80] and taking into consideration the GRK2 specificity for Gαq/11, Olefsky et al. investigated the G-protein signaling desensitization by GRK2. Confirming the working hypothesis, inhibition of GRK2 by antibody microinjection, dominant-negative GRK2 expression, or siRNA-mediated GRK2 knockdown enhanced 3T3-L1 adipocytes response to insulin stimulation in terms of GLUT4 translocation and activation of glucose transport [81]. Conversely, in the rescue experiments, overexpression of GRK2 inhibits insulin-stimulated glucose transport, validating GRK2 as an endogenous protein inhibitor of insulin signaling and glucose uptake [81]. Yet, the GRK2 desensitizing effects on Gαq/11 signaling downstream of IR is not completely equivalent to the GPCR paradigm as expression of a kinase-defective GRK2 mutant showed increased glucose uptake, suggesting a kinase-independent mechanism. As endogenous GRK2 co-precipitates with Gαq/11 in an insulin-dependent manner, further experiments demonstrated that the amino (N′)-termini of GRKs that contain an RGS-like domain are necessary for the inhibitory function of GRK2 on insulin-stimulated GLUT4 translocation.

2.2.6 GRK/β-Arrestin System and Other RTKs

Clearly, the GRK/β-arrestin system modulates signaling and biological activities downstream of the IGF-1R and IR. In addition, the activity of several other RTKs is also controlled by different GRK isoforms, either alone or in a β-arrestin-dependent manner (for extensive review see [1] and Table 1). EGFR and its cognate ligand EGF have been shown to recruit β-arrestin1 in a ligand-dependent manner [52] and a C-terminal β-arrestin1 fragment which cannot direct receptor endocytosis, impairs EGF-induced MAPK activation, suggesting β-arrestin1's signaling involvement. There are also other studies indicating that inhibition of β-arrestin1 had no effect on MAPK activation [12, 49]. However, ligand-activated EGFR led to translocation of GRK2 to the plasma membrane in a Gβγ subunit-dependent manner and increased p42/44 phosphorylation [1, 82].

Similarly, in the platelet-derived growth factor (PDGF) system, β-arrestin1 and GRK2 were associated with the receptor in a ligand-dependent manner [83], however this association depends upon the formation of a complex between the PDGFR and a GPCR, the endothelial differentiation gene 1 receptor (EDG-1R). PDGF binds to its receptor, the PDGFR trans-activates the EDG-1R, which causes β-arrestin1 translocation to the plasma membrane and subsequent complex internalization via clathrin-mediated endocytosis [84]. GRK2 recruitment to PDGFR was demonstrated to increase the phosphorylation of PDGFR serines and initiate a ligand-dependent inhibitory feedback on the receptor kinase activity and its downstream signaling [1]. Reciprocally, GRK2 was also shown to be activated following interaction with an activated PDGFR. In a similar manner to IGF-1R [66], ligand-induced ubiquitination of the PDGFR was enhanced in cells over-expressing GRK2 without increasing its downregulation [85]. More importantly, this study suggested that specificity of GRK2 for RTKs may be controlled by the ability to recruit and activate the G-protein signaling.

2.3 GRK's Role in Malignancy

Whilst recognizing RTK's essential role in initiating, maintaining, and promoting the malignant phenotype, and secondly, identifying GRK's role in routing downstream signaling, one must question what the GRK's roles are in cancer, and whether they may provide a suitable therapeutic target.

It is becoming increasingly clear that GRK's cellular role is by no means limited to promoting β-arrestin binding to activated

GPCRs. Instead, GRKs are multi-domain proteins with diverse cellular functions, and in particular, GRK2 is being recognized as a key node in signal transduction pathways [86] downstream of both GPCRs and RTKs. Emerging evidence points at GRK2 as an important cell cycle regulator. GRK2 knockout mice are embryonic lethal [87] and the mechanism goes beyond cardiac-specific abnormalities, as the complete GRK2 KO embryos display generalized growth retardation as well as some other developmental abnormalities as opposed to the viable and normal growth phenotype of the GRK2 cardiac-specific deletion [88]. The growth retardation of GRK2 KO embryos strongly suggests that the protein plays a role in basic cellular functions such as growth, proliferation, and differentiation [86]. Of note, zebrafish models using knockdown of the GRK2 ortholog that have shown a similar developmental growth arrest to murine models can be partially restored by expression of a kinase-inactive GRK2 mutant [89], reinforcing the important GRK2 roles on the growth phenotype, both kinase dependent and independent. In a HEK293T system, response to EGF relied on GRK2 to potentiate MAPK activation [90], as in normal osteoblasts; a dominant negative GRK2 mutant (K220R) reduced MAPK activation in response to IGF-1 and EGF, which translated into a blunted cellular proliferation [91].

There are a few studies investigating GRK expression and function in the context of cancer [92]. King et al. reported an increased expression of GRK2 protein in a malignant human ovarian granulosa tumor cell line as well as in patient-derived tissue samples. These tumor cells express significantly less GRK4 α/β protein and higher levels of GRK2 and GRK4 γ/δ protein as compared to nonmalignant human granulosa cells [93]. Likewise, increased GRK2 was observed in differentiated thyroid carcinoma (DTC), with a significant decrease in GRK5 expression [94]. Functional studies demonstrated that growth of prostate tumor xenografts were retarded in mice following GRK2 inhibition by GRK2ct [95]. GRK2 acts to inhibit TGF-mediated growth arrest and apoptosis in human hepatocarcinoma cells [96], however this action is likely to be cell type specific as GRK2 seems to reduce PDGF-induced proliferation of thyroid cancer cell lines [97].

GRKs are also emerging as important nodes in modulation of signaling controlling cell migration. GRK2 can play a role in the organization of actin and microtubule networks and in adhesion dynamics, through interaction with substrates such as the GIT1 scaffold or the cytoplasmic α-tubulin deacetylase histone deacetylase 6 (HDAC6). Overall the emerging effect of GRK2 modulation on cell migration is not straightforward, and seems to depend upon cell type and physiological context (for review see [98]). In a physiologically normal context, GRK2 was demonstrated to promote migration toward fibronectin in numerous epithelial cell lines and fibroblasts, in a kinase-independent fashion [99]. In contrast, in mesenchymal-derived cells such as immune T cells, GRK2 silencing increases chemotaxis and signaling in response to CCL4 [100]. In this context, GRK2 plays a role more intuitive of GPCR desensitization, in the integral turnover of GPCR chemokine receptors at the leading edge of a migrating cell [86, 101]. The role GRKs play in migration is clearly very context-dependent; however their clear upregulation in certain malignant cancers warrants exploration of their potential in metastatic control.

2.4 RTK/GPCR Functional Hybrid Model

The instances examined here account for two separate processes. First, transactivation or receptor crosstalk is an indirect method by which an RTK can utilize GPCR components. Many of the RTKs use this platform, whereby their ligand-induced activation can in turn activate a GPCR or vice versa. The second scenario, highlighted in this chapter for the case of the IGF-1R, is the direct utilization of GPCR components by an RTK, completely independent of a GPCR. In this respect, in addition to its classical kinase activity, the IGF-1R has been recognized to operate as a prototypical GPCR with all functional characteristics: (1) G-protein signaling activation [50, 52], (2) GRK-dependent phosphorylation of the receptor serine residues [66], (3) β-arrestin binding to the phosphorylated serine residues [61, 63, 66], (4) desensitization of G-protein signaling, (5) activation of the second signaling wave, originating from β-arrestins [63, 66], and (6) receptor endocytosis with subsequent recycling or degradation [61, 66]. Altogether this strongly supports the updating of the IGF-1R from a prototypical RTK to an RTK/GPCR functional hybrid. This model takes into consideration that the IGF-1R can initiate both G-protein signaling and classical kinase signaling. In this scenario, the regulatory role of β-arrestin, on receptor signaling activation [63] could be interpreted as desenzitization of the G-protein signaling, kinase signaling attenuation through endocytosis in connection with a new wave of β-arrestin-dependent MAPK activation [62, 76, 77]. This paradigm is endorsed by the key mechanism switching between downstream signaling pathways as well as between trafficking routes: phosphorylation of specific serine residues by the GRKs [62, 78, 79] (Fig. 2).

Featuring a GPCR-like pattern within the RTK perspective could explain the impossible behavior of the "kinase-only" IGF-1R, such as kinase-independent signaling or kinase-independent downregulation. Far from being simply a theoretical exercise, such an updating would have at least two major implications. First, highlighting the evidence of non-tyrosine-kinase signaling, so far neglected in targeting strategies, reveals the shortcomings of a kinase inhibitor in this system as well as strategies to counteract them (for review see [44]). On the bright side, this also points to new possibilities in anti-IGF-1R therapeutic strategies. In the model, we propose that the receptor conformation that activates the kinase cascade can be distinct from that which interacts with β-arrestins, thus indicating that IGF-1R signaling could be activated and/or downregulated in a "biased manner" via β-arrestins, even by IGF-1R inhibitors or GRK modulators. In addition, recognizing the β-arrestin/GRK system as a central modulator of the intracellular signaling may open new perspectives in the search for molecular-designed treatments of cancer. In particular, proteins that modify IGF-1R (as well as other major RTKs) function have potential as biomarkers in diagnosis and in evaluating the outcome of therapy. Such proteins also have potential to be new targets and may ultimately be better targets than the IGF-1R itself.

3   Conclusions

Today, targeting the IGF-1R and components of its signaling pathway in different forms of cancer is a major research area. Although clearly insufficient to explain the complexities of IGF-1R signaling, the classical RTK "kinase only" paradigm has been used thus far in selecting anti-IGF-1R agents. The present review highlights the facts that in addition to the classical kinase pathway, IGF-1R activity and its biological effects are controlled by the prototypical components of the GPCR signaling pathway including the GRK/arrestin system. In this context, the complexity of IGF-1R behavior following exposure to agonists or inhibitors reinforces the need to understand the relationships between different signaling pathways and between signaling and biological effects. Only an updating of the working model and a true appreciation of signaling complexities across receptor subfamilies, can unearth an effective anti-IGF-1R therapeutic and make use of these crucial GPCR "borrowed" components. This stands true not only for the IGF-1R but also for other RTKs, whose aberrant activity is associated with ageing, diabetes, metabolic syndrome, cancer, and Alzheimer's disease, to name but a few, and therefore such an updating cannot be underappreciated in drug development.

Acknowledgements

Research support for Leonard Girnita's group: Swedish Research Council, Swedish Cancer Society, Children Cancer Society, Crown Princess Margareta's Foundation for the Visually Impaired, Welander Finsen Foundation, King Gustaf V Jubilee Foundation, Stockholm Cancer Society, the Stockholm County, and Karolinska Institutet.

References

1. Hupfeld CJ, Olefsky JM (2007) Regulation of receptor tyrosine kinase signaling by GRKs and beta-arrestins. Annu Rev Physiol 69:561–577

2. Aaronson SA (1991) Growth-factors and cancer. Science 254(5035):1146–1153

3. Ullrich A, Schlessinger J (1990) Signal transduction by receptors with tyrosine kinase-activity. Cell 61(2):203–212

4. Heldin CH (1995) Dimerization of cell-surface receptors in signal-transduction. Cell 80(2):213–223

5. Weiss A, Schlessinger J (1998) Switching signals on or off by receptor dimerization. Cell 94(3):277–280

6. Heldin CH, Ostman A (1996) Ligand-induced dimerization of growth factor receptors: variations on the theme. Cytokine Growth Factor Rev 7(1):3–10

7. Lemmon MA, Schlessinger J (1994) Regulation of signal-transduction and signal diversity by receptor oligomerization. Trends Biochem Sci 19(11):459–463

8. Lemmon MA, Schlessinger J (2010) Cell signaling by receptor tyrosine kinases. Cell 141(7):1117–1134

9. Girnita L, Worrall C, Takahashi S, Seregard S, Girnita A (2014) Something old, something new and something borrowed: emerging paradigm of insulin-like growth factor type 1 receptor (IGF-1R) signaling regulation. Cell Mol Life Sci 71(13):2403–2427

10. Waterfield MD, Scrace GT, Whittle N, Stroobant P, Johnsson A, Wasteson A, Westermark B, Heldin CH, Huang JS, Deuel TF (1983) Platelet-derived growth factor is structurally related to the putative transforming protein p28sis of simian sarcoma virus. Nature 304(5921):35–39

11. Doolittle RF, Hunkapiller MW, Hood LE, Devare SG, Robbins KC, Aaronson SA, Antoniades HN (1983) Simian sarcoma virus onc gene, v-sis, is derived from the gene (or genes) encoding a platelet-derived growth factor. Science 221(4607):275–277

12. Ullrich A, Coussens L, Hayflick JS, Dull TJ, Gray A, Tam AW, Lee J, Yarden Y, Libermann TA, Schlessinger J, Downward J, Mayes ELV, Whittle N, Waterfield MD, Seeburg PH (1984) Human epidermal growth-factor receptor CDNA sequence and aberrant expression of the amplified gene in A431 epidermoid carcinoma-cells. Nature 309(5967):418–425

13. Roberts PJ, Der CJ (2007) Targeting the Raf-MEK-ERK mitogen-activated protein kinase cascade for the treatment of cancer. Oncogene 26(22):3291–3310

14. Wong WM (1999) Trastuzumab: anti-HER2 antibody for treatment of metastatic breast cancer. Cancer Pract 7(1):48–50

15. Abdel-Rahman O (2015) Targeting platelet-derived growth factor (PDGF) signaling in gastrointestinal cancers: preclinical and clinical considerations. Tumor Biol 36(1):21–31

16. Ashman LK, Griffith R (2013) Therapeutic targeting of c-KIT in cancer. Expert Opin Inv Drug 22(1):103–115

17. Baserga R (1995) The insulin-like growth factor I receptor: a key to tumor growth? Cancer Res 55(2):249–252

18. Jones JI, Clemmons DR (1995) Insulin-like growth-factors and their binding-proteins—biological actions. Endocr Rev 16(1):3–34

19. Ullrich A, Gray A, Tam AW, Yangfeng T, Tsubokawa M, Collins C, Henzel W, Lebon T, Kathuria S, Chen E, Jacobs S, Francke U, Ramachandran J, Fujitayamaguchi Y (1986) Insulin-like growth factor-I receptor primary structure—comparison with insulin-receptor suggests structural determinants that define functional specificity. EMBO J 5(10):2503–2512

20. Girnita A, Zheng H, Gronberg A, Girnita L, Stahle M (2012) Identification of the cathelicidin peptide LL-37 as agonist for the type I insulin-like growth factor receptor. Oncogene 31(3):352–365

21. Raizada MK (1993) Insulin receptor-related receptor—an orphan with neurotrophic neuromodulatory potential. Endocrinology 133(1):1–2

22. Soos MA, Whittaker J, Lammers R, Ullrich A, Siddle K (1990) Receptors for insulin and insulin-like growth factor-I can form hybrid dimers—characterization of hybrid receptors in transfected cells. Biochem J 270(2):383–390

23. Favelyukis S, Till JH, Hubbard SR, Miller WT (2001) Structure and autoregulation of the insulin-like growth factor 1 receptor kinase. Nat Struct Biol 8(12):1058–1063

24. Liu JP, Baker J, Perkins AS, Robertson EJ, Efstratiadis A (1993) Mice carrying null mutations of the genes encoding insulin-like growth factor-I (Igf-1) and type-1 Igf receptor (Igf1r). Cell 75(1):59–72

25. Kitamura T, Kahn CR, Accili E (2003) Insulin receptor knockout mice. Annu Rev Physiol 65:313–332

26. Efstratiadis A (1998) Genetics of mouse growth. Int J Dev Biol 42(7):955–976

27. Sell C, Dumenil G, Deveaud C, Miura M, Coppola D, DeAngelis T, Rubin R, Efstratiadis A, Baserga R (1994) Effect of a null mutation of the insulin-like growth factor I receptor gene on growth and transformation of mouse embryo fibroblasts. Mol Cell Biol 14(6):3604–3612

28. Baserga R, Peruzzi F, Reiss K (2003) The IGF-1 receptor in cancer biology. Int J Cancer 107(6):873–877

29. Girnita A, All-Ericsson C, Economou MA, Astrom K, Axelson M, Seregard S, Larsson O, Girnita L (2006) The insulin-like growth factor-I receptor inhibitor picropodophyllin causes tumor regression and attenuates mechanisms involved in invasion of uveal melanoma cells. Clin Cancer Res 12(4): 1383–1391

30. Ulanet DB, Ludwig DL, Kahn CR, Hanahan D (2010) Insulin receptor functionally enhances multistage tumor progression and conveys intrinsic resistance to IGF-1R targeted therapy. Proc Natl Acad Sci U S A 107(24):10791–10798

31. Soos MA, Siddle K (1989) Immunological relationships between receptors for insulin and insulin-like growth factor-I—evidence for structural heterogeneity of insulin-like growth factor-I receptors involving hybrids with insulin-receptors. Biochem J 263(2): 553–563

32. Moxham CP, Duronio V, Jacobs S (1989) Insulin-like growth factor-I receptor beta-subunit heterogeneity—evidence for hybrid tetramers composed of insulin-like growth factor-I and insulin-receptor heterodimers. J Biol Chem 264(22):13238–13244

33. Pandini G, Frasca F, Mineo R, Sciacca L, Vigneri R, Belfiore A (2002) Insulin/insulin-like growth factor I hybrid receptors have different biological characteristics depending on the insulin receptor isoform involved. J Biol Chem 277(42):39684–39695

34. Belfiore A (2007) The role of insulin receptor isoforms and hybrid insulin/IGF-I receptors in human cancer. Curr Pharm Des 13(7): 671–686

35. Vigneri P, Frasca F, Sciacca L, Pandini G, Vigneri R (2009) Diabetes and cancer. Endocr Relat Cancer 16(4):1103–1123

36. Girnita L, Wang M, Xie Y, Nilsson G, Dricu A, Wejde J, Larsson O (2000) Inhibition of N-linked glycosylation down-regulates insulin-like growth factor-1 receptor at the cell surface and kills Ewing's sarcoma cells: therapeutic implications. Anticancer Drug Des 15(1):67–72

37. Wang M, Xie Y, Girnita L, Nilsson G, Dricu A, Wejde J, Larsson O (1999) Regulatory role of mevalonate and N-linked glycosylation in proliferation and expression of the EWS/FLI-1 fusion protein in Ewing's sarcoma cells. Exp Cell Res 246(1):38–46

38. Girnita A, Girnita L, del Prete F, Bartolazzi A, Larsson O, Axelson M (2004) Cyclolignans as inhibitors of the insulin-like growth factor-1 receptor and malignant cell growth. Cancer Res 64(1):236–242

39. Baserga R (2005) The insulin-like growth factor-I receptor as a target for cancer therapy. Expert Opin Ther Targets 9(4):753–768

40. Gualberto A, Pollak M (2009) Emerging role of insulin-like growth factor receptor inhibitors in oncology: early clinical trial results and future directions. Oncogene 28(34):3009–3021

41. Furukawa J, Miyake H, Fujisawa M (2012) Antisense oligonucleotide targeting Insulin-like growth factor-1 receptor (IGF-1R) enhances paclitaxel sensitivity in a castrate-resistant and paclitaxel-resistant prostate cancer model. Eur Urol Suppl 11(1):E234

42. Girnita L, Girnita A, Brodin B, Xie Y, Nilsson G, Dricu A, Lundeberg J, Wejde J, Bartolazzi A, Wiman KG, Larsson O (2000) Increased expression of insulin-like growth factor I receptor in malignant cells expressing aberrant p53: functional impact. Cancer Res 60(18):5278–5283

43. Beauchamp MC, Yasmeen A, Knafo A, Gotlieb WH (2010) Targeting insulin and insulin-like growth factor pathways in epithelial ovarian cancer. J Oncol 2010:257058

44. Crudden C, Ilic M, Suleymanova N, Worrall C, Girnita A, Girnita L (2015) The dichotomy of the Insulin-like growth factor 1 receptor: RTK and GPCR: friend or foe for cancer treatment? Growth Horm IGF Res 25(1): 2–12

45. Natarajan K, Berk BC (2006) Crosstalk coregulation mechanisms of G protein-coupled receptors and receptor tyrosine kinases. Methods Mol Biol 332:51–77

46. Luttrell L, Kilgour E, Larner J, Romero G (1990) A pertussis toxin-sensitive G-protein mediates some aspects of insulin action in BC3H-1 murine myocytes. J Biol Chem 265(28):16873–16879

47. Heyworth CM, Grey AM, Wilson SR, Hanski E, Houslay MD (1986) The action of islet activating protein (pertussis toxin) on insulin ability to inhibit adenylate-cyclase and activate cyclic-AMP phosphodiesterases in hepatocytes. Biochem J 235(1):145–149

48. Rothenberg PL, Kahn CR (1988) Insulin inhibits pertussis toxin-catalyzed ADP-ribosylation of G-proteins—evidence for a novel interaction between insulin-receptors and G-proteins. J Biol Chem 263(30):15546–15552

49. Imamura T, Vollenweider P, Egawa K, Clodi M, Ishibashi K, Nakashima N, Ugi S, Adams JW, Brown JH, Olefsky JM (1999) G alpha-q/11 protein plays a key role in insulin-induced glucose transport in 3T3-L1 adipocytes. Mol Cell Biol 19(10):6765–6774

50. Luttrell LM, van Biesen T, Hawes BE, Koch WJ, Touhara K, Lefkowitz RJ (1995) G beta gamma subunits mediate mitogen-activated protein kinase activation by the tyrosine kinase insulin-like growth factor 1 receptor. J Biol Chem 270(28):16495–16498

51. Hallak H, Seiler AEM, Green JS, Ross BN, Rubin R (2000) Association of heterotrimeric G(i) with the insulin-like growth factor-I receptor—Release of G(beta gamma) sub-units upon receptor activation. J Biol Chem 275(4):2255–2258

52. Dalle S, Ricketts W, Imamura T, Vollenweider P, Olefsky JM (2001) Insulin and insulin-like growth factor I receptors utilize different G protein signaling components. J Biol Chem 276(19):15688–15695

53. Waters C, Pyne S, Pyne NJ (2004) The role of G-protein coupled receptors and associated proteins in receptor tyrosine kinase signal transduction. Semin Cell Dev Biol 15(3):309–323

54. Rakhit S, Pyne S, Pyne NJ (2001) Nerve growth factor stimulation of p42/p44 mitogen-activated protein kinase in PC12 cells: role of G(i/o), G protein-coupled receptor kinase 2, beta-arrestin I, and endocytic processing. Mol Pharmacol 60(1):63–70

55. Pyne NJ, Pyne S (2011) Receptor tyrosine kinase-G-protein-coupled receptor signalling platforms: out of the shadow? Trends Pharmacol Sci 32(8):443–450

56. Lin FT, Daaka Y, Lefkowitz RJ (1998) beta-arrestins regulate mitogenic signaling and clathrin-mediated endocytosis of the insulin-like growth factor I receptor. J Biol Chem 273(48):31640–31643

57. Sehat B, Andersson S, Vasilcanu R, Girnita L, Larsson O (2007) Role of ubiquitination in IGF-1 receptor signaling and degradation. PLoS One 2(4):e340

58. Vecchione A, Marchese A, Henry P, Rotin D, Morrione A (2003) The Grb10/Nedd4 complex regulates ligand-induced ubiquitination and stability of the insulin-like growth factor I receptor. Mol Cell Biol 23(9):3363–3372

59. Larsson O, Girnita A, Girnita L (2005) Role of insulin-like growth factor 1 receptor signalling in cancer. Br J Cancer 92(12):2097–2101

60. Girnita L, Girnita A, Larsson O (2003) Mdm2-dependent ubiquitination and degradation of the insulin-like growth factor 1 receptor. Proc Natl Acad Sci U S A 100(14):8247–8252

61. Girnita L, Shenoy SK, Sehat B, Vasilcanu R, Girnita A, Lefkowitz RJ, Larsson O (2005) {beta}-Arrestin is crucial for ubiquitination and down-regulation of the insulin-like growth factor-1 receptor by acting as adaptor for the MDM2 E3 ligase. J Biol Chem 280(26):24412–24419

62. Lefkowitz RJ, Shenoy SK (2005) Transduction of receptor signals by beta-arrestins. Science 308(5721):512–517

63. Girnita L, Shenoy SK, Sehat B, Vasilcanu R, Vasilcanu D, Girnita A, Lefkowitz RJ, Larsson O (2007) Beta-arrestin and Mdm2 mediate IGF-1 receptor-stimulated ERK activation and cell cycle progression. J Biol Chem 282(15):11329–11338

64. Zheng H, Shen H, Oprea I, Worrall C, Stefanescu R, Girnita A, Girnita L (2012) beta-Arrestin-biased agonism as the central mechanism of action for insulin-like growth factor 1 receptor-targeting antibodies in Ewing's sarcoma. Proc Natl Acad Sci U S A 109(50):20620–20625

65. Vasilcanu R, Vasilcanu D, Sehat B, Yin S, Girnita A, Axelson M, Girnita L (2008) Insulin-like growth factor type-I receptor-dependent phosphorylation of extracellular signal-regulated kinase 1/2 but not Akt (protein kinase B) can be induced by picropodophyllin. Mol Pharmacol 73(3):930–939

66. Zheng H, Worrall C, Shen H, Issad T, Seregard S, Girnita A, Girnita L (2012) Selective recruitment of G protein-coupled receptor kinases (GRKs) controls signaling of the insulin-like growth factor 1 receptor. Proc Natl Acad Sci U S A 109(18):7055–7060

67. Chow JC, Condorelli G, Smith RJ (1998) Insulin-like growth factor-1 receptor internalization regulates signaling via the Shc/mitogen-activated protein kinase pathway, but not the insulin receptor substrate-1 pathway. J Biol Chem 273(8):4672–4680

68. Morrison DK, Davis RJ (2003) Regulation of map kinase signaling modules by scaffold proteins in mammals. Annu Rev Cell Dev Biol 19:91–118

69. McDonald PH, Chow CW, Miller WE, Laporte SA, Field ME, Lin FT, Davis RJ, Lefkowitz RJ (2000) Beta-arrestin 2: a receptor-regulated MAPK scaffold for the activation of JNK3. Science 290(5496): 1574–1577

70. Sacks DB (2006) The role of scaffold proteins in MEK/ERK signalling. Biochem Soc Trans 34:833–836

71. Povsic TJ, Kohout TA, Lefkowitz RJ (2003) beta-arrestin1 mediates insulin-like growth factor 1 (IGF-1) activation of phosphatidylinositol 3-kinase (PI3K) and anti-apoptosis. J Biol Chem 278(51):51334–51339

72. Zhande R, Mitchell JJ, Wu J, Sun XJ (2002) Molecular mechanism of insulin-induced degradation of insulin receptor substrate 1. Mol Cell Biol 22(4):1016–1026

73. Rui LY, Yuan MS, Frantz D, Shoelson S, White MF (2002) SOCS-1 and SOCS-3 block insulin signaling by ubiquitin-mediated degradation of IRS1 and IRS2. J Biol Chem 277(44):42394–42398

74. Dalle S, Imamura T, Rose DW, Worrall DS, Ugi S, Hupfeld CJ, Olefsky JM (2002) Insulin induces heterologous desensitization of G-protein-coupled receptor and insulin-like growth factor I signaling by downregulating beta-arrestin-1. Mol Cell Biol 22(17): 6272–6285

75. Luan B, Zhao J, Wu HY, Duan BY, Shu GW, Wang XY, Li DS, Jia WP, Kang JH, Pei G (2009) Deficiency of a beta-arrestin-2 signal complex contributes to insulin resistance. Nature 457(7233):1146–1149

76. Shenoy SK, Drake MT, Nelson CD, Houtz DA, Xiao K, Madabushi S, Reiter E, Premont RT, Lichtarge O, Lefkowitz RJ (2006) beta-arrestin-dependent, G protein-independent ERK1/2 activation by the beta2 adrenergic receptor. J Biol Chem 281(2):1261–1273

77. Lefkowitz RJ (2004) Historical review: a brief history and personal retrospective of seven-transmembrane receptors. Trends Pharmacol Sci 25(8):413–422

78. Shenoy SK, Lefkowitz RJ (2003) Multifaceted roles of beta-arrestins in the regulation of seven-membrane-spanning receptor trafficking and signalling. Biochem J 375(Pt 3): 503–515

79. DeWire SM, Ahn S, Lefkowitz RJ, Shenoy SK (2007) Beta-arrestins and cell signaling. Annu Rev Physiol 69:483–510

80. Usui I, Imamura T, Huang J, Satoh H, Olefsky JM (2003) Cdc42 is a rho GTPase family member that can mediate insulin signaling to glucose transport in 3T3-L1 adipocytes. J Biol Chem 278(16):13765–13774

81. Usui I, Imamura T, Satoh H, Huang J, Babendure JL, Hupfeld CJ, Olefsky JM (2004) GRK2 is an endogenous protein inhibitor of the insulin signaling pathway for glucose transport stimulation. EMBO J 23(14):2821–2829

82. Gao JX, Li JL, Ma L (2005) Regulation of EGF-induced ERK/MAPK activation and EGFR internalization by G protein-coupled receptor kinase 2. Acta Biochim Biophys Sin 37(8):525–531

83. Alderton F, Rakhit S, Kong KC, Palmer T, Sambi B, Pyne S, Pyne NJ (2001) Tethering of the platelet-derived growth factor ss receptor to G-protein-coupled receptors—a novel platform for integrative signaling by these receptor classes in mammalian cells. J Biol Chem 276(30):28578–28585

84. Hobson JP, Rosenfeldt HM, Barak LS, Olivera A, Poulton S, Caron MG, Milstien S, Spiegel S (2001) Role of the sphingosine-1-phosphate receptor EDG-1 in PDGF-induced cell motility. Science 291(5509):1800–1803

85. Freedman NJ, Kim LK, Murray JP, Exum ST, Brian L, Wu JH, Peppel K (2002) Phosphorylation of the platelet-derived growth factor receptor-beta and epidermal growth factor receptor by G protein-coupled receptor kinase-2—mechanisms for selectivity of desensitization. J Biol Chem 277(50):48261–48269

86. Penela P, Murga C, Ribas C, Lafarga V, Mayor F (2010) The complex G protein-coupled receptor kinase 2 (GRK2) interactome unveils new physiopathological targets. Br J Pharmacol 160(4):821–832

87. Jaber M, Koch WJ, Rockman H, Smith B, Bond RA, Sulik KK, Ross J Jr, Lefkowitz RJ, Caron MG, Giros B (1996) Essential role of beta-adrenergic receptor kinase 1 in cardiac development and function. Proc Natl Acad Sci U S A 93(23):12974–12979

88. Matkovich SJ, Marreez Y, Diwan A, Odley AM, Koch WJ, Schwartz RJ, Brunskill EW, Dorn GW (2006) Cardiac-specific ablation of GRK2 re-defines its roles in heart development and beta-adrenergic signaling. Circulation 114(18):159

89. Jiang X, Yang P, Ma L (2009) Kinase activity-independent regulation of cyclin pathway by GRK2 is essential for zebrafish early development. Proc Natl Acad Sci U S A 106(25): 10183–10188

90. Wan KF, Sambi BS, Tate R, Waters C, Pyne NJ (2003) The inhibitory gamma subunit of the type 6 retinal cGMP phosphodiesterase functions to link c-Src and G-protein-coupled receptor kinase 2 in a signaling unit

that regulates p42/p44 mitogen-activated protein kinase by epidermal growth factor. J Biol Chem 278(20):18658–18663

91. Bliziotes M, Gunness M, Zhang XW, Nissenson R, Wiren K (2000) Reduced G-protein-coupled-receptor kinase 2 activity results in impairment of osteoblast function. Bone 27(3):367–373

92. Metaye T, Gibelin H, Perdrisot R, Kraimps JL (2005) Pathophysiological roles of G-protein-coupled receptor kinases. Cell Signal 17(8): 917–928

93. King DW, Steinmetz R, Wagoner HA, Hannon TS, Chen LY, Eugster EA, Pescovitz OH (2003) Differential expression of GRK isoforms in nonmalignant and malignant human granulosa cells. Endocrine 22(2): 135–141

94. Metaye T, Menet E, Guilhot J, Kraimps JL (2002) Expression and activity of G protein-coupled receptor kinases in differentiated thyroid carcinoma. J Clin Endocr Metab 87(7): 3279–3286

95. Bookout AL, Finney AE, Guo RS, Peppel K, Koch WJ, Daaka Y (2003) Targeting G beta gamma signaling to inhibit prostate tumor formation and growth. J Biol Chem 278(39): 37569–37573

96. Ho J, Cocolakis E, Dumas VM, Posner BI, Laporte PA, Lebrun JJ (2005) The G protein-coupled receptor kinase-2 is a TGF beta-inducible antagonist of TGF beta signal transduction. EMBO J 24(18):3247–3258

97. Metaye T, Levillain P, Kraimps JL, Perdrisot R (2008) Immunohistochemical detection, regulation and antiproliferative function of G-protein-coupled receptor kinase 2 in thyroid carcinomas. J Endocrinol 198(1): 101–110

98. Penela P, Nogues L, Mayor F Jr (2014) Role of G protein-coupled receptor kinases in cell migration. Curr Opin Cell Biol 27:10–17

99. Penela P, Ribas C, Aymerich I, Eijkelkamp N, Barreiro O, Heijnen CJ, Kavelaars A, Sanchez-Madrid F, Mayor F (2008) G protein-coupled receptor kinase 2 positively regulates epithelial cell migration. EMBO J 27(8):1206–1218

100. Vroon A, Heijnen CJ, Lombardi MS, Cobelens PM, Mayor F, Caron MG, Kavelaars A (2004) Reduced GRK2 level in T cells potentiates chemotaxis and signaling in response to CCL4. J Leukocyte Biol 75(5): 901–909

101. Vroon A, Heijnen CJ, Kavelaars A (2006) GRKs and arrestins: regulators of migration and inflammation. J Leukocyte Biol 80(6): 1214–1221

102. Conway AM, Rakhit S, Pyne S, Pyne NJ (1999) Platelet-derived-growth-factor stimulation of the p42/p44 mitogen-activated protein kinase pathway in airway smooth muscle: role of pertussis-toxin-sensitive G-proteins, c-Src tyrosine kinases and phosphoinositide 3-kinase. Biochem J 337(Pt 2):171–177

103. Zhang BH, Ho V, Farrell GC (2001) Specific involvement of G(alpha i2) with epidermal growth factor receptor signaling in rat hepatocytes, and the inhibitory effect of chronic ethanol. Biochem Pharmacol 61(8): 1021–1027

104. Piiper A, StryjekKaminska D, Zeuzem S (1997) Epidermal growth factor activates phospholipase C-gamma(1) via G(il-2) proteins in isolated pancreatic acinar membranes. Am J Physiol 272(5):G1276–G1284

105. Zeng HY, Zhao DZ, Yang SP, Datta K, Mukhopadhyay D (2003) Heterotrimeric G alpha(q)/G alpha(11) proteins function upstream of vascular endothelial growth factor (VEGF) receptor-2 (KDR) phosphorylation in vascular permeability factor/VEGF signaling. J Biol Chem 278(23): 20738–20745

106. Gavard J, Gutkind JS (2006) VEGF controls endothelial-cell permeability by promoting the beta-arrestin-dependent endocytosis of VE-cadherin. Nat Cell Biol 8(11): 1223–1234

107. Rieck PW, Cholidis S, Hartmann C (2001) Intracellular signaling pathway of FGF-2-modulated corneal endothelial cell migration during wound healing in vitro. Exp Eye Res 73(5):639–650

108. Sa G, Fox PL (1994) Basic fibroblast growth factor-stimulated endothelial-cell movement is mediated by a pertussis-toxin-sensitive pathway regulating phospholipase-A(2) activity. J Biol Chem 269(5):3219–3225

Chapter 8

Differential Control of Potassium Channel Activity by GRK2

Adi Raveh, Liora Guy-David, and Eitan Reuveny

Abstract

Extending their accepted role in downregulating GPCRs from the cell membrane following GPCR activation, GRK shows an additional novel role, to rapidly control GPCRs activation of effectors that depend on the G protein βγ subunits (Gβγ), independent of their catalytic activity. GPCR-coupled potassium channels (GIRK) are found in excitable tissues such as neurons, heart, and endocrine organs, where they are known to decrease cells' excitability following their activation by Gi/o-coupled GPCRs. In these tissues, GIRK participate in signaling systems that demand a precise temporal control, such as the regulation of heart rate and synaptic activity. While GPCRs activation can be prolonged by agonists, a constrained temporal response of GIRK channel activity can be achieved by GRKs capable of binding Gβγ subunit (GRK2 and 3). Simultaneously with GPCR activation, GRK2 binds the free Gβγ subunits through its pleckstrin homology domain immediately ceasing GIRK channel activity, in a process of fast desensitization. GIRK fast desensitization occurs with the mass action of cytosolic GRK2 recruited to the cell membrane upon receptor activation which appears simultaneously with channel current desensitization. Interestingly, GRK-mediated desensitization of GIRK currents is mediated by many but not all different Gi/o-linked GPCRs. The question whether a GPCR-mediated GRK fast desensitization relies on a specific Gβγ subunits pair coupled to a specific receptor, or on a direct precoupling of GRK to a specific subset of the GPCRs is still an open question.

Key words G-protein-coupled potassium channel, G-protein-coupled receptor kinase, Desensitization

1 Introduction

1.1 G-Protein-Coupled K+ (GIRK) Channels

Numerous neurotransmitters exert their inhibitory effect by the activation of Gi/o-coupled G-protein-coupled receptors (GPCRs), which in turn activate G-protein-coupled K+ (GIRK) channels. GIRK channels are mainly found in excitable tissues such as neurons, heart atrial cells, and endocrine tissues, where they hyperpolarize the cell membrane upon activation to reduce excitability [1]. Their postsynaptic localization and unique activation mechanism endows GIRK channels with a dominant role in the slow regulation of synaptic excitability [2]. In addition, GIRK channels (also known as IK(ACh)) play a pivotal role in the cholinergic regulation of the heart beat [3–5]. GPCR activation stimulates the exchange of GTP for the GDP that is associated with the Gα of the trimeric

Vsevolod V. Gurevich et al. (eds.), *G Protein-Coupled Receptor Kinases*, Methods in Pharmacology and Toxicology,
DOI 10.1007/978-1-4939-3798-1_8, © Springer Science+Business Media New York 2016

G protein, leading to dissociation of Gα-GTP and Gβγ (for review, see [6]). G-protein Gβγ subunits were identified as the key G-protein component that mediates GIRK channel activation [7–13]. More recently Gα subunits were also implicated in channel regulation, by controlling basal channel activity and the robustness of GPCR-mediated activation [14–18].

At the molecular level, the GIRK channel subfamily is comprised of four distinct subunits (GIRK1-4/Kir3.1-4) that form functional channels, either as a homotetramers (mainly GIRK2 in selected areas of the brain) or various heterotetramers, depending on the specific tissue [1]. Many studies have shown that animals missing one or more of the channel subunits have various cardiac [19], metabolic [20], or neuronal abnormalities (for review see [21]). In addition, excess of channel gene has also been shown to affect neuronal function. These genetic studies highlight not only the importance of GIRK channels in normal physiological processes, but also the need to avoid excessive GIRK activity to keep neuronal functionality intact.

1.2 Fast Desensitization Ensures the Precise Timing and Magnitude of GIRK Activity

GIRK is the effector of different GPCRs, some of these are activated by ligands that are retained in the synaptic cleft for prolonged time, such as opioids and adenosine [22–24]. Thus, different mechanisms are needed for limiting the response time of their effectors thus avoiding excessive GIRK activity over time. This need becomes even clearer considering that GIRK is involved in different organ systems where precise timing is the main concern. For example, in atrial cells GIRK channels are an integral part of the pacemaking mechanism. Therefore, any fault in GIRK signal termination might affect the pacemaker cycle and consequently the heart beat [25, 26]. It was indeed shown that rapid specific inhibition of GIRK channel activity in response to atrial stretch increased the heart rate [27].

In the central nervous system (CNS), a timed and accurate neuronal signaling is essential, even in response to a prolonged presence of GPCR agonists. For example, in *locus ceruleus* neurons, Blanchet and Luscher [28] demonstrated that a prolonged activation of the μ-opioid receptor (μ-OR) leads to the inhibition of GIRK function. The μOR-mediated inhibition was constant over time at presynaptic locations whereas postsynaptic inhibition, mediated by GIRK activation, exhibited strong time-dependent desensitization of the response, indicating that the GIRK activity is further regulated downstream of the μOR receptors. GIRK current desensitization was observed in GABAergic neurons in the ventral tegmental area (VTA) [29], as well as in hippocampal neurons [30–32]. In addition, distinct GIRK desensitization was detected for adenosine, serotonin, and baclofen responses in pyramidal neurons of the neocortex [24, 33].

One mode of regulation of GIRK response over time originates from the kinetic properties of the G-protein activation/deactivation cycle, i.e., the rates of GDP–GTP exchange and GTP hydrolysis by Gα [24, 34, 35], which limits the amount of heterotrimeric G protein available for activation during prolonged agonist exposure. In addition, the response to an activated receptor can be downregulated by different proteins acting downstream of the G proteins, to reduce overall receptor-mediated effector responses. This mode of fast ("acute"/"short-term") desensitization can be mediated by several proteins [36], one of which is the GRK2.

2   Regulation of GIRK by GRKs

2.1 Fast GIRK Desensitization Is Mediated by GRK2

The role of GRK2 in GPCR desensitization has been long attributed to its enzymatic activity, namely, phosphorylation of active GPCRs. GPCR phosphorylation is then followed by the recruitment of arrestin to initiate clathrin-mediated endocytosis that decreases the density of receptors on the cell surface. This process of receptor downregulation involves several steps and is considered to be slow (minutes–hours), as compared to the electrical activity in excitable tissues, and is therefore referred to as slow/long-term desensitization. Thus, it cannot account for the fast desensitization of GIRK currents that occurs within seconds following channel activation [28]. Work from our laboratory described a new, nonenzymatic, role of GRK2 that can mediate fast desensitization [37]. In this mode GRK2 acts downstream of the receptor, to titer the active G-protein levels that can potentially activate the GIRK channel (Fig. 1). This mode of desensitization does not involve the GPCR phosphorylation by GRK2, as it is induced also by GRK2/K220R that lacks kinase catalytic activity [38] and is associated only with GRK molecules that are capable of binding the Gβγ subunits of the G protein.

2.2 GIRK Fast Desensitization by GRK2 Involves Gβγ Binding

The fast desensitization by GRK2 starts concomitantly with receptor activation by an agonist. Receptor activation leads to the dissociation of Gβγ subunits from the Gα subunit. At the same time that Gβγ is free to interact with the Gβγ-binding domains on the channel and gating it, GRK2 starts its role in fast desensitization. GRK2 binds Gβγ subunits via its C-terminal Pleckstrin homology (PH) domain [39], which competitively reduces the amounts of the Gβγ subunits available to gate the channel. This leads to GIRK closure in the process of fast desensitization [37]. GRK2 binds Gβ at the interface of Gβγ with Gα [39, 40] at the spot where different Gβ subunits are identical at all amino acids, and Gβ genes sequence is highly conserved throughout species and subunits [39, 40].

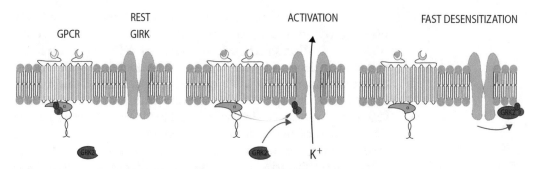

Fig. 1 A cartoon describing the mechanism by which GRK2 is regulating GIRK current desensitization. At rest, the GPCR is coupled with G-protein trimer. Upon ligand application, Gβγ dimer is released from Gα subunit to activate GIRK channels. In the presence of GRK2, upon ligand application, Gβγ dimer is quickly sequestered by GRK2 and GIRK current is then desensitized in a rapid manner (adapted from ref. [37])

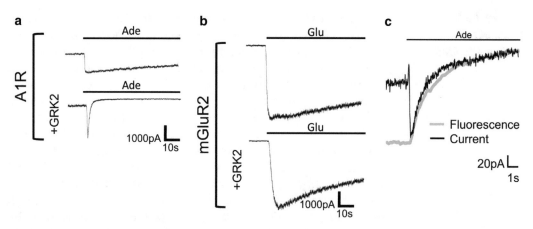

Fig. 2 GIRK current desensitization in HEK293 cells transfected with A1R or mGluR2 in the presence and absence of GRK2. (**a**) Adenosine-evoked currents desensitization is significantly increased when GRK2 is over-expressed. (**b**) Glutamate-invoked currents desensitization is not affected by overexpression of GRK2. (**c**) Recruitment of GRK2-GFP to the membrane following A1R activation occurs simultaneously with GIRK current desensitization (adapted from ref. [37])

While we and others observed a significant GRK2 membrane recruitment from the cytosol following receptor activation [37, 41] and simultaneous with GIRK desensitization [37] (Fig. 2), another GRK2 population is also known to be at the membrane even before receptor activation [42–44]. In addition, it is also possible that GRK2 is already precoupled to GIRK [45] and undergoes an orientation/conformation change upon activation. All these might contribute to the immediate competition with the channels for Gβγ subunits, and enable virtually instantaneous fast desensitization.

GRK2 competition for Gβγ with the channel is enabled due to the fact that GRK2 has a higher affinity for Gβγ than does the channel. Indeed, the binding studies have shown that Gβγ subunits bind recombinant GIRK1 or GIRK4 subunits with dissociation constants of ~125 nM and ~50 nM, respectively [46], whereas Gβγ affinity for GRK2 is ~20 nM [41, 47].

Several lines of evidence support the binding of Gβγ as the mechanism of GIRK desensitization by GRK2: (1) GRK2 mutants with impaired Gβγ binding capability, GRK2/R587Q [48] and GRK2/K663E;K665E;K667E [49], failed to accelerate GIRK desensitization; (2) constituently active, Gβγ-independent, GIRK mutants GIRK1/S170P;GIRK4/S176P [50] were insensitive to GRK2; (3) the interaction between YFP-tagged Gβ1 and mCherry-tagged GRK2 increased following A1R activation in a time course typical to GIRK desensitization as was shown by FRET measurements [37]. In addition, (4) GRK isoforms that lack the ability to bind Gβγ subunits were incapable of desensitizing GIRK currents.

2.3 Receptor Specificity of GRK2 Response Allowing a Differential GIRK Regulation

It was shown that GRK2 is involved in the fast desensitization of GIRK currents induced by a variety, but not all, GPCRs. GRK2 desensitizes GIRK current responses of adenosine A1 receptors [37], μ-opioid receptors [37], muscarinic acetylcholine M2 receptors [51], GABA$_B$ receptors [32], and α2 adrenergic receptors [52].

However, GRK2 failed to desensitize the responses of metabotropic glutamate receptors 2 [37], muscarinic acetylcholine M4 receptors [37], and adenosine A3 receptors [52].

The mechanism that provides GRK2 with the differential control over GIRK currents induced only by specific receptors and not by the others is still unknown. One possibility might result from a precoupling of GRK2 just to a subset of the receptors. However, GIRK currents gated by α2 adrenergic receptor mutants (R225A, K320A, K358A) with impaired GRK2 binding [53] were not different from the wild type receptor in their fast desensitization and in its GRK2 membrane recruitment [52]. Likewise, fluorescence recovery after photobleaching (FRAP) experiments measure the mobility of GRK2 within the membrane milieu, using membrane-associated GRK2 (myristoylated GRK2-GFP, myrGRK2-GFP), showed that the fluorescence recovery of myrGRK2-GFP is much faster than that of the α2AR, which implies that prior to activation the two molecules are mostly not precoupled (Fig. 3). Following ligand application, a significant reduction in myrGRK2-GFP mobility was observed only in the presence of α2AR. Abolishing GRK2 binding to the receptor using the α2AR mutant did not alter the myrGRK2-GFP mobility, confirming again that direct binding of GRK2 to α2AR is not necessary for this process.

Another possibility is differential ability of GPCRs to recruit cytosolic GRK2 to the membrane upon activation. It was already shown that GRK2 membrane recruitment is receptor-specific [54]. Indeed, we showed that current desensitization happens

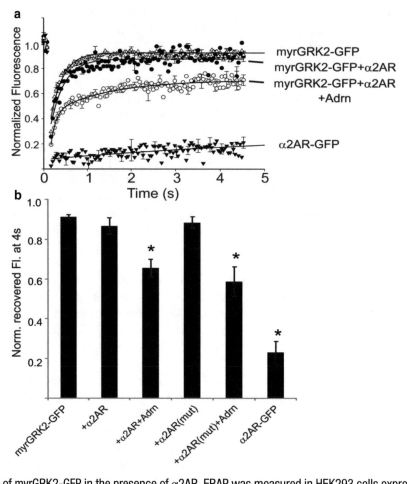

Fig. 3 FRAP of myrGRK2-GFP in the presence of α2AR. FRAP was measured in HEK293 cells expressing either myrGRK2-GFP or α2AR-GFP. (**a**) Average fluorescence recovery traces of the different groups measured. (**b**) Average normalized fluorescence recovery at 4 s (*P* < 0.005) of myrGRK2-GFP, in the presence of either wt-α2AR or α2AR-mut before and after adrenalin application

simultaneously with the recruitment of cytosolic GFP-tagged GRK2 to the membrane, using TIRF microscopy [37], and that GIRK currents mediated by the GPCRs that induced GRK2 recruitment were the ones sensitive to GRK2 fast desensitization [37]. However, follow-up experiments showed that this is not always the case, as additional GPCRs could recruit GRK2 to the membrane upon their activation, but their GIRK currents were insensitive to GRK2 desensitization (muscarinic acetylcholine receptors 4 (M4R) and adenosine A3 receptors (A3R)) [52] (Table 1). Of note, while there is no complete overlap between the processes of GRK membrane recruitment and regulation of GIRK desensitization, all GPCRs that were found by us to induce GIRK desensitization were also able to promote apparent membrane recruitment. In order to verify whether these two processes are independent, an extensive screen, studying more GPCRs, should be conducted.

Table 1
Specificity of GRK2 response to different GPCRs

GPCR	GIRK current desensitization	GRK2-GFP membrane association
A1R	V	V
A3R	X	V
α2AR	V	V
M4R	X	V
μOR	V	V
mGluR2	X	X

The effect of different GPCRs activation on GRK2-GFP membrane recruitment and on GIRK currents gating is detailed

Last possibility is that the specific composition of the G-protein subunits constituting the activated G-protein trimer is involved in setting regulation specificity. In such case, receptors that are capable of inducing GIRK desensitization release Gβγ subtypes that bind GIRK channels with moderate affinity, while GPCRs that do not induce GIRK desensitization release Gβγ subtypes that bind GIRK channels strongly. The tighter association of the former with the GIRK channels precludes their sequestration by GRK2, thus maintaining the channels in an open state. It is known that heterotrimeric G proteins with different subunit composition display different affinity for distinct GRK subtypes [54–56]. If activated receptor specifically activates downstream G proteins subsets with high GRK2 binding affinity [57–61], its activated GIRK current will be sensitive to GRK2-mediated desensitization.

3   Conclusion

Based on our continued studies of the differential control of GIRK channel activity by GRK2 (Fig. 1), it appears that a pool of GRK2 molecules resides next to the membrane but mostly not in complex with GPCRs or GIRK channels. Upon activation of GPCRs, GRK2 may sequester Gβγ that were uncoupled from GPCRs. We propose a balance between affinities of Gβγ subunits for GRKs and for GIRK channels. Therefore, probably not all available Gβ subunits are present in specific GPCR-G-protein-GIRK complexes. The activation of GIRK currents seems not to be selective for β subunits (as previously reported). But in contrast, enhancement of GIRK current desensitization by GRK2 can only be conducted effectively when GRK is able to compete with the channel for the specific G-protein resources. A change in affinities balance, for example knocking out a specific β subunit, or forced coupling to other βγ subunits, can affect the efficiency of GRK2 to sequester βγ subunits, thus slow down or even abolish current desensitization. This may also explain why some GPCRs do not promote GIRK current desensitization enhancement by GRK2, possibly having preferred coupling to a different set of Gβγ subunits. The selectivity of Gβγ complex for the GPCRs, the GIRK channels, and the GRK2 may probably result from the sum of specificities of α, β, and γ subunits [62–65].

Several questions still need to be answered to completely understand the molecular mechanism of GRK2-mediated fast desensitization process. While the desensitization of GIRK current by GRK2 competition binding of Gβγ is well characterized now, the exact molecular mechanism that differentially sets GRK2 sensitivity of GIRK currents induced by some receptors but not by the others is still unclear. In addition, the exact relation between the GIRK desensitization and GRK2 membrane recruitment is unclear. Is the membrane recruitment of cytosolic GRK2 an indispensable part of GIRK current desensitization or the membrane basal distribution of GRK2 molecules is sufficient? It would be also important to know whether there is a heterologous aspect of GRK2 fast desensitization, letting GRK2 activated by one active GPCR to desensitize the signaling pathway of a second one.

Another open question is whether GRK2 can regulate also other effector systems that are regulated by Gβγ subunits. For example, will GRK2 be able to regulate the activity of voltage-gated calcium channels [66, 67] by competitively removing Gβγ inhibition of these channels via its own Gβγ binding capability?

Another aspect that is missing, in order to evaluate better the importance GRK2 under physiological conditions, is the implication of lack of GRK2 activity on heart or CNS physiology. This is mainly due the fact that a full knockout of GRK2 is lethal [68]. To overcome this problem, more experiments should be done using GRK2 conditional knockout mice or stereotactic injection that target GRK2 expression in specific organs. Such experiments might supply answers about the physiological importance of GRK2 desensitization in the system level.

Acknowledgement

This work was supported by grants from the Israeli Science Foundation 207/09 and 1248/15 to ER.

References

1. Hibino H, Inanobe A, Furutani K, Murakami S, Findlay I, Kurachi Y (2010) Inwardly rectifying potassium channels: their structure, function, and physiological roles. Physiol Rev 90(1):291–366

2. Luscher C, Slesinger PA (2010) Emerging roles for G protein-gated inwardly rectifying potassium (GIRK) channels in health and disease. Nat Rev Neurosci 11(5):301–315

3. Loewi O (1921) On the humoral propagation of cardiac nerve action. Pflugers Arch 189:239–242

4. Harris EJ, Hutter OF (1956) The action of acetylcholine on the movements of potassium ions in the sinus venosus of the frog. J Physiol 133:58P–59P

5. Trautwein W, Dudel J (1958) Zum mechanismus der membranwirkung des acetylcholin an der herzmuskelfaser. Pflugers Arch 266:324–334

6. Gilman AG (1987) G proteins: transducers of receptor-generated signals. Annu Rev Biochem 56:615–649

7. Ito H, Tung RT, Sugimoto T, Kobayashi I, Takahashi K, Katada T, Ui M, Kurachi Y (1992) On the mechanism of G protein beta gamma subunit activation of the muscarinic K+ channel in guinea pig atrial cell membrane. Comparison with the ATP-sensitive K+ channel. J Gen Physiol 99(6):961–983

8. Logothetis DE, Kurachi Y, Galper J, Neer EJ, Clapham DE (1987) The beta gamma subunits of GTP-binding proteins activate the muscarinic K+ channel in heart. Nature 325(6102):321–326

9. Nair LA, Inglese J, Stoffel R, Koch WJ, Lefkowitz RJ, Kwatra MM, Grant AO (1995) Cardiac muscarinic potassium channel activity is attenuated by inhibitors of G beta gamma. Circ Res 76(5):832–838

10. Reuveny E, Slesinger PA, Inglese J, Morales JM, Iniguez-Lluhi JA, Lefkowitz RJ, Bourne HR, Jan YN, Jan LY (1994) Activation of the cloned muscarinic potassium channel by G protein beta gamma subunits. Nature 370(6485):143–146

11. Wickman KD, Iniguez-Lluhl JA, Davenport PA, Taussig R, Krapivinsky GB, Linder ME, Gilman AG, Clapham DE (1994) Recombinant G-protein beta gamma-subunits activate the muscarinic-gated atrial potassium channel. Nature 368(6468):255–257

12. Yamada M, Ho YK, Lee RH, Kontanill K, Takahashill K, Katadall T, Kurachi Y (1994) Muscarinic K+ channels are activated by beta gamma subunits and inhibited by the GDP-bound form of alpha subunit of transducin. Biochem Biophys Res Commun 200(3):1484–1490

13. Yamada M, Jahangir A, Hosoya Y, Inanobe A, Katada T, Kurachi Y (1993) GK* and brain G beta gamma activate muscarinic K+ channel through the same mechanism. J Biol Chem 268(33):24551–24554

14. Berlin S, Keren-Raifman T, Castel R, Rubinstein M, Dessauer CW, Ivanina T, Dascal N (2010) G alpha(i) and G betagamma jointly regulate the conformations of a G betagamma effector, the neuronal G protein-activated K+ channel (GIRK). J Biol Chem 285(9):6179–6185

15. Berlin S, Tsemakhovich VA, Castel R, Ivanina T, Dessauer CW, Keren-Raifman T, Dascal N (2011) Two distinct aspects of coupling between Galpha(i) protein and G protein-activated K+ channel (GIRK) revealed by fluorescently labeled Galpha(i3) protein subunits. J Biol Chem 286(38):33223–33235

16. Peleg S, Varon D, Ivanina T, Dessauer CW, Dascal N (2002) G(alpha)(i) controls the gating of the G protein-activated K(+) channel, GIRK. Neuron 33(1):87–99

17. Rubinstein M, Peleg S, Berlin S, Brass D, Dascal N (2007) Galphai3 primes the G protein-activated K+ channels for activation by coexpressed Gbetagamma in intact Xenopus oocytes. J Physiol 581(Pt 1):17–32

18. Rubinstein M, Peleg S, Berlin S, Brass D, Keren-Raifman T, Dessauer CW, Ivanina T, Dascal N (2009) Divergent regulation of GIRK1 and GIRK2 subunits of the neuronal G protein gated K+ channel by GalphaiGDP and Gbetagamma. J Physiol 587(Pt 14):3473–3491

19. Wickman K, Nemec J, Gendler SJ, Clapham DE (1998) Abnormal heart rate regulation in GIRK4 knockout mice. Neuron 20(1):103–114

20. Perry CA, Pravetoni M, Teske JA, Aguado C, Erickson DJ, Medrano JF, Lujan R, Kotz CM, Wickman K (2008) Predisposition to late-onset obesity in GIRK4 knockout mice. Proc Natl Acad Sci U S A 105(23):8148–8153

21. Pravetoni M, Wickman K (2008) Behavioral characterization of mice lacking GIRK/Kir3 channel subunits. Genes Brain Behav 7(5):523–531

22. Dunwiddie TV, Masino SA (2001) The role and regulation of adenosine in the central nervous system. Annu Rev Neurosci 24:31–55

23. Przewlocka B, Lason W, Przewlocki R (1992) Time-dependent changes in the activity of opioid systems in the spinal cord of monoarthritic rats—a release and in situ hybridization study. Neuroscience 46(1):209–216

24. Sickmann T, Alzheimer C (2003) Short-term desensitization of G-protein-activated, inwardly rectifying K+ (GIRK) currents in pyramidal neurons of rat neocortex. J Neurophysiol 90(4):2494–2503

25. Mighiu AS, Heximer SP (2012) Controlling parasympathetic regulation of heart rate: a gatekeeper role for RGS proteins in the sinoatrial node. Front Physiol 3:204

26. Jan LY, Jan YN (2000) Heartfelt crosstalk: desensitization of the GIRK current. Nat Cell Biol 2(9):E165–E167

27. Han S, Wilson SJ, Bolter CP (2010) Tertiapin-Q removes a mechanosensitive component of muscarinic control of the sinoatrial pacemaker in the rat. Clin Exp Pharmacol Physiol 37(9):900–904

28. Blanchet C, Luscher C (2002) Desensitization of mu-opioid receptor-evoked potassium currents: initiation at the receptor, expression at the effector. Proc Natl Acad Sci U S A 99(7):4674–4679

29. Cruz HG, Ivanova T, Lunn ML, Stoffel M, Slesinger PA, Luscher C (2004) Bi-directional effects of GABA(B) receptor agonists on the mesolimbic dopamine system. Nat Neurosci 7(2):153–159

30. Sodickson DL, Bean BP (1996) GABAB receptor-activated inwardly rectifying potassium current in dissociated hippocampal CA3 neurons. J Neurosci 16(20):6374–6385

31. Schwenk J, Metz M, Zolles G, Turecek R, Fritzius T, Bildl W, Tarusawa E, Kulik A, Unger A, Ivankova K, Seddik R, Tiao JY, Rajalu M, Trojanova J, Rohde V, Gassmann M, Schulte U, Fakler B, Bettler B (2010) Native GABA(B) receptors are heteromultimers with a family of auxiliary subunits. Nature 465(7295): 231–235

32. Turecek R, Schwenk J, Fritzius T, Ivankova K, Zolles G, Adelfinger L, Jacquier V, Besseyrias V, Gassmann M, Schulte U, Fakler B, Bettler B (2014) Auxiliary GABAB receptor subunits uncouple G protein betagamma subunits from effector channels to induce desensitization. Neuron 82(5):1032–1044

33. Sodickson DL, Bean BP (1998) Neurotransmitter activation of inwardly rectifying potassium current in dissociated hippocampal CA3 neurons: interactions among multiple receptors. J Neurosci 18(20): 8153–8162

34. Chuang HH, Yu M, Jan YN, Jan LY (1998) Evidence that the nucleotide exchange and hydrolysis cycle of G proteins causes acute desensitization of G-protein gated inward rectifier K^+ channels. Proc Natl Acad Sci U S A 95(20):11727–11732

35. Leaney JL, Benians A, Brown S, Nobles M, Kelly D, Tinker A (2004) Rapid desensitization of G protein-gated inwardly rectifying K(+) currents is determined by G protein cycle. Am J Physiol Cell Physiol 287(1):C182–C191

36. Raveh A, Turecek R, Bettler B (2015) Mechanisms of fast desensitization of GABA(B) receptor-gated currents. Adv Pharmacol 73:145–165

37. Raveh A, Cooper A, Guy-David L, Reuveny E (2010) Nonenzymatic rapid control of GIRK channel function by a G protein-coupled receptor kinase. Cell 143(5):750–760

38. Kong G, Penn R, Benovic JL (1994) A beta-adrenergic receptor kinase dominant negative mutant attenuates desensitization of the beta 2-adrenergic receptor. J Biol Chem 269(18): 13084–13087

39. Tesmer VM, Kawano T, Shankaranarayanan A, Kozasa T, Tesmer JJ (2005) Snapshot of activated G proteins at the membrane: the Galphaq-GRK2-Gbetagamma complex. Science 310(5754):1686–1690

40. Lodowski DT, Pitcher JA, Capel WD, Lefkowitz RJ, Tesmer JJ (2003) Keeping G proteins at bay: a complex between G protein-coupled receptor kinase 2 and Gbetagamma. Science 300(5623):1256–1262

41. Pitcher JA, Inglese J, Higgins JB, Arriza JL, Casey PJ, Kim C, Benovic JL, Kwatra MM, Caron MG, Lefkowitz RJ (1992) Role of beta gamma subunits of G proteins in targeting the beta-adrenergic receptor kinase to membrane-bound receptors. Science 257(5074):1264–1267

42. Aragay AM, Ruiz-Gomez A, Penela P, Sarnago S, Elorza A, Jimenez-Sainz MC, Mayor F Jr (1998) G protein-coupled receptor kinase 2 (GRK2): mechanisms of regulation and physiological functions. FEBS Lett 430(1–2): 37–40

43. Garcia-Higuera I, Penela P, Murga C, Egea G, Bonay P, Benovic JL, Mayor F Jr (1994) Association of the regulatory beta-adrenergic receptor kinase with rat liver microsomal membranes. J Biol Chem 269(2):1348–1355

44. Murga C, Penela P, Zafra F, Mayor F Jr (1998) The subcellular and cellular distribution of G protein-coupled receptor kinase 2 in rat brain. Neuroscience 87(3):631–637

45. Rishal I, Keren-Raifman T, Yakubovich D, Ivanina T, Dessauer CW, Slepak VZ, Dascal N (2003) Na + promotes the dissociation between Galpha GDP and Gbeta gamma, activating G protein-gated K+ channels. J Biol Chem 278(6):3840–3845

46. Krapivinsky G, Krapivinsky L, Wickman K, Clapham DE (1995) G beta gamma binds directly to the G protein-gated K+ channel, IKACh. J Biol Chem 270(49):29059–29062

47. Wu G, Benovic JL, Hildebrandt JD, Lanier SM (1998) Receptor docking sites for G-protein betagamma subunits. Implications for signal regulation. J Biol Chem 273(13):7197–7200

48. Carman CV, Barak LS, Chen C, Liu-Chen LY, Onorato JJ, Kennedy SP, Caron MG, Benovic JL (2000) Mutational analysis of Gbetagamma and phospholipid interaction with G protein-coupled receptor kinase 2. J Biol Chem 275(14):10443–10452

49. Touhara K, Koch WJ, Hawes BE, Lefkowitz RJ (1995) Mutational analysis of the pleckstrin homology domain of the beta-adrenergic

receptor kinase. Differential effects on G beta gamma and phosphatidylinositol 4,5-bisphosphate binding. J Biol Chem 270(28):17000–17005

50. Sadja R, Smadja K, Alagem N, Reuveny E (2001) Coupling Gbetagamma-dependent activation to channel opening via pore elements in inwardly rectifying potassium channels. Neuron 29(3):669–680

51. Shui Z, Khan IA, Tsuga H, Haga T, Boyett MR (1998) Role of receptor kinase in short-term desensitization of cardiac muscarinic K+ channels expressed in Chinese hamster ovary cells. J Physiol 507(Pt 2):325–334

52. Guy-David L, Reuveny E (2013) A novel mechanism for acquiring GPCR effector selectivity. Biophys J 104(2):538a

53. Pao CS, Benovic JL (2005) Structure/function analysis of alpha2A-adrenergic receptor interaction with G protein-coupled receptor kinase 2. J Biol Chem 280(12):11052–11058

54. Pitcher JA, Freedman NJ, Lefkowitz RJ (1998) G protein-coupled receptor kinases. Annu Rev Biochem 67:653–692

55. Daaka Y, Pitcher JA, Richardson M, Stoffel RH, Robishaw JD, Lefkowitz RJ (1997) Receptor and G betagamma isoform-specific interactions with G protein-coupled receptor kinases. Proc Natl Acad Sci U S A 94(6): 2180–2185

56. Muller S, Hekman M, Lohse MJ (1993) Specific enhancement of beta-adrenergic receptor kinase activity by defined G-protein beta and gamma subunits. Proc Natl Acad Sci U S A 90(22):10439–10443

57. Albert PR, Robillard L (2002) G protein specificity: traffic direction required. Cell Signal 14(5):407–418

58. Gudermann T, Schoneberg T, Schultz G (1997) Functional and structural complexity of signal transduction via G-protein-coupled receptors. Annu Rev Neurosci 20:399–427

59. Hou Y, Azpiazu I, Smrcka A, Gautam N (2000) Selective role of G protein gamma subunits in receptor interaction. J Biol Chem 275(50):38961–38964

60. Hou Y, Chang V, Capper AB, Taussig R, Gautam N (2001) G Protein beta subunit types differentially interact with a muscarinic receptor but not adenylyl cyclase type II or phospholipase C-beta 2/3. J Biol Chem 276(23):19982–19988

61. Richardson M, Robishaw JD (1999) The alpha2A-adrenergic receptor discriminates between Gi heterotrimers of different beta-gamma subunit composition in Sf9 insect cell membranes. J Biol Chem 274(19): 13525–13533

62. Kleuss C, Scherubl H, Hescheler J, Schultz G, Wittig B (1993) Selectivity in signal transduction determined by gamma subunits of heterotrimeric G proteins. Science 259(5096): 832–834

63. Liu YF, Jakobs KH, Rasenick MM, Albert PR (1994) G protein specificity in receptor-effector coupling. Analysis of the roles of G0 and Gi2 in GH4C1 pituitary cells. J Biol Chem 269(19):13880–13886

64. Schwindinger WF, Betz KS, Giger KE, Sabol A, Bronson SK, Robishaw JD (2003) Loss of G protein gamma 7 alters behavior and reduces striatal alpha(olf) level and cAMP production. J Biol Chem 278(8):6575–6579

65. Schwindinger WF, Giger KE, Betz KS, Stauffer AM, Sunderlin EM, Sim-Selley LJ, Selley DE, Bronson SK, Robishaw JD (2004) Mice with deficiency of G protein gamma3 are lean and have seizures. Mol Cell Biol 24(17): 7758–7768

66. Dunlap K, Fischbach GD (1978) Neurotransmitters decrease the calcium component of sensory neurone action potentials. Nature 276(5690):837–839

67. Tedford HW, Zamponi GW (2006) Direct G protein modulation of Cav2 calcium channels. Pharmacol Rev 58(4):837–862

68. Jaber M, Koch WJ, Rockman H, Smith B, Bond RA, Sulik KK, Ross J Jr, Lefkowitz RJ, Caron MG, Giros B (1996) Essential role of beta-adrenergic receptor kinase 1 in cardiac development and function. Proc Natl Acad Sci U S A 93(23):12974–12979

Part IV

Physiological and Pathophysiological Mechanisms Regulated by GRKs

Chapter 9

Critical Role of GRK2 in the Prevention of Chronic Pain

Faiza Baameur, Pooja Singhmar, Cobi J. Heijnen, and Annemieke Kavelaars

Abstract

Chronic pain is an incapacitating condition that arises from diverse origins, including inflammatory disorders, nerve damage, chemotherapy, and diabetes, implicating numerous signaling mechanisms. The pain response involves multiple cell types including neurons, microglia, and astrocytes. Recently our group and others have elucidated a crucial role for G protein coupled receptor kinase 2 (GRK2) in the development and maintenance of chronic pain using mice with global and cell specific deletion of GRK2 in vivo. The studies summarized here indicate that GRK2 controls multiple pathways in order to regulate severity and duration of pain in a cell-specific manner. For instance, reduced GRK2 in nociceptive neurons leads to increased G protein coupled receptor signaling and increased pain in response to a chemokine. Low GRK2 in nociceptors leads to transition to chronic pain by promoting biased cAMP signaling to Epac/PKCε/ERK- mediated pathway. Via mechanisms that remain to be elucidated, low monocyte GRK2 leads to IL-10 deficiency and prolonged inflammatory pain. The clinical relevance of these findings is discussed in the light of the observed decrease of GRK2 in nociceptors, glia and leukocytes in response to nerve injury in rodents and in patients and rodents with inflammatory conditions such as arthritis or multiple sclerosis.

Key words GRK2, Neuropathy, Chronic pain, Inflammation, Hyperalgesia, Nociceptor

Abbreviations

6-Bnz-cAMP	N^6-Benzoyladenosine cAMP
8-Br-cAMP	8-Bromoadenosine cAMP
8-pCPT	8-(4-Chlorophenylthio)-2'-O-methyladenosine cAMP
asODN	Antisense oligodeoxynucleotide
cAMP	Cyclic adenosine monophosphate
CCL2/3	Chemokine (C-C motif) ligand 2/3
CCR1/5	CC-chemokine receptor 1/5
cdk1	Cyclin-dependent kinase 1
CFA	Complete Freund's adjuvant
DRG	Dorsal root ganglion
Epac	Exchange protein directly activated by cAMP
EPI	Epinephrine

Vsevolod V. Gurevich et al. (eds.), *G Protein-Coupled Receptor Kinases*, Methods in Pharmacology and Toxicology, DOI 10.1007/978-1-4939-3798-1_9, © Springer Science+Business Media New York 2016

ERK	Extracellular signal-regulated kinase
GDNF	Glial cell-derived neurotrophic factor
GLAST	Glutamate aspartate transporter
GPCR	G-protein-coupled receptor
GRK	G-protein-coupled receptor kinase
HI	Hypoxic–ischemic
IFNγ	Interferon γ
IL-1R	Interleukin 1 receptor
IL-1β	Interleukin-1β
LPS	Lipopolysaccharide
LysM	Lysozyme M
MAPK	Mitogen-activated protein kinase
miRNA	MicroRNA
MS	Multiple sclerosis
mTOR	Mechanistic target of rapamycin
NGF	Nerve growth factor
PBMC	Peripheral blood mononuclear cells
PGE2	Prostaglandin E2
PKA/C	Protein kinase A or C
RA	Rheumatoid arthritis
ROS	Reactive oxygen species
SNS	Small sensory neuron
TAM	Tamoxifen
TNFα	Tumor necrosis factor α
TRPV1	Transient receptor potential cation channel V1
WT	Wild type
α/βAR	α or β adrenergic receptor
ΨRACK	PKCε activator

1   Introduction

The G-protein-coupled receptor kinase (GRK) family of kinases consists of seven members (GRK1–7); these kinases phosphorylate agonist-stimulated G protein-coupled receptors (GPCRs) to initiate a receptor desensitization pathway leading to termination of signaling. GRKs also regulate the activity of downstream signaling pathways by directly interacting with a number of signaling kinases including protein kinase C (PKC), Akt, PI3K, p38/MAPK, ERK1/2, and c-Src [1–6], as well as with cytoskeletal proteins, e.g. α-actinin, tubulin, and ezrin [7–11]. Changes in expression levels of GRKs greatly affect cellular signaling and function; therefore, expression levels of GRKs should be minutely regulated for the maintenance of homeostasis. It has been well-established that intracellular GRK levels are altered in multiple pathological conditions and these changes in the level of GRKs can have a major impact on cardiovascular functioning, blood pressure, immune system, tumor proliferation, opiate, and dopamine sensitivity, to cite a few [12–23]. More recent evidence indicates that changes in GRK expression levels also affect metabolic pathways and contribute to type 2 diabetes [24]. Here, we will review the role of GRKs, and in particular of GRK2, in inflammatory and neuropathic pain. We will also describe regulation of intracellular GRK2 levels by inflammatory processes.

2 Pain

Pain is defined as "an unpleasant sensory and emotional experience associated with actual or potential tissue damage or described in terms of such damage" by the International Association for the Study of Pain (IASP) [25]. In other words, pain is a normal physiological response associated with a specific injury, inflammation, or disease. Acute, transient pain is adaptive and subsides when the underlying cause gets treated or spontaneously resolves. However, in many cases pain lasts longer than its usefulness as a protective mechanism and turns into chronic pain thereby becoming a problem in itself. Chronic pain can persist for months to years and severely affects quality of life. Nearly 25 million adult Americans suffer from chronic pain and another 23 million from severe pain [26]. Chronic pain is associated with multiple pathological conditions and disorders; examples include post-herpetic neuralgia, chronic low back pain, and neuropathic pain, which can be induced by inflammation, trauma, diabetes, or chemotherapy. Patients suffering from chronic pain often develop increased sensitivity to painful stimuli and perceive normally innocuous stimuli as painful; sensitization of peripheral sensory neurons is thought to play a key role in these phenomena. The sensory pathway involved in pain signaling consists of a primary sensory neuron (nociceptor) with its nerve endings in the periphery where it senses potential or actual tissue-damaging stimuli (Fig. 1). It transmits the information through the axon to the cell body located in the dorsal root ganglion (DRG). Subsequently, a central nerve terminal carries the information to secondary pain neurons in the dorsal horn of the spinal cord followed by transmission of the signal to the brain. Several mediators (e.g. prostaglandin E2 (PGE2), epinephrine (EPI), chemokines (CCL3) and cytokines) produced at the site of inflammation or damage bind to their cognate GPCR and non-GPCR receptors on nociceptors to increase their excitability, causing hyperalgesia; a phenomenon known as peripheral sensitization. Especially in the case of chronic pain, inflammatory mediators produced in the spinal cord further sensitize the pain signaling pathway and this process is referred to as central sensitization (Fig. 1).

Peripheral and central sensitization modulates pain transmission by posttranslational modifications or transcriptional activation of different targets, including ion channels that facilitate neuronal

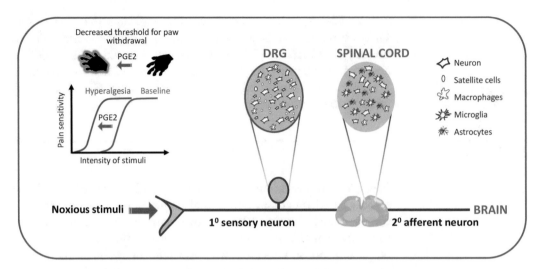

Fig. 1 A schematic overview of pain pathway. Noxious thermal, mechanical, or chemical stimuli are detected by peripheral endings of afferent nociceptive neurons and carried to second-order afferent neurons in the spinal cord dorsal horn from where the signal is propagated to brain [69, 121, 122]. The cell bodies of primary nociceptors are located in the dorsal root ganglion along with other non-neuronal cells like satellite cells and infiltrating macrophages. Microglia and astrocytes in the spinal cord can sensitize the pain pathway by local production of inflammatory mediators. Local inflammation in the paw leading to release of mediators such as PGE2, ATP, IL-1β, TNFα, NGF, or injection of these mediators themselves sensitizes the primary nociceptors leading to increased sensitivity (hyperalgesia) to various stimuli, including heat and mechanical stimulation. In animal models, the change in threshold to elicit paw withdrawal in response to application of ascending force intensities using von Frey hairs gives a measure of mechanical hyperalgesia. The decrease in latency to withdrawal from a heat source (laser beam) in the Hargreaves test is an indicator of heat hyperalgesia

activation. Evidence from numerous studies has implicated the second messenger cAMP in the process of sensitization of sensory neurons; several inflammatory mediators signal via Gs-coupled receptors to increase intracellular cAMP [27, 28]. Elevated cAMP levels lead in turn to activation of the downstream sensors protein kinase A (PKA) and exchange protein directly activated by cAMP (Epac). While PKA is involved in the acute phase of pain sensitivity and enhances neuronal excitability [29, 30] without affecting the development of chronic hyperalgesia [31, 32], Epac1 on the other hand enhances and prolongs hyperalgesia through activation of the small G protein Rap1. In non-peptidergic neurons, Epac1 signals to PKCε to induce chronic hyperalgesia [31, 33, 34].

Intrathecal administration of GPCR agonists like substance P (via neurokinin-1 receptors), monocyte chemoattractant protein 1 (via CCR2 receptors), PGE2 (via EP receptors), EPI (via adrenergic receptors), 5-hydroxytryptamine (via 5-HT receptors), and A2 adenosine receptor agonist target DRG and spinal cord to induce hyperalgesia in rodents [35–39]. These same mediators also enhance pain sensitivity when they are applied peripherally, e.g. in the paw. Conversely, antagonists to these GPCRs inhibit behavioral symptoms of pain [38, 40–42].

It is likely that GRKs modulate the pain response as they regulate the responsiveness of GRCR signaling by initiating their desensitization. In addition, as mentioned above, GRKs interact with several downstream GPCR signaling molecules and regulate their activity via phosphorylation-dependent or independent mechanisms; e.g. GRK2 modulates non-GPCR pathways like MAPK by interacting with p38 and MEK1/2 directly [43]. These kinases are all known to play a role in pain signaling and, thus, represent another potential pathway, by which GRKs can regulate pain [43].

3 Role of GRKs in Pain

In view of the prominent role of GPCR signaling in pain, we started to investigate the role of GRKs in pain using GRK knockout mouse models. So far, most of these studies have focused on GRK2. To investigate the role of GRK2 in the development and course of pain, hemizygous GRK2 knockout (GRK2+/−) mice with approximately 50% reduction in all tissues, were used. Homozygous GRK2 knockout mice are embryonically lethal [44].

It has been well established that local injection of inflammatory mediators, such as carrageenan, IL-1β, CCL3, or PGE2, in the hind paw, results in increased sensitivity toward normally non-noxious mechanical and thermal stimuli as quantified using von Frey hairs and the Hargreaves test, respectively. Under baseline conditions, the pain threshold for mechanical or thermal stimuli is similar in GRK2+/− and wild type (WT) mice, indicating that GRK2 does not contribute to the basal sensitivity to pain. The transient sensitization to pain in response to local inflammation was increased for some, but not all inflammatory stimuli in GRK2+/− as compared to WT mice. For example, the transient increase in pain sensitivity induced by PGE2 or the chemokine CCL3 was augmented, whereas hyperalgesia induced by IL-1β was not affected by hemizygous deletion of GRK2. We will come back to this aspect later. The most prominent effect of partial deletion of GRK2 was that upon the induction of transient local inflammation in the paw, with both thermal and mechanical hyperalgesia markedly prolonged (Table 1) [31, 45, 46]. Inflammation-induced hyperalgesia lasted up to 21 days in GRK2+/− mice as compared to the transient/acute hyperalgesia in WT mice, which lasted less than 1 or up to 3–4 days, depending on the stimulus (Table 1). This means that GRK2 determines the severity and duration of the increased sensitivity to pain that occurs upon inflammation. The prolongation of the pain response in GRK2-deficient mice was not the result of lifelong adaptation to the decreased GRK2 protein level, since prolongation of the pain response was similar in mice with tamoxifen-inducible deletion of GRK2 (TAM-GRK2+/−). Use of the tamoxifen-inducible deletion of GRK2 also allowed for comparison of the effect of partial versus complete deletion of GRK2

Table 1
Effects of GRK2 deficiency in specific cells on hyperalgesia induced by various stimuli (h: hour; d: day; w: week; vs: versus)

Model system	Agent/receptor	Thermal hyperalgesia vs WT	Mechanical hyperalgesia vs WT	References
GRK2+/–	IL-1β/IL-1R1 and IL-1R2	8–15 d vs 1–2 d		[45, 46]
	Carrageenan	More pronounced during first 24 h >20 d vs 3 d	More pronounced during first 24 h 30 d vs 3 d	[46]
	CCL3/CCR1 and CCR5	More pronounced during first 24 h >10 d vs 1 d	More pronounced and prolonged	[46]
	Epinephrine/βAR	18–21 d vs 3–4 d	21 d vs 3–4 d	[47]
	PGE2/EP4	>21 d vs 6 h		[31]
TAM-GRK2+/– and TAM-GRK2–/–	Epinephrine/βAR		21 d vs 3–4 d	[47]
	PGE2/EP4	>3 d vs 1 d		[31]
SNS-GRK2+/– and SNS-GRK2–/–	IL-1β/IL-1R1 and IL-1R2	No difference		[45, 46]
	Carrageenan	Enhanced during first 24 h 8–10 d vs 2–4 d		[46]
	CCL3/CCR1 and CCR5	Enhanced during first 12 h but not prolonged		[46]
	PGE2/EP4	4–6 d vs 4–6 h		[31]
	L-902688/EP4	3 d vs 4 h		[31]
	Sulprostone/EP1 and EP3	No hyperalgesia		[31]
	8-Br-cAMP/Epac1 and PKA	4–6 d vs 6 h		[31]
	8-pCPT/Epac1	8 d vs 6 h		[31]
	6-Bnz-cAMP/PKA	No difference		[31]
	Epinephrine/βAR	21 d vs 3 d	21 d vs 4 d	[47]
LysMGRK2+/– vs LysMGRK2–/–	IL-1β/IL-1R1 and IL-1R2	>8 d vs 6–24 h	15 d vs 1 d	[45, 46, 90]
	Carrageenan	>30 d vs 2–4 d		[46]
	CCL3/CCR1 and CCR5	15 d vs 1 d		[46]
	Epinephrine/βAR	10 d vs 3 d	10 d vs 2–3 d	[47]
GFAP-GRK2+/–	IL-1β/IL-1R1 and IL-1R2	No difference		[45, 46]
	Carrageenan	No difference		[46]
	CCL3/CCR1 and CCR5	No difference		[46]
	Epinephrine/βAR		No difference	[47]

on the course of the pain response (Table 1) [47]. Interestingly, there was no additive effect of homozygous versus hemizygous deletion of GRK2. For example, treatment with the adrenergic receptor agonist EPI prolonged mechanical hyperalgesia in TAM-GRK2+/− as well as in TAM-GRK2−/− mice to 21 days as compared to 3 days in WT mice [47]. It is of interest to note that there was no further prolongation of hyperalgesia when comparing the effect of homo- to hemizygous deletion of GRK2. Thus, even a partial reduction in GRK2 is sufficient for the maximal effect, and this is of interest in view of the changes in the level of GRK2 that are observed in the context of, e.g. chronic inflammation (see below).

There is evidence that another member of the GRK family, GRK6, can also regulate the pain response, in particular, in the context of colonic inflammation and in the case of intraplantar cytokine-induced hyperalgesia [48–50].

Ferrari et al. used intrathecal administration of antisense oligodeoxynucleotides (asODN) to reduce GRK2 mRNA in sensory neurons in the DRG, although it should be noted that this approach likely also reduces GRK2 in other cells in the DRG as well as in cells in the spinal cord. Similar to our results in GRK2+/− mice, intrathecal injection of asODN against GRK2 enhanced and prolonged hyperalgesia induced by PGE2, carrageenan, and EPI [51]. Surprisingly, hyperalgesia induced by PGE2 administration even 1 week post asODN administration when GRK2 levels had recovered was still prolonged. Low GRK2 likely leads to neuroplastic changes in the nociceptors, which predisposes the animals to a latent hyper-responsiveness state resulting in chronic pain upon subsequent exposure to a stimulus that normally would induce only transient pain [51]. This phenomenon is defined as hyperalgesic priming [52]. It is unclear at present how transient reduction of GRK2 causes hyperalgesic priming and the long-lasting consequences for the duration of pain.

There is evidence that GRK2 deficiency not only alters the duration of the pain response, but also modifies in vivo inflammatory disease activity. For example, GRK2+/− mice show an advanced onset but decreased severity of experimental autoimmune encephalomyelitis [53]. The course of arthritis in mice is also altered by hemizygous deletion of GRK2; it aggravates this inflammatory disease [54]. Moreover, depletion of GRK2 in myeloid cells resulted in marked increase of lipopolysaccharide (LPS)-induced cytokines and chemokines production [55].

However, in our model of inflammatory pain, there is no evidence for an effect of GRK2 deletion on duration or severity of local inflammation in the paw, into which the sensitizing inflammatory stimulus was injected. For example, GRK2 levels did not affect either carrageenan or CCL3-induced paw inflammation, as no significant differences were observed in myeloperoxidase activity (neutrophil infiltration), IL-1β, CCL3, and TNFα mRNA levels, or paw thickness between WT and GRK2+/– mice [45, 46]. Moreover, depletion of mice from granulocytes did not affect the prolongation of the pain response in GRK2-deficient mice [46].

From studies in models of chronic pain induced by chronic inflammation or peripheral nerve injury, it is known that spinal cord microglial activation contributes to the persistence of hyperalgesia [56, 57]. Interestingly, the same is true for the prolonged pain response in GRK2-deficient mice. Specifically, Iba-1+ microglia in spinal cord of GRK2-deficient mice displayed a more activated phenotype relative to WT mice in the intraplantar carrageenan model of paw inflammation [46]. Furthermore, the prolonged thermal hyperalgesia induced by intraplantar injection of IL-1β into the hind paws of GRK2+/– mice was associated with persistent spinal cord microglial activation and increased mRNA levels of IL-1β, cathepsin S (fractalkine-releasing enzyme), and CX3CR1 (fractalkine receptor) in lumbar but not thoracic spinal cord in GRK2+/– mice. Intrathecal treatment to target the dorsal root ganglia and spinal cord with minocycline, an inhibitor of microglia/macrophage activation, prevented the prolongation of carrageenan, IL-1β- or CCL3-induced thermal hyperalgesia but did not reduce the maximal response in GRK2-deficient mice, suggesting spinal cord microglial/macrophage activity is required to maintain the prolonged hyperalgesic state in GRK2+/– mice in response to these stimuli [45]. In a rat model of trigeminal neuropathic pain, GRK2 was shown to be decreased in the medullary dorsal horn neurons. Administration of a calpain inhibitor, minocycline, or an astrocyte inhibitor, prevented downregulation of GRK2 and blocked the development of the neuropathic pain [58].

Additionally, injection of either a CX3CR1 antibody, IL-1 receptor antagonist (IL-1RA) or soluble TNF receptor (inhibitor of TNF signaling) reversed the prolonged inflammatory hyperalgesia in GRK2-deficient mice. Together these findings demonstrate that the prolonged hyperalgesia in GRK2-deficient mice is associated with persistent activation of a microglia-dependent local inflammatory pathway in the spinal cord, while peripheral inflammatory activity in the paw is not affected.

The MAPKinase p38 is an important regulator of microglial activity and cytokine production [59–61]. Consistent with a key role for p38 in spinal cord microglial activation and local cytokine production, the prolonged inflammatory hyperalgesia in GRK2-deficient mice was reversed by intrathecal administration of two different p38 inhibitors. The inhibitors also reduced microglial activation in the spinal cord [45, 62]. Administration of the p38 inhibitor also showed promise in a human study of neuropathic pain [63]; moreover, intrathecal administration of p38 inhibitors has been shown to inhibit spinal cord microglial activation and chronic neuropathic pain [62, 64, 65]. In a mouse model of painful diabetic neuropathy, inhibition of p38 was effective in preventing mechanical hyperalgesia [66].

In a rat model of complex regional pain syndrome type I following ischemia–reperfusion, treatment with either an α2-adrenergic receptor agonist (dexmedetomidine) or a serotonin reuptake inhibitor (paroxetine) normalized GRK2 expression levels in the superior cervical ganglion and prevented the development of mechanical hyperalgesia [67, 68]. In summary, hemizygous GRK2 knockout mice show prolonged hyperalgesia. Moreover, in response to specific GPCR ligands, hyperalgesia is increased in GRK2-deficient mice (see also below) [45–47].

Pain response involves multiple cell types and pain enhancement or suppression can occur at different levels. Glia (microglia and astrocytes) interacts with neurons to modulate their excitability and release inflammatory factors like cytokines and chemokines, which in turn act on neurons. To further understand the mechanisms via which GRK2 deficiency increases and prolongs hyperalgesia, the contribution of GRK2 in different cell types was determined using conditional knockout mice with cell-specific deletions of GRK2 in peripheral sensory neurons, monocytes/macrophages, and astrocytes (Fig. 1).

3.1 Neuronal GRK2 Deficiency

Different sets of sensory neurons respond to different stimuli and contribute to inflammatory, neuropathic, spontaneous, or chemotherapy pain. Small-diameter neurons in DRG (0.4–1.2 μm) are unmyelinated and belong to the family of C-afferent fibers, and contribute to 85% of the DRG nociceptive neurons [69, 70]. C-fibers are divided into peptidergic neurons (NGF and/or GDNF-positive IB4-negative) and non-peptidergic (GDNF-negative IB4-positive) neurons. In addition, large diameter neurons in the DRG also contribute to pain signaling. Distribution of GRK2 varies in different neuronal subtypes in the DRG. It is highly expressed in IB4(+) small diameter neurons, and levels are much lower in medium and large diameter neurons. Approximately 90% of the small diameter neurons expresses sodium channel $Na_v1.8$. $Na_v1.8$-positive small sensory neurons (also known as SNS) play a major role in inflammatory pain [71]. Therefore, to determine specific role of GRK2 in sensory neurons in determining the duration and severity of inflammatory pain, GRK2 was knocked down in $Na_v1.8+$ small-diameter peripheral sensory neurons using a Cre-Lox recombination system (SNS-GRK2+/− mice) [31, 46].

As briefly mentioned above, global GRK2 deficiency in all cells not only prolongs but also increases hyperalgesia induced by the GPCR ligands CCL3, PGE2, and EPI. In contrast, the response to IL-1β (a non-GPCR ligand) was prolonged but not increased. GRK2 deficiency in $Na_v1.8+$ nociceptors was sufficient to increase hyperalgesia induced by CCL3 and PGE2. One potential explanation for this observation would be that GRK2 deficiency leads to

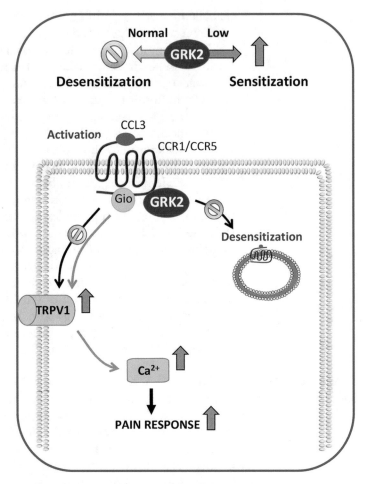

Fig. 2 GRK2 deficiency enhances CCL3-induced hyperalgesia through classical regulation of GPCR activity by GRK2. GRK2 regulates cellular responses by phosphorylating specific agonist-occupied GPCRs leading to termination of signaling by receptor desensitization. CCR1 and CCR5 activation by the chemokine CCL3 sensitizes TRPV1 channels in nociceptors leading to hyperalgesia. Low GRK2 leads to prolonged pain response by increasing CCL3-induced calcium signaling through the GPCRs CCR1/5 thereby enhancing TRPV1 sensitization [46]

impaired desensitization of the GPCRs for these ligands, resulting in increased signaling. Indeed, the existing evidence indicates that for CCL3, which binds to CCR1 and CCR5, this is the case. CCR1 and CCR5 receptors couple to $G_{i/o}$ proteins [72, 73], and activation of these receptors by CCL3 induces an increase in intracellular calcium concentrations [74]. Notably, the CCL3-induced calcium response was larger in primary sensory neurons from GRK2+/− relative to WT mice [46, 75]. CCL3 is thought to induce thermal hyperalgesia via sensitizing the temperature- and capsaicin-sensitive ion channel transient receptor potential V1 (TRPV1) (Fig. 2). Interestingly, in the absence of CCL3, reduced levels of GRK2 did not affect TRPV1 signaling, which is consistent with the normal thermal sensitivity of GRK2-deficient mice under baseline conditions. However, CCL3-induced TRPV1 sensitization was potentiated in GRK2+/− relative to WT mice [46]. Moreover, injection of the TRPV1 antagonist capsazepine before CCL3 administration reversed the acute thermal hyperalgesia in both WT and GRK2+/− mice [46]. These findings indicate that low nociceptor GRK2 causes an increase in CCR1/CCR5 sensitivity leading to increased sensitization of TRPV1 and increased thermal hyperalgesia. Consistent with a role of decreased sensitization in the aggravation of hyperalgesia in mice with low nociceptor GRK2, the pain response to IL-1β, which is not a GPCR ligand, was not affected. It is known that IL-1β promotes hyperalgesia via a p38/MAPK-dependent pathway in neurons leading to increased tetrodotoxin-resistant sodium currents causing thermal hypersensitivity. Notably, there is evidence that GRK2 directly inhibits p38/MAPK activation, independently of GPCR signaling, GRK2 deficiency is thought to promote cytokine production via this pathway [5]. Nevertheless, reduced levels of nociceptor GRK2 did not lead to an increase in the p38-mediated sensitization of these neurons by IL-1β treatment [45], indicating that the regulation of p38 activity by GRK2 may represent a cell-specific phenomenon.

The Gs-coupled β adrenergic receptors (βAR) were the first identified receptors regulated by GRK2 [76, 77]; their activation leads to increased cellular cAMP, and in vitro studies have clearly shown that decreased GRK2 leads to increased and prolonged β-adrenergic agonist-induced cAMP responses. In both global GRK2+/− and SNS-GRK2+/− mice, thermal and mechanical hyperalgesia induced by the adrenergic receptor agonist EPI were increased and prolonged (Table 1) [47]. ICI-118551 (βAR inverse agonist) but not phentolamine (αAR antagonist) reversed the EPI-induced mechanical hyperalgesia in both WT and GRK2-deficient mice indicating that βAR are responsible for mediating EPI-induced hyperalgesia in both genotypes [47]. PGE2, another GPCR ligand that signals via cAMP, also induced an enhanced and prolonged heat hyperalgesia in GRK2+/− as well as in SNS-GRK2+/− mice as compared to WT mice. The prolonged hyperalgesia in GRK2+/− mice in response to PGE2 was not caused by a change in the use of PGE2 receptor subtypes (Table 1) [31]. One potential explanation for these findings would be that GRK2 deficiency results in impaired desensitization of the βAR and EP receptors. Surprisingly, however, the prolongation of the pain response in SNS-GRK2+/− mice was also observed after intraplantar injection of 8-Br-cAMP, which induces hyperalgesia independently of GPCR stimulation [31]. Thus, it is unlikely that deficient GPCR desensitization is the main factor underlying the prolongation of the pain response in GRK2-deficient mice. Further studies into the underlying mechanism point toward a switch in cAMP signaling toward downstream kinases in mice with low GRK2 in nociceptors [29, 31].

It is well established that cAMP signals to PKA to enhance pain sensitivity [27, 29, 31]. Indeed, in WT mice, inhibition of the activation of the cAMP sensor protein kinase A (PKA) by H89 prevented EPI- and PGE2-induced mechanical hyperalgesia. However, EPI- and PGE2-induced hyperalgesia was not affected by inhibition of PKA in GRK2-deficient mice. Conversely, inhibition of PKCε by TAT-PKCεv1-2 or MEK by U0126 prevented EPI- and PGE2-induced hyperalgesia in SNS-GRK2+/− mice but not in their WT littermates [31, 47]. It has been shown that activation of the alternative cAMP-sensor Epac by intraplantar injection of its specific agonist 8-pCPT (8-(4-chlorophenylthio)-2′-O-methyladenosine 3′,5′-cyclic monophosphate monosodium) leads to prolonged pain via a PKCε- and ERK-dependent pathway as well [31, 78, 79]. Based on these findings, we propose a model, in which reduced GRK2 levels induce a switch in cAMP signaling from a PKA- to an Epac1-mediated PKCε/ERK-dependent pathway [31] as illustrated in Fig. 3.

In support of this model, SNS-GRK2+/− mice injected with the Epac-specific agonist 8-pCPT, or the Epac/PKA agonist 8-Br-cAMP (cell-permeable cAMP analog) also exhibited prolonged thermal and mechanical hyperalgesia relative to WT control mice (Table 1). However, when the PKA-specific cAMP analog 6-Bnz-cAMP was used, there was no prolongation of the pain response in GRK2-deficient mice (Table 1) [31]. Interestingly, a similar shift in cAMP-induced pain signaling from a PKA- to a PKCε-dependent pathway has been described before in a model of hyperalgesic priming by Levine and co-workers. In this model, transient hyperalgesia induced by, e.g. carrageenan or the PKCε activator ΨεRACK results in a long-lasting change in the nociceptor including a prolongation of hyperalgesia in response to subsequent exposure to PGE2 [33, 36]. This switch in signaling from PKA to PKCε was accompanied by a marked reduction in nociceptor GRK2 (in the case of carrageenan priming) or an increase in Epac1 (in the case of priming with ΨεRACK) expression levels in the DRG [33, 36, 80]. In vivo interventions to either increase intracellular GRK2 levels via administration of HSV (Herpes Simplex Virus) amplicons expressing GRK2 or to decrease Epac1 using asODN prevented the prolongation of the PGE2 response in primed mice [33, 81]. The model that emerges from studies in GRK2-deficient mice and in the model of priming is that the balance between GRK2 and Epac1 levels in primary nociceptors plays a key role in determining how cAMP signaling induces hyperalgesia. When GRK2 and Epac1 are normal, cAMP-inducing mediators will use PKA pathway to induce transient pain. When GRK2 is low and/or Epac1 is high, cAMP will also signal to an Epac1- and PKCε-mediated pathway that causes prolonged pain. In line with this model, DRG Epac1 levels are increased and GRK2 levels are decreased in the complete Freund's adjuvant model of chronic pain; increasing GRK2 or reducing Epac1 using the strategies mentioned above inhibits complete Freund's adjuvant (CFA)-induced hyperalgesia [33, 81].

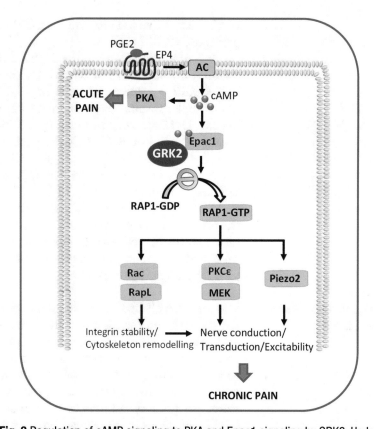

Fig. 3 Regulation of cAMP signaling to PKA and Epac1 signaling by GRK2. Under normal conditions, cAMP signals to protein kinase A leading to a transient increase in sensitivity to pain [29, 123]. cAMP can also signal to the cAMP sensor Epac1. GRK2 interacts with Epac1 and acts as an endogenous inhibitor of Epac1-to-RAP1 signaling. GRK2 deficiency in nociceptors prolongs hyperalgesia in response to cAMP-inducing agents like PGE2 by facilitating cAMP-to-Epac1 signaling [31, 33, 46]. Epac1 serves as guanine nucleotide exchange factor and catalyzes the exchange of GDP for GTP for Rap1 and Rap2, resulting in activation of these small GTP-binding proteins [124, 125]. Epac1 leads to hyperalgesia via activation of PKCε- and ERK-dependent signaling pathways [78]. Epac1 is also reported to sensitive Piezo2-dependent mechanical currents thereby contributing to hyperalgesia [34]. Rap1 crosstalks with RhoGTPases (Rho and Rac) and RapL to modulate cell adhesion and cell-to-cell junctions, which can interfere with integrin signaling and thereby contribute to pain [82]

Epac1 mRNA and protein expression levels are increased in models of chronic neuropathic pain caused by spinal nerve transection or chronic constriction injury of the sciatic nerve. The neuropathic pain that develops in these models is markedly attenuated in Epac1−/− and Epac1+/− mice as compared to their WT littermates. It is not completely clear at present how Epac1 activation leads to chronic pain. Proposed pathways include PKCε-mediated sensitization of specific ion channels, and/or sensitization of the mechanosensitive ion channel Piezo2 through an Epac1-mediated pathway [34, 82] (Fig. 3).

It is of interest to note that PGE2-induced thermal hyperalgesia in WT mice resolved within 4–6 h, and within 4–8 days in SNS-GRK2+/– mice, whereas in GRK2+/– mice it lasted 21 days. Similar results were obtained with 8-pCPT and 8-Br-cAMP (Table 1) [31]. In addition, CCL3-induced hyperalgesia was increased in SNS-GRK2-deficient mice, but not prolonged like in global GRK2-deficient mice. Moreover, carrageenan-induced hyperalgesia was less persistent in SNS-GRK2+/– as compared to GRK2+/– animals (Table 1) [46]. These findings indicate that low GRK2 in cell types other than the primary nociceptors contribute to the prolonged pain response observed in mice with global reduction of GRK2. The most likely candidates are astrocytes and microglia/monocytes that are known to contribute to pain signaling (Fig. 1) [46].

3.2 Astrocyte GRK2 Deficiency

It is well established that spinal cord astrocytes play a key role in the chronic pain that develops in models of neuropathic pain such as that induced by surgical damage to peripheral nerves or chemotherapy [83–86]. Astrocytes can regulate pain via multiple pathways, including production of chemokines and cytokines, and the uptake of glutamate. GRK2 is expressed in astrocytes and in vitro studies of primary cultures of murine astrocytes have shown that GRK2 deficiency in astrocytes increases the level of the membrane glutamate transporter GLAST, leading to increased glutamate uptake in GRK2-deficient astrocytes as compared to WT astrocytes [87]. GRK2 also regulates the response of astrocytes to the chemokine CCL2; GRK2 deficiency increases CCL2 signaling to Akt and ERK1/2. Conversely, culture of WT astrocytes with the pro-inflammatory cytokine IL-1β increases endogenous GRK2, which in turn led to a decrease in the CCL2-induced activation of Akt and of ERK1/2 [88]. In addition, although both chemokine and glutamate signaling are thought to contribute to persistent pain, we did not detect a role for astrocyte GRK2 in regulation of the pain response. The course of hyperalgesia induced by PGE2, carrageenan, EPI, CCL3, or IL-1β was not affected by cell-specific deletion of GRK2 in astrocytes [45–47].

3.3 Monocyte/ Macrophage GRK2 Deficiency

The prolonged hyperalgesic response of mice with global GRK2 deficiency is associated with persistent inflammatory activity in the spinal cord, as evidenced by microglial/macrophage activation and production of inflammatory mediators such as IL-1β and TNFα in the spinal cord [45, 46, 89]. In addition, chronic neuropathic pain in rats and chronic inflammatory pain in mice are associated with a decrease in GRK2 in spinal cord microglia/macrophages [45]. We did not directly assess the contribution of resting microglial GRK2 to the pain response. However, we determined the contribution of

GRK2 in systemic monocytes/macrophages to inflammatory pain using mice with reduced GRK2 specifically in lysozyme M (LysM)-positive myeloid cells. The LysM promoter is active in monocytes, macrophages, and granulocytes; however, the LysM promoter is not active in resting microglia [46]. It was already known that granulo-cytes do not contribute to the prolonged pain response in GRK2-deficient mice [46] and, therefore, LysM-GRK2-deficient mice represent an excellent model to study the role of GRK2 in systemic monocytes/macrophages in the regulation of pain. In response to intraplantar IL-1β, LysMGRK2+/− mice exhibited prolonged ther-mal and mechanical hyperalgesia up to 15 days relative to their WT littermates, which resolved within 24 h (Table 1) [45, 46, 90]. Similarly, thermal hyperalgesia induced by carrageenan or CCL3 was prolonged up to 20 and 10 days respectively in LysM-GRK2+/− mice as compared to 2–4 days in carrageenan-treated and 1 day in CCL3-treated WT mice (Table 1). In addition, EPI-induced hyper-algesia in LysM-GRK2+/− mice was prolonged as compared to control mice (Table 1) [47]. The prolonged hyperalgesia in LysMGRK2+/− mice was associated with increased and prolonged spinal cord microglial activation; specifically, the microglia/macro-phage activation M1 marker CD16/32 (pro-inflammatory) was sig-nificantly higher in the LysM-GRK2+/− relative to WT mice, whereas the M2 markers CD206 and arginase I (anti-inflammatory) were significantly lower; thus shifting the equilibrium toward a more pro-inflammatory pathway, which was associated with increased local TNFα and IL-1β production and ongoing p38 activity [46].

Spinal cord microglia of LysM-GRK2+/− mice had lower lev-els of miRNA-124 and increased expression of the transcription factor CCAAT-enhancer-binding protein-α in response to IL-1β as compared to WT mice [90]. In fact, administration of miRNA-124 normalized the M1/M2 balance and prevented the prolongation of IL-1β-induced hyperalgesia in GRK2-deficient mice [90].

As described above, spinal cord microglial GRK2 levels were completely normal in LysM-GRK2+/− mice with prolonged inflammatory hyperalgesia, indicating that the ongoing microglial activity in the spinal cord of LysM-GRK2+/− mice was a direct consequence of low GRK2 in monocytes/macrophages rather than caused by abnormal GRK2 in the microglia themselves [45, 46, 90]. This hypothesis is supported by the intriguing finding that transfer of WT monocytes to LysM-GRK2+/− mice normalizes the duration of inflammatory hyperalgesia. Conversely, depletion of peripheral macrophages in WT mice without depleting microg-lia prolonged inflammatory hyperalgesia. Thus, monocytes/mac-rophages are required for the normal resolution of inflammatory pain and either the absence of monocytes/macrophages or reduced levels of GRK2 in monocytes/macrophages prevent normal reso-lution of hyperalgesia leading to chronic pain.

In search for the underlying mechanisms, it has been shown that production of the anti-inflammatory cytokine IL-10 was decreased in GRK2+/− macrophages as compared to WT, while production of the pro-inflammatory cytokines IL-1β and TNFα was increased. Importantly, transfer of IL-10−/− monocytes to LysM-GRK2+/− mice did not prevent the persistent IL-1β-induced hyperalgesia [91]. Moreover, intrathecal injection of IL-10 inhibited IL-1β-induced thermal hyperalgesia in LysM-GRK2+/− mice, while administration of anti-IL-10 antibody delayed the resolution of IL-1β or carrageenan-induced hyperalgesia in WT mice [91]. These results indicate that peripheral monocytes/macrophages with normal levels of GRK2 produce IL-10, which is crucial for signaling in spinal cord and DRG for resolution of inflammatory hyperalgesia.

4   Regulation of GRK Levels

The findings summarized above indicate that changes in GRK2 protein level in specific cell types can have marked consequences for the development of chronic pain. This raises the question how GRK2 levels in cells are controlled.

In the context of pain, various studies have been performed. For example, we showed that persistent inflammatory pain was associated with decreased levels of GRK2 in lumbar spinal cord microglia/macrophages [45]. Moreover, in a rat model of chronic neuropathic pain induced by chronic constriction injury of the sciatic nerve, it has been shown that GRK2 expression levels were reduced in spinal cord microglia/macrophages [46]. Neuropathic pain induced by spinal nerve transection was associated with reduced GRK2 in spinal cord neurons [46, 92]. This reduction in neuronal GRK2 developed downstream of IL-1β signaling, because GRK2 was unchanged in mice deficient in the IL-1β receptor (IL-1R−/−). Consistently, IL-1β treatment of cultured spinal cord slices ex vivo also reduced expression of GRK2. Notably, IL-1R1-deficient mice were protected against nerve injury-induced mechanical hyperalgesia, which may indicate that the IL-1β-induced decrease in GRK2 expression contributes to the development of chronic hyperalgesia in this model [92, 93]. Further, intraplantar injection into the hind paw of the inflammatory agents CFA or carrageenan in mice led to a decrease in GRK2 protein levels in lumbar but not thoracic DRG neurons, in sciatic nerve fibers, and in spinal microglia/macrophages of these animals during inflammatory pain [33, 45]. Collectively, these findings indicate that inflammation induces a decrease in GRK2 in spinal cord and dorsal root ganglia that contributes to chronic neuropathic and inflammatory pain. Finally, not only GRK2 but also GRK6 levels were shown to be reduced in the dorsal horn of the lumbar spinal cord in a rat chronic constriction injury model, which was associated with both mechanical and heat hyperalgesia [94].

Additional evidence for regulation of GRK levels by inflammation comes from studies in humans with painful inflammatory disorders. For example, in peripheral blood mononuclear cells (PBMCs) of patients with rheumatoid arthritis (RA), GRK activity was markedly reduced relative to healthy controls. There was a significant decrease (~50%) in GRK2 protein levels with no changes in the mRNA levels, indicating that these changes represent posttranscriptional events. Moreover, a decrease in GRK2 levels was also observed in PBMC from patients with multiple sclerosis (MS) during all stages of the disease [19, 95]. The change in GRK2 protein levels in patients with autoimmune disease is thought to be due to the inflammatory process in multiple sclerosis, as GRK2 levels are not affected in leukocytes from patients who suffered neurological insults such as stroke [19]. In addition, the inflammatory response following cardiopulmonary bypass correlated with a significant decrease in both GRK2 and 6 expression levels in PBMCs [96]. In vitro treatment of PBMCs from healthy individuals with IL-6 or IFN-γ caused a significant decrease in GRK2 protein levels [20].

To assess whether the observed changes in GRK2 levels in humans with chronic inflammatory diseases are cause or consequence of the disease, animal models were used. In the adjuvant-induced model of rheumatoid arthritis in rats it was shown that GRK2, 3, and 6 protein levels were markedly reduced in splenocytes and mesenteric lymph nodes at the peak of the inflammation as compared to controls. Similarly, induction of experimental autoimmune encephalitis, an animal model of multiple sclerosis resulted in a decrease in splenocyte GRK2 levels. The role of inflammation and reactive oxygen species in the downregulation of GRK2 is further supported by studies in a model of cerebral hypoxic–ischemic (HI) insults. Reperfusion after a hypoxic ischemic insult is accompanied by generation of reactive oxygen species (ROS) and nitric oxide and a marked production of chemokines, which recruit immune cells and pro-inflammatory cytokines, including IL-1β, IL-6, and TNFα [97–100]. In the neonatal rat brain, HI was shown to cause a decrease in GRK2 protein levels with no changes in mRNA levels 24–48 h post HI, while arrestin2 protein and mRNA levels were increased 6–12 h following HI [101]. Decrease in GRK2 activity and protein levels was also described in an earlier study in an ischemic dog model following cardiac artery ligation. GRK2 activity as measured by its ability to desensitize β2 adrenergic receptor in arrhythmogenic subepicardial border zone tissue was decreased as compared to non-ischemic remote-site subepicardial tissue from the same animal [102]. It should be noted that there are also examples where inflammation is associated with an increase in cellular GRK2 levels. For example, expression of both GRK2 and GRK5 was markedly increased in neutrophils from patients with sepsis relative to controls [103]. In vitro, treatment of control neutrophils and macrophages with cytokines, lipopolysaccharide, or other Toll-like receptor agonists in vitro also increased expression of GRK2 [103–105]. It is likely that this apparent discrepancy can be explained by cell-specific changes in GRK2 in the context of inflammation. Peripheral blood mononuclear cells consist predominantly of lymphocytes with a smaller contribution of monocytes and an absence of neutrophils, the cell types in which an increase, rather than a decrease in GRK2 was reported.

Interestingly, in patients with RA or MS as well as in animal models, GRK protein levels were decreased, while mRNA levels were not altered. This indicates that the decrease in GRK2 protein level that was observed in the context of inflammation is regulated at the post-transcriptional level. This is consistent with in vitro studies from our group, showing that inflammatory mediators and oxidative stress reduce GRK2 via multiple pathways that are all independent of a change in GRK2 mRNA levels [19, 20, 106–108]. As an example of ROS-induced regulation of GRK2 protein levels, we observed that exposure of T lymphocytes to H_2O_2 led to a ~50% decrease in GRK2 protein levels as well as its activity as measured by the ability of GRK2 to phosphorylate rhodopsin in vitro. No changes in mRNA levels of GRK2 were detected under these conditions suggesting that the decreased levels of the protein was posttranscriptionally regulated (Fig. 4). Indeed, GRK2 was shown to be degraded via a calpain-mediated pathway presumably via a putative PEST region comprising residues 591–615 [106, 109]. Stimulation of calpain by reactive oxygen species activated the cdk1/mTOR pathway, which inhibits GRK translation [109]. Moreover, this study revealed that exposure of T cells to H_2O_2 led to a decrease in isoproterenol-stimulated β2AR internalization, consistent with a decrease in GRK2 protein levels and activity. It is also known that H_2O_2 treatment leads to activation of MAPK and PKC [110]; however, inhibition of these proteins in T lymphocytes did not prevent the decrease in GRK2 protein levels. In agreement with these findings, GRK2 expression levels were significantly decreased in cultures of hippocampal slices deprived of oxygen and glucose and this was associated with an increase in GRK2 phosphorylation at Ser670. Surprisingly, inhibition of ERK did not abolish degradation, nor decreased Ser670 phosphorylation but inhibition of PI3K prevented both its phosphorylation and degradation [111]. There are also examples of regulation of GRK at the mRNA level. Activity of the GRK2 promoter was shown to be reduced in vascular smooth muscle cells by the cytokines IFN-γ, TNFα, and IL-1β [112].

In summary, chronic inflammation in vivo is associated with changes in GRK2 protein levels in multiple cells and tissues. The reduction of GRK2 observed in the context of inflammation is most likely due to increased degradation and reduced translation rather than to changes in transcription.

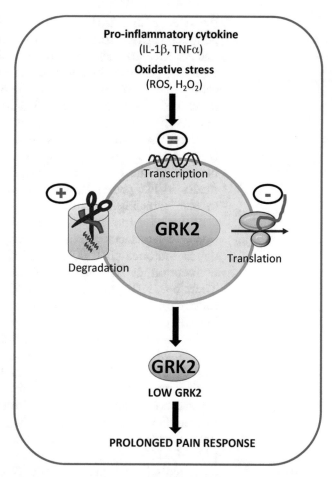

Fig. 4 Regulation of GRK2 expression in the context of inflammation. During chronic inflammation, cytokines like IL-1β and reactive oxygen species (ROS) reduce GRK2 protein levels via posttranscriptional mechanisms, including increased GRK2 degradation and reduced translation. We propose that low GRK2 levels in neurons and in inflammatory cells including monocytes enhance and prolong the pain response thereby promoting development of chronic pain

5   Conclusions

In this review, we summarized the evidence that GRK2 is a key regulator of pain; impaired GRK2 activity increases and prolongs the duration of pain. In other words, the GRK2 deficiency promotes transition to chronic pain. Interestingly, there are clear cell- and stimulus-specific mechanisms, via which adequate levels of GRK2 prevent transition to chronic pain. Although there is some evidence for a classical role of GRK2-mediated receptor desensitization in the regulation of the pain response, the findings compiled here mostly point to an alternative mechanism underlying pain regulation by GRK2. The best studied at the mechanistic level is the change in cAMP-dependent pain signaling that occurs in peripheral nociceptors when GRK2 is low; GRK2 deficiency in primary nociceptors allows activation of an Epac1-mediated cAMP signaling pathway in addition to the classical PKA-dependent route. At present, we do not know whether low GRK2 also promotes cAMP signaling to Epac1 with consequences for pathology outside the nervous system. Within the nervous system, however, we know that activation of nociceptor Epac1 signaling when GRK2 is low markedly prolongs pain. This is an important observation, because of the central role of cAMP signaling, downstream of mediators like prostaglandins, adenosine, and adrenergic agonists, in pain signaling. It is also important because it identifies the GRK2/Epac1 interface as a potential novel target for the prevention and treatment of chronic pain, especially since existing evidence indicates that GRK2 and Epac1 do not contribute to nociception in the absence of inflammation or tissue damage. Therefore, interfering with the GRK2-Epac1 pathway would not impact the acute, transient pain that serves a protective purpose, but will only affect the sensitization to pain that occurs in pathological conditions. However, we should not forget that GRK2 controls a wide array of pathophysiological responses and global stimulation of GRK2 activity or a global increase in GRK2 protein levels (if we had ways to accomplish this) are unlikely to be without adverse unwanted effects. It is already known, for example, that increased expression of GRK2 in the cardiovascular system in experimental animals leads to cardiac and blood pressure abnormalities [12–14, 113]. In addition, type 2 diabetes is associated with increased GRK2 expression and GRK2 deficiency protects against diet-induced obesity and type 2 diabetes [114, 115]. However, it is conceivable that local overexpression of GRK2 in nociceptors in an area affected by chronic pain using a virally mediated targeting could be developed clinically [33]. Indeed, a phase I clinical trial indicating the potential feasibility of such approach to locally overexpress an anti-nociceptive protein (enkephalin) has been completed [116]. Recently, specific Epac inhibitors that are active in vivo have been developed, and our preliminary data indicate that these inhibitors alleviate chronic pain in multiple models (unpublished results). In addition, so far no adverse effects of these inhibitors have been described in two preclinical studies: lethal rickettsiosis, and prevention of pancreatic tumor metastases [117–119].

The second key pathway via which low GRK2 promotes transition to chronic pain involves the initially unexpected cell type: the peripheral monocyte/infiltrating macrophage. Until recently, monocytes/macrophages were thought to have primarily adverse effects on pain. Our findings demonstrate that monocytes/macrophages with normal levels of GRK2 that are capable of producing adequate levels of IL-10 are required for the normal resolution of transient pain. The exact mechanism, via which GRK2 regulates IL-10 production by monocytes in the context of inflammatory pain, remains unclear; further studies are needed. It was already known that exogenously administered IL-10 can reduce pain in animal models, but the importance of endogenous IL-10 was only uncovered by our studies in GRK2-deficient mice [91]. Unfortunately, although exogenous IL-10 has pain-relieving effects in animal studies, these beneficial effects are transient. Our data further support the need for additional studies to develop more stable IL-10 analogues or ways to locally increase IL-10 production, e.g. as is being done by Watkins and colleagues [120]. An additional question is whether patients at risk for transitioning from acute to chronic pain have reduced monocyte GRK2 levels and/or impaired capacity to produce IL-10. Prospective clinical studies in patients undergoing surgery, patients suffering from Herpes zoster infection, or cancer patients treated with chemotherapy, of which a substantial subset is known to transition to chronic pain, should be performed to address this translational question.

Finally, even though mechanisms governing onset and maintenance of chronic neuropathic pain are not fully elucidated given the complexity of the various triggers, major breakthroughs have taken place. Clearly, GRK2 expression and activity play a central role in these pathways. In an effort to develop effective therapeutic strategies to relieve chronic neuropathic pain, one should target pathways that specifically inhibit the cAMP-Epac1 route, increase GRK2 or promote its activity (no current means available), or promote the anti-inflammatory pathway via delivery of IL-10.

Acknowledgements

The work of Drs. Kavelaars and Heijnen is supported by grants NS 073939, NS 074999, CA 183736, and CA 193522 from the National Institutes of Health and a STAR grant from the University of Texas System.

References

1. Winstel R, Freund S, Krasel C, Hoppe E, Lohse MJ (1996) Protein kinase cross-talk: membrane targeting of the beta-adrenergic receptor kinase by protein kinase C. Proc Natl Acad Sci U S A 93(5):2105–2109

2. Salcedo A, Mayor F Jr, Penela P (2006) Mdm2 is involved in the ubiquitination and degradation of G-protein-coupled receptor kinase 2. EMBO J 25(20):4752–4762

3. Liu S, Premont RT, Kontos CD, Zhu S, Rockey DC (2005) A crucial role for GRK2 in regulation of endothelial cell nitric oxide synthase function in portal hypertension. Nat Med 11(9):952–958

4. Naga Prasad SV, Laporte SA, Chamberlain D, Caron MG, Barak L, Rockman HA (2002) Phosphoinositide 3-kinase regulates beta2-adrenergic receptor endocytosis by AP-2 recruitment to the receptor/beta-arrestin complex. J Cell Biol 158(3):563–575

5. Peregrin S, Jurado-Pueyo M, Campos PM, Sanz-Moreno V, Ruiz-Gomez A, Crespo P, Mayor F Jr, Murga C (2006) Phosphorylation of p38 by GRK2 at the docking groove unveils a novel mechanism for inactivating p38MAPK. Curr Biol 16(20):2042–2047

6. Penela P, Ribas C, Aymerich I, Eijkelkamp N, Barreiro O, Heijnen CJ, Kavelaars A, Sanchez-

Madrid F, Mayor F Jr (2008) G protein-coupled receptor kinase 2 positively regulates epithelial cell migration. EMBO J 27(8):1206–1218

7. Cant SH, Pitcher JA (2005) G protein-coupled receptor kinase 2-mediated phosphorylation of ezrin is required for G protein-coupled receptor-dependent reorganization of the actin cytoskeleton. Mol Biol Cell 16(7):3088–3099

8. Carman CV, Som T, Kim CM, Benovic JL (1998) Binding and phosphorylation of tubulin by G protein-coupled receptor kinases. J Biol Chem 273(32):20308–20316

9. Pitcher JA, Hall RA, Daaka Y, Zhang J, Ferguson SS, Hester S, Miller S, Caron MG, Lefkowitz RJ, Barak LS (1998) The G protein-coupled receptor kinase 2 is a microtubule-associated protein kinase that phosphorylates tubulin. J Biol Chem 273(20):12316–12324

10. Freeman JL, Pitcher JA, Li X, Bennett V, Lefkowitz RJ (2000) alpha-Actinin is a potent regulator of G protein-coupled receptor kinase activity and substrate specificity in vitro. FEBS Lett 473(3):280–284

11. Yi XP, Gerdes AM, Li F (2002) Myocyte redistribution of GRK2 and GRK5 in hypertensive, heart-failure-prone rats. Hypertension 39(6):1058–1063

12. Ungerer M, Bohm M, Elce JS, Erdmann E, Lohse MJ (1993) Altered expression of beta-adrenergic receptor kinase and beta 1-adrenergic receptors in the failing human heart. Circulation 87(2):454–463

13. Iaccarino G, Keys JR, Rapacciuolo A, Shotwell KF, Lefkowitz RJ, Rockman HA, Koch WJ (2001) Regulation of myocardial betaARK1 expression in catecholamine-induced cardiac hypertrophy in transgenic mice overexpressing alpha1B-adrenergic receptors. J Am Coll Cardiol 38(2):534–540

14. Gros R, Chorazyczewski J, Meek MD, Benovic JL, Ferguson SS, Feldman RD (2000) G-Protein-coupled receptor kinase activity in hypertension : increased vascular and lymphocyte G-protein receptor kinase-2 protein expression. Hypertension 35(1 Pt 1):38–42

15. Martini JS, Raake P, Vinge LE, DeGeorge BR Jr, Chuprun JK, Harris DM, Gao E, Eckhart AD, Pitcher JA, Koch WJ (2008) Uncovering G protein-coupled receptor kinase-5 as a histone deacetylase kinase in the nucleus of cardiomyocytes. Proc Natl Acad Sci U S A 105(34):12457–12462

16. Kaur G, Kim J, Kaur R, Tan I, Bloch O, Sun MZ, Safaee M, Oh MC, Sughrue M, Phillips J, Parsa AT (2013) G-protein coupled receptor kinase (GRK)-5 regulates proliferation of glioblastoma-derived stem cells. J Clin Neurosci 20(7):1014–1018

17. Metaye T, Menet E, Guilhot J, Kraimps JL (2002) Expression and activity of g protein-coupled receptor kinases in differentiated thyroid carcinoma. J Clin Endocrinol Metab 87(7):3279–3286

18. Nakaya M, Tajima M, Kosako H, Nakaya T, Hashimoto A, Watari K, Nishihara H, Ohba M, Komiya S, Tani N, Nishida M, Taniguchi H, Sato Y, Matsumoto M, Tsuda M, Kuroda M, Inoue K, Kurose H (2013) GRK6 deficiency in mice causes autoimmune disease due to impaired apoptotic cell clearance. Nat Commun 4:1532

19. Vroon A, Kavelaars A, Limmroth V, Lombardi MS, Goebel MU, Van Dam AM, Caron MG, Schedlowski M, Heijnen CJ (2005) G protein-coupled receptor kinase 2 in multiple sclerosis and experimental autoimmune encephalomyelitis. J Immunol 174(7):4400–4406

20. Lombardi MS, Kavelaars A, Schedlowski M, Bijlsma JW, Okihara KL, Van de Pol M, Ochsmann S, Pawlak C, Schmidt RE, Heijnen CJ (1999) Decreased expression and activity of G-protein-coupled receptor kinases in peripheral blood mononuclear cells of patients with rheumatoid arthritis. FASEB J 13(6):715–725

21. Mak JC, Chuang TT, Harris CA, Barnes PJ (2002) Increased expression of G protein-coupled receptor kinases in cystic fibrosis lung. Eur J Pharmacol 436(3):165–172

22. Gainetdinov RR, Bohn LM, Sotnikova TD, Cyr M, Laakso A, Macrae AD, Torres GE, Kim KM, Lefkowitz RJ, Caron MG, Premont RT (2003) Dopaminergic supersensitivity in G protein-coupled receptor kinase 6-deficient mice. Neuron 38(2):291–303

23. Ferrer-Alcon M, La Harpe R, Garcia-Sevilla JA (2004) Decreased immunodensities of micro-opioid receptors, receptor kinases GRK 2/6 and beta-arrestin-2 in postmortem brains of opiate addicts. Brain Res Mol Brain Res 121(1–2):114–122

24. Garcia-Guerra L, Nieto-Vazquez I, Vila-Bedmar R, Jurado-Pueyo M, Zalba G, Diez J, Murga C, Fernandez-Veledo S, Mayor F Jr, Lorenzo M (2010) G protein-coupled receptor kinase 2 plays a relevant role in insulin resistance and obesity. Diabetes 59(10):2407–2417

25. Merskey H, Bogduk N (eds) (1994) Part III: pain terms, a current list with definitions and notes on usage. Classification of chronic pain, 2nd edn. IASP Press, Seattle, pp 209–214

26. Nahin RL (2015) Estimates of pain prevalence and severity in adults: United States, 2012. J Pain 16(8):769–780

27. Lolignier S, Eijkelkamp N, Wood JN (2015) Mechanical allodynia. Pflugers Arch 467(1):133–139

28. Wu LJ, Steenland HW, Kim SS, Isiegas C, Abel T, Kaang BK, Zhuo M (2008) Enhancement of presynaptic glutamate release and persistent inflammatory pain by increasing neuronal cAMP in the anterior cingulate cortex. Mol Pain 4:40

29. Hucho T, Levine JD (2007) Signaling pathways in sensitization: toward a nociceptor cell biology. Neuron 55(3):365–376

30. Song XJ, Wang ZB, Gan Q, Walters ET (2006) cAMP and cGMP contribute to sensory neuron hyperexcitability and hyperalgesia in rats with dorsal root ganglia compression. J Neurophysiol 95(1):479–492

31. Eijkelkamp N, Wang H, Garza-Carbajal A, Willemen HL, Zwartkruis FJ, Wood JN, Dantzer R, Kelley KW, Heijnen CJ, Kavelaars A (2010) Low nociceptor GRK2 prolongs prostaglandin E2 hyperalgesia via biased cAMP signaling to Epac/Rap1, protein kinase Cepsilon, and MEK/ERK. J Neurosci 30(38):12806–12815

32. Parada CA, Reichling DB, Levine JD (2005) Chronic hyperalgesic priming in the rat involves a novel interaction between cAMP and PKCepsilon second messenger pathways. Pain 113(1–2):185–190

33. Wang H, Heijnen CJ, van Velthoven CT, Willemen HL, Ishikawa Y, Zhang X, Sood AK, Vroon A, Eijkelkamp N, Kavelaars A (2013) Balancing GRK2 and EPAC1 levels prevents and relieves chronic pain. J Clin Invest 123(12):5023–5034

34. Eijkelkamp N, Linley JE, Torres JM, Bee L, Dickenson AH, Gringhuis M, Minett MS, Hong GS, Lee E, Oh U, Ishikawa Y, Zwartkuis FJ, Cox JJ, Wood JN (2013) A role for Piezo2 in EPAC1-dependent mechanical allodynia. Nat Commun 4:1682

35. Shi X, Guo TZ, Wei T, Li WW, Clark DJ, Kingery WS (2015) Facilitated spinal neuropeptide signaling and upregulated inflammatory mediator expression contribute to post-fracture nociceptive sensitization. Pain 156(10):1852–1863

36. Ferrari LF, Araldi D, Levine JD (2015) Distinct terminal and cell body mechanisms in the nociceptor mediate hyperalgesic priming. J Neurosci 35(15):6107–6116

37. Ferrari LF, Bogen O, Reichling DB, Levine JD (2015) Accounting for the delay in the transition from acute to chronic pain: axonal and nuclear mechanisms. J Neurosci 35(2):495–507

38. Aley KO, Messing RO, Mochly-Rosen D, Levine JD (2000) Chronic hypersensitivity for inflammatory nociceptor sensitization mediated by the epsilon isozyme of protein kinase C. J Neurosci 20(12):4680–4685

39. Bogen O, Dina OA, Gear RW, Levine JD (2009) Dependence of monocyte chemoattractant protein 1 induced hyperalgesia on the isolectin B4-binding protein versican. Neuroscience 159(2):780–786

40. Meert TF, Vissers K, Geenen F, Kontinen VK (2003) Functional role of exogenous administration of substance P in chronic constriction injury model of neuropathic pain in gerbils. Pharmacol Biochem Behav 76(1):17–25

41. White FA, Sun J, Waters SM, Ma C, Ren D, Ripsch M, Steflik J, Cortright DN, Lamotte RH, Miller RJ (2005) Excitatory monocyte chemoattractant protein-1 signaling is up-regulated in sensory neurons after chronic compression of the dorsal root ganglion. Proc Natl Acad Sci U S A 102(39):14092–14097

42. Dina OA, McCarter GC, de Coupade C, Levine JD (2003) Role of the sensory neuron cytoskeleton in second messenger signaling for inflammatory pain. Neuron 39(4):613–624

43. Ribas C, Penela P, Murga C, Salcedo A, Garcia-Hoz C, Jurado-Pueyo M, Aymerich I, Mayor F Jr (2007) The G protein-coupled receptor kinase (GRK) interactome: role of GRKs in GPCR regulation and signaling. Biochim Biophys Acta 1768(4):913–922

44. Jaber M, Koch WJ, Rockman H, Smith B, Bond RA, Sulik KK, Ross J Jr, Lefkowitz RJ, Caron MG, Giros B (1996) Essential role of beta-adrenergic receptor kinase 1 in cardiac development and function. Proc Natl Acad Sci U S A 93(23):12974–12979

45. Willemen HL, Eijkelkamp N, Wang H, Dantzer R, Dorn GW 2nd, Kelley KW, Heijnen CJ, Kavelaars A (2010) Microglial/macrophage GRK2 determines duration of peripheral IL-1beta-induced hyperalgesia: contribution of spinal cord CX3CR1, p38 and IL-1 signaling. Pain 150(3):550–560

46. Eijkelkamp N, Heijnen CJ, Willemen HL, Deumens R, Joosten EA, Kleibeuker W, den Hartog IJ, van Velthoven CT, Nijboer C, Nassar MA, Dorn GW 2nd, Wood JN, Kavelaars A (2010) GRK2: a novel cell-specific regulator of severity and duration of inflammatory pain. J Neurosci 30(6):2138–2149

47. Wang H, Heijnen CJ, Eijkelkamp N, Garza Carbajal A, Schedlowski M, Kelley KW, Dantzer R, Kavelaars A (2011) GRK2 in sensory neurons regulates epinephrine-induced signalling and duration of mechanical hyperalgesia. Pain 152(7):1649–1658

48. Eijkelkamp N, Heijnen CJ, Lucas A, Premont RT, Elsenbruch S, Schedlowski M, Kavelaars A (2007) G protein-coupled receptor kinase 6 controls chronicity and severity of dextran sodium sulphate-induced colitis in mice. Gut 56(6):847–854

49. Eijkelkamp N, Heijnen CJ, Elsenbruch S, Holtmann G, Schedlowski M, Kavelaars A (2009) G protein-coupled receptor kinase 6 controls post-inflammatory visceral hyperalgesia. Brain Behav Immun 23(1):18–26

50. Eijkelkamp N, Heijnen CJ, Carbajal AG, Willemen HL, Wang H, Minett MS, Wood JN, Schedlowski M, Dantzer R, Kelley KW, Kavelaars A (2012) G protein-coupled receptor kinase 6 acts as a critical regulator of cytokine-induced hyperalgesia by promoting phosphatidylinositol 3-kinase and inhibiting p38 signaling. Mol Med 18:556–564

51. Ferrari LF, Bogen O, Alessandri-Haber N, Levine E, Gear RW, Levine JD (2012) Transient decrease in nociceptor GRK2 expression produces long-term enhancement in inflammatory pain. Neuroscience 222:392–403

52. Reichling DB, Levine JD (2009) Critical role of nociceptor plasticity in chronic pain. Trends Neurosci 32(12):611–618

53. Haerter K, Vroon A, Kavelaars A, Heijnen CJ, Limmroth V, Espinosa E, Schedlowski M, Elsenbruch S (2004) In vitro adrenergic modulation of cellular immune functions in experimental autoimmune encephalomyelitis. J Neuroimmunol 146(1–2):126–132

54. Tarrant TK, Rampersad RR, Esserman D, Rothlein LR, Liu P, Premont RT, Lefkowitz RJ, Lee DM, Patel DD (2008) Granulocyte chemotaxis and disease expression are differentially regulated by GRK subtype in an acute inflammatory arthritis model (K/BxN). Clin Immunol 129(1):115–122

55. Patial S, Saini Y, Parvataneni S, Appledorn DM, Dorn GW 2nd, Lapres JJ, Amalfitano A, Senagore P, Parameswaran N (2011) Myeloid-specific GPCR kinase-2 negatively regulates NF-kappaB1p105-ERK pathway and limits endotoxemic shock in mice. J Cell Physiol 226(3):627–637

56. DeLeo JA, Tanga FY, Tawfik VL (2004) Neuroimmune activation and neuroinflammation in chronic pain and opioid tolerance/hyperalgesia. Neuroscientist 10(1):40–52

57. Milligan ED, Watkins LR (2009) Pathological and protective roles of glia in chronic pain. Nat Rev Neurosci 10(1):23–36

58. Won KA, Kim MJ, Yang KY, Park JS, Lee MK, Park MK, Bae YC, Ahn DK (2014) The glial-neuronal GRK2 pathway participates in the development of trigeminal neuropathic pain in rats. J Pain 15(3):250–261

59. Noguchi K, Okubo M (2011) Leukotrienes in nociceptive pathway and neuropathic/inflammatory pain. Biol Pharm Bull 34(8):1163–1169

60. Ji RR, Gereau RW, Malcangio M, Strichartz GR (2009) MAP kinase and pain. Brain Res Rev 60(1):135–148

61. Gao YJ, Ji RR (2010) Chemokines, neuronal-glial interactions, and central processing of neuropathic pain. Pharmacol Ther 126(1):56–68

62. Willemen HL, Campos PM, Lucas E, Morreale A, Gil-Redondo R, Agut J, Gonzalez FV, Ramos P, Heijnen C, Mayor F Jr, Kavelaars A, Murga C (2014) A novel p38 MAPK docking-groove-targeted compound is a potent inhibitor of inflammatory hyperalgesia. Biochem J 459(3):427–439

63. Anand P, Shenoy R, Palmer JE, Baines AJ, Lai RY, Robertson J, Bird N, Ostenfeld T, Chizh BA (2011) Clinical trial of the p38 MAP kinase inhibitor dilmapimod in neuropathic pain following nerve injury. Eur J Pain 15(10):1040–1048

64. Ji RR, Suter MR (2007) p38 MAPK, microglial signaling, and neuropathic pain. Mol Pain 3:33

65. Wen YR, Tan PH, Cheng JK, Liu YC, Ji RR (2011) Microglia: a promising target for treating neuropathic and postoperative pain, and morphine tolerance. J Formos Med Assoc 110(8):487–494

66. Cheng HT, Dauch JR, Oh SS, Hayes JM, Hong Y, Feldman EL (2010) p38 mediates mechanical allodynia in a mouse model of type 2 diabetes. Mol Pain 6:28

67. Tang J, Dong J, Yang L, Gao L, Zheng J (2015) Paroxetine alleviates rat limb post-ischemia induced allodynia through GRK2 upregulation in superior cervical ganglia. Int J Clin Exp Med 8(2):2065–2076

68. Dong J, Yang L, Tang J, Zheng J (2015) Dexmedetomidine alleviates rat post-ischemia induced allodynia through GRK2 upregulation in superior cervical ganglia. Auton Neurosci 187:76–83

69. Woolf CJ, Ma Q (2007) Nociceptors—noxious stimulus detectors. Neuron 55(3):353–364

70. Gold MS, Gebhart GF (2010) Nociceptor sensitization in pain pathogenesis. Nat Med 16(11):1248–1257

71. Das V (2015) An introduction to pain pathways and pain "targets". Prog Mol Biol Transl Sci 131:1–30

72. Gilliland CT, Salanga CL, Kawamura T, Trejo J, Handel TM (2013) The chemokine receptor CCR1 is constitutively active, which leads to G protein-independent, beta-arrestin-mediated internalization. J Biol Chem 288(45):32194–32210

73. Scholten DJ, Canals M, Maussang D, Roumen L, Smit MJ, Wijtmans M, de Graaf C, Vischer HF, Leurs R (2012) Pharmacological modulation of chemokine receptor function. Br J Pharmacol 165(6):1617–1643

74. Nardelli B, Tiffany HL, Bong GW, Yourey PA, Morahan DK, Li Y, Murphy PM, Alderson RF (1999) Characterization of the signal transduction pathway activated in human monocytes and dendritic cells by MPIF-1, a specific ligand for CC chemokine receptor 1. J Immunol 162(1):435–444

75. Vroon A, Heijnen CJ, Lombardi MS, Cobelens PM, Mayor F Jr, Caron MG, Kavelaars A (2004) Reduced GRK2 level in T cells potentiates chemotaxis and signaling in response to CCL4. J Leukoc Biol 75(5):901–909

76. Sterne-Marr R, Leahey PA, Bresee JE, Dickson HM, Ho W, Ragusa MJ, Donnelly RM, Amie SM, Krywy JA, Brookins-Danz ED, Orakwue SC, Carr MJ, Yoshino-Koh K, Li Q, Tesmer JJ (2009) GRK2 activation by receptors: role of the kinase large lobe and carboxyl-terminal tail. Biochemistry 48(20):4285–4293

77. Pao CS, Barker BL, Benovic JL (2009) Role of the amino terminus of G protein-coupled receptor kinase 2 in receptor phosphorylation. Biochemistry 48(30):7325–7333

78. Hucho TB, Dina OA, Levine JD (2005) Epac mediates a cAMP-to-PKC signaling in inflammatory pain: an isolectin B4(+) neuron-specific mechanism. J Neurosci 25(26):6119–6126

79. Wang C, Gu Y, Li GW, Huang LY (2007) A critical role of the cAMP sensor Epac in switching protein kinase signalling in prostaglandin E2-induced potentiation of P2X3 receptor currents in inflamed rats. J Physiol 584(Pt 1):191–203

80. Kandasamy R, Price TJ (2015) The pharmacology of nociceptor priming. Handb Exp Pharmacol 227:15–37

81. Singhmar P, Huo X, Eijkelkamp N, Berciano SR, Baameur F, Mei FC, Zhu Y, Cheng X, Hawke D, Mayor F, Jr., Murga C, Heijnen CJ, Kavelaars A (2016) Critical role for Epac1 in inflammatory pain controlled by GRK2-mediated phosphorylation of Epac1. Proceedings of the National Academy of Sciences of the United States of America. doi:10.1073/pnas.1516036113

82. Dina OA, Parada CA, Yeh J, Chen X, McCarter GC, Levine JD (2004) Integrin signaling in inflammatory and neuropathic pain in the rat. Eur J Neurosci 19(3):634–642

83. Gao YJ, Ji RR (2010) Targeting astrocyte signaling for chronic pain. Neurotherapeutics 7(4):482–493

84. Morioka N, Zhang FF, Nakamura Y, Kitamura T, Hisaoka-Nakashima K, Nakata Y (2015) Tumor necrosis factor-mediated downregulation of spinal astrocytic connexin43 leads to increased glutamatergic neurotransmission and neuropathic pain in mice. Brain Behav Immun 49:293–310

85. Ji XT, Qian NS, Zhang T, Li JM, Li XK, Wang P, Zhao DS, Huang G, Zhang L, Fei Z, Jia D, Niu L (2013) Spinal astrocytic activation contributes to mechanical allodynia in a rat chemotherapy-induced neuropathic pain model. PLoS One 8(4):e60733

86. Yoon SY, Robinson CR, Zhang H, Dougherty PM (2013) Spinal astrocyte gap junctions contribute to oxaliplatin-induced mechanical hypersensitivity. J Pain 14(2):205–214

87. Nijboer CH, Heijnen CJ, Degos V, Willemen HL, Gressens P, Kavelaars A (2013) Astrocyte GRK2 as a novel regulator of glutamate transport and brain damage. Neurobiol Dis 54:206–215

88. Kleibeuker W, Jurado-Pueyo M, Murga C, Eijkelkamp N, Mayor F Jr, Heijnen CJ, Kavelaars A (2008) Physiological changes in GRK2 regulate CCL2-induced signaling to ERK1/2 and Akt but not to MEK1/2 and calcium. J Neurochem 104(4):979–992

89. Winkelstein BA, Rutkowski MD, Sweitzer SM, Pahl JL, DeLeo JA (2001) Nerve injury proximal or distal to the DRG induces similar spinal glial activation and selective cytokine expression but differential behavioral responses to pharmacologic treatment. J Comp Neurol 439(2):127–139

90. Willemen HL, Huo XJ, Mao-Ying QL, Zijlstra J, Heijnen CJ, Kavelaars A (2012) MicroRNA-124 as a novel treatment for persistent hyperalgesia. J Neuroinflammation 9:143

91. Willemen HL, Eijkelkamp N, Garza Carbajal A, Wang H, Mack M, Zijlstra J, Heijnen CJ, Kavelaars A (2014) Monocytes/macrophages control resolution of transient inflammatory pain. J Pain 15(5):496–506

92. Kleibeuker W, Gabay E, Kavelaars A, Zijlstra J, Wolf G, Ziv N, Yirmiya R, Shavit Y, Tal M, Heijnen CJ (2008) IL-1 beta signaling is required for mechanical allodynia induced by nerve injury and for the ensuing reduction in spinal cord neuronal GRK2. Brain Behav Immun 22(2):200–208

93. Kleibeuker W, Ledeboer A, Eijkelkamp N, Watkins LR, Maier SF, Zijlstra J, Heijnen CJ, Kavelaars A (2007) A role for G protein-coupled receptor kinase 2 in mechanical allodynia. Eur J Neurosci 25(6):1696–1704

94. Zhou Y, Huang X, Wu H, Xu Y, Tao T, Xu G, Cheng C, Cao S (2013) Decreased expression and role of GRK6 in spinal cord of rats after chronic constriction injury. Neurochem Res 38(10):2168–2179

95. Giorelli M, Livrea P, Trojano M (2004) Post-receptorial mechanisms underlie functional disregulation of beta2-adrenergic receptors in lymphocytes from Multiple Sclerosis patients. J Neuroimmunol 155(1–2):143–149

96. Hagen SA, Kondyra AL, Grocott HP, El-Moalem H, Bainbridge D, Mathew JP, Newman MF, Reves JG, Schwinn DA, Kwatra MM (2003) Cardiopulmonary bypass decreases G protein-coupled receptor kinase activity and expression in human peripheral blood mononuclear cells. Anesthesiology 98(2):343–348

97. Bona E, Andersson AL, Blomgren K, Gilland E, Puka-Sundvall M, Gustafson K, Hagberg H (1999) Chemokine and inflammatory cell response to hypoxia-ischemia in immature rats. Pediatr Res 45(4 Pt 1):500–509

98. Liu F, McCullough LD (2013) Inflammatory responses in hypoxic ischemic encephalopathy. Acta Pharmacol Sin 34(9):1121–1130

99. van den Tweel ER, Nijboer C, Kavelaars A, Heijnen CJ, Groenendaal F, van Bel F (2005) Expression of nitric oxide synthase isoforms and nitrotyrosine formation after hypoxia-ischemia in the neonatal rat brain. J Neuroimmunol 167(1–2):64–71

100. van den Tweel ER, Kavelaars A, Lombardi MS, Nijboer CH, Groenendaal F, van Bel F, Heijnen CJ (2006) Bilateral molecular changes in a neonatal rat model of unilateral hypoxic-ischemic brain damage. Pediatr Res 59(3):434–439

101. Lombardi MS, van den Tweel E, Kavelaars A, Groenendaal F, van Bel F, Heijnen CJ (2004) Hypoxia/ischemia modulates G protein-coupled receptor kinase 2 and beta-arrestin-1 levels in the neonatal rat brain. Stroke 35(4):981–986

102. Yu X, Zhang M, Kyker K, Patterson E, Benovic JL, Kem DC (2000) Ischemic inactivation of G protein-coupled receptor kinase and altered desensitization of canine cardiac beta-adrenergic receptors. Circulation 102(20):2535–2540

103. Arraes SM, Freitas MS, da Silva SV, de Paula Neto HA, Alves-Filho JC, Auxiliadora Martins M, Basile-Filho A, Tavares-Murta BM, Barja-Fidalgo C, Cunha FQ (2006) Impaired neutrophil chemotaxis in sepsis associates with GRK expression and inhibition of actin assembly and tyrosine phosphorylation. Blood 108(9):2906–2913

104. Loniewski K, Shi Y, Pestka J, Parameswaran N (2008) Toll-like receptors differentially regulate GPCR kinases and arrestins in primary macrophages. Mol Immunol 45(8):2312–2322

105. Alves-Filho JC, Freitas A, Souto FO, Spiller F, Paula-Neto H, Silva JS, Gazzinelli RT, Teixeira MM, Ferreira SH, Cunha FQ (2009) Regulation of chemokine receptor by Toll-like receptor 2 is critical to neutrophil migration and resistance to polymicrobial sepsis. Proc Natl Acad Sci U S A 106(10):4018–4023

106. Lombardi MS, Kavelaars A, Penela P, Scholtens EJ, Roccio M, Schmidt RE, Schedlowski M, Mayor F Jr, Heijnen CJ (2002) Oxidative stress decreases G protein-coupled receptor kinase 2 in lymphocytes via a calpain-dependent mechanism. Mol Pharmacol 62(2):379–388

107. Lombardi MS, Kavelaars A, Cobelens PM, Schmidt RE, Schedlowski M, Heijnen CJ (2001) Adjuvant arthritis induces down-regulation of G protein-coupled receptor kinases in the immune system. J Immunol 166(3):1635–1640

108. Vroon A, Heijnen CJ, Kavelaars A (2006) GRKs and arrestins: regulators of migration and inflammation. J Leukoc Biol 80(6):1214–1221

109. Cobelens PM, Kavelaars A, Heijnen CJ, Ribas C, Mayor F Jr, Penela P (2007) Hydrogen peroxide impairs GRK2 translation via a calpain-dependent and cdk1-mediated pathway. Cell Signal 19(2):269–277

110. Abe MK, Kartha S, Karpova AY, Li J, Liu PT, Kuo WL, Hershenson MB (1998) Hydrogen peroxide activates extracellular signal-regulated kinase via protein kinase C, Raf-1, and MEK1. Am J Respir Cell Mol Biol 18(4):562–569

111. Lombardi MS, Vroon A, Sodaar P, van Muiswinkel FL, Heijnen CJ, Kavelaars A (2007) Down-regulation of GRK2 after oxygen and glucose deprivation in rat hippocampal slices: role of the PI3-kinase pathway. J Neurochem 102(3):731–740

112. Ramos-Ruiz R, Penela P, Penn RB, Mayor F Jr (2000) Analysis of the human G protein-coupled receptor kinase 2 (GRK2) gene promoter: regulation by signal transduction systems in aortic smooth muscle cells. Circulation 101(17):2083–2089

113. Woodall MC, Ciccarelli M, Woodall BP, Koch WJ (2014) G protein-coupled receptor kinase 2: a link between myocardial contractile function and cardiac metabolism. Circ Res 114(10):1661–1670

114. Mayor F Jr, Lucas E, Jurado-Pueyo M, Garcia-Guerra L, Nieto-Vazquez I, Vila-Bedmar R, Fernandez-Veledo S, Murga C (2011) G Protein-coupled receptor kinase 2 (GRK2): a novel modulator of insulin resistance. Arch Physiol Biochem 117(3):125–130

115. Vila-Bedmar R, Cruces-Sande M, Lucas E, Willemen HL, Heijnen CJ, Kavelaars A, Mayor F Jr, Murga C (2015) Reversal of diet-induced obesity and insulin resistance by inducible genetic ablation of GRK2. Sci Signal 8(386):ra73

116. Wolfe D, Wechuck J, Krisky D, Mata M, Fink DJ (2009) A clinical trial of gene therapy for chronic pain. Pain Med 10(7):1325–1330

117. Chen H, Wild C, Zhou X, Ye N, Cheng X, Zhou J (2014) Recent advances in the discovery of small molecules targeting exchange proteins directly activated by cAMP (EPAC). J Med Chem 57(9):3651–3665

118. Gong B, Shelite T, Mei FC, Ha T, Hu Y, Xu G, Chang Q, Wakamiya M, Ksiazek TG, Boor PJ, Bouyer DH, Popov VL, Chen J, Walker DH, Cheng X (2013) Exchange protein directly activated by cAMP plays a critical role in bacterial invasion during fatal rickettsioses. Proc Natl Acad Sci U S A 110(48):19615–19620

119. Almahariq M, Tsalkova T, Mei FC, Chen H, Zhou J, Sastry SK, Schwede F, Cheng X (2013) A novel EPAC-specific inhibitor suppresses pancreatic cancer cell migration and invasion. Mol Pharmacol 83(1):122–128

120. Kwilasz AJ, Grace PM, Serbedzija P, Maier SF, Watkins LR (2015) The therapeutic potential of interleukin-10 in neuroimmune diseases. Neuropharmacology 96(Pt A):55–69

121. Basbaum AI, Bautista DM, Scherrer G, Julius D (2009) Cellular and molecular mechanisms of pain. Cell 139(2):267–284

122. Kuner R (2010) Central mechanisms of pathological pain. Nat Med 16(11):1258–1266

123. Eijkelkamp N, Singhmar P, Heijnen CJ, Kavelaars A (2015) Sensory neuron cAMP signaling in chronic pain. Cyclic Nucleotide Signaling 13:113

124. de Rooij J, Zwartkruis FJ, Verheijen MH, Cool RH, Nijman SM, Wittinghofer A, Bos JL (1998) Epac is a Rap1 guanine-nucleotide-exchange factor directly activated by cyclic AMP. Nature 396(6710):474–477

125. Kawasaki H, Springett GM, Mochizuki N, Toki S, Nakaya M, Matsuda M, Housman DE, Graybiel AM (1998) A family of cAMP-binding proteins that directly activate Rap1. Science 282(5397):2275–2279

Chapter 10

Roles of GRK Dysfunction in Alzheimer's Pathogenesis

William Z. Suo

Abstract

G protein-coupled receptors (GPCRs) mediate a wide variety of physiological functions. GPCR signaling, once activated, is subsequently dampened by receptor desensitization, a procedure initiated by a group of kinases, including GPCR kinases (GRKs). GRK2 upregulation and GRK5 deficiency were reported to occur in Alzheimer's disease. GRK2 accumulation was proposed to participate in cerebral vascular pathology, whereas GRK5 deficiency is believed to mediate the Alzheimer's cholinergic neuronal dysfunction and degeneration via the impaired M2/M4 muscarinic receptor desensitization. The GRK dysfunction can be experimentally caused by ß-amyloid, while the subsequent cerebral vascular dysfunction and cholinergic deficiency in turn may worsen the ß-amyloidogenesis. Therefore, the GRK dysfunction appears to link the ß-amyloid accumulation to the cerebrovascular degeneration and the cholinergic degeneration in Alzheimer's disease. Given that the ß-amyloid hypothesis, the cholinergic hypothesis, and the cerebrovascular hypothesis are all important mainstream hypotheses that are actively pursued to explain the Alzheimer's pathogenesis, further exploration of their relations may reveal therapeutic strategies that can break their pathogenic links.

Key words G protein, Neurodegeneration, Kinase, Cholinergic, Cerebrovasculature, Alzheimer, Pathogenesis

1 Introduction

Alzheimer's disease (AD) affects 5.4 million Americans, and this number is projected to double by 2020. AD is one of the most persistent and devastating dementias with little or no effective disease-modifying therapies. The cost of care for this particular patient population is disproportionately high, since they require expensive support. According to the Alzheimer's Association, the cost of care was $183 billion in 2010, which did not include 14.9 million in services provided by unpaid caregivers. Therefore, advances with translational potentials are highly appreciable and desperately needed.

AD is a neurodegenerative disorder, clinically characterized by progressive loss of memory and other cognitive functions, and pathologically—by accumulation of senile plaques (SPs) and neurofibrillary tangles (NFTs) in the limbic system and

Vsevolod V. Gurevich et al. (eds.), *G Protein-Coupled Receptor Kinases*, Methods in Pharmacology and Toxicology, DOI 10.1007/978-1-4939-3798-1_10, © Springer Science+Business Media New York 2016

association cortices [1–4]. There have been many hypotheses for AD, such as cholinergic hypothesis, amyloid hypothesis, tau hypothesis, glucose metabolism hypothesis, inflammatory hypothesis, cerebrovascular hypothesis, oxidative stress hypothesis, and aluminum hypothesis [5–15]. Indeed, each hypothesis has its own supportive evidence and explains certain aspects of the disease process, yet links or relations between these different hypotheses remain to be revealed before a unifying hypothesis is born. Numerous reviews have been written to summarize advances in the mainstream hypotheses; this chapter instead briefly describes recent progress related to the dysfunction of G protein-coupled receptor (GPCR) kinase-2/5 (GRK2/GRK5) in AD, and discusses its relation to other hypotheses and the relevant future perspectives.

2 Characteristics of GRK2/5 Distribution and Function

2.1 GRK Family

GRK is a small family (seven members) of serine/threonine protein kinases first discovered through its role in receptor desensitization [16–18]. GRK family members can be subdivided into three main groups based on sequence homology: rhodopsin kinase or visual GRK subfamily (GRK1/GRK7), the ß-adrenergic receptor kinases subfamily (GRK2/GRK3), and the GRK4 subfamily (GRK4/GRK5/GRK6). These kinases share certain characteristics but are distinct enzymes with specific regulatory properties.

All GRK members contain a centrally located 263-266 amino acid (a.a.) catalytic domain flanked by large amino- and carboxyl-terminal regulatory domains [19]. The amino-terminal domains share a common size (~185 a.a.) and demonstrate a fair degree of structural homology. These characteristics have led to the speculation that amino-terminal domains may perform a common function in all GRK members, potentially that of receptor recognition. The primary function of GRK is to desensitize activated GPCRs via a negative regulative process comprising phosphorylation of the activated receptor, uncoupling the receptor-G-protein binding and initiation of the receptor internalization. GRK phosphorylates GPCR primarily when the receptor is activated (agonist occupied). The receptor phosphorylation triggers binding of arrestins, which blocks the activation of G proteins, leading to rapid homologous desensitization [19–21]. As a result of the arrestin binding, the phosphorylated receptor is targeted for clathrin-mediated endocytosis, a process that classically serves to resensitize and recycle receptor back to the plasma membrane; or alternatively sorts the receptor to the degradation pathway [22].

2.2 GRK2/5 Expression and Distribution

Among seven GRK members, GRK2, 3, 5, and 6 are ubiquitously expressed in various mammalian tissues, which is in contrast to

GRK1, 4, and 7 that are confined to specific organs. For example, GRK2/5 mRNA is detectable in most tissues, whereas GRK1 and 7 are limited to retinal rods and cones, respectively, and GRK4 is only present in testis, cerebellum, and kidney [23, 24]. On the other hand, although GRK2/5 can be detected in most tissues, their levels in different tissues vary significantly. GRK2 is mostly enriched in the leukocytes and the frontal cortex whereas heart, lung, and kidney have much lower GRK2 expression [25]. In contrast, the highest levels of GRK5 were found in heart, lung, and placenta whereas brain and kidney express much lower levels of GRK5.

As compared to cardiovascular tissues, GRK5 content in the brain is minimal [23, 24]. This low content of GRK5 in brain is in part because majority of the cortical areas has little GRK5 expression, except for the limbic system [26]. The message of this kinase was found to be moderately expressed in several limbic regions namely the cingulate cortex, the septohippocampal nucleus, the anterior thalamic nuclei, dentate gyrus of Ammon's horn, and the medial habenula. Notably within these subregions that express GRK5, the lateral septum was found to have the highest GRK5 message. Therefore, this characteristic distribution of GRK5 in brain discloses its unique functional relation to the limbic system.

In addition to the tissue-specific distribution patterns, increased GRK5 expression has been reported in relation to overexpression of tazarotene-induced gene 1 (a tumor suppressor gene) or α-synuclein, and in adriamycin-resistant tumor cells or hypothyroid animals, as well as in AngII-treated vascular smooth muscle cells and macrophage inflammatory protein-2 (MIP-2)-treated in polymorphonuclear leukocytes (PMNs) [27–32]. In general, there is a dearth of systematic studies that specifically address how GRK5 expression may be regulated under different circumstances, including the normal responses to various physiological stimuli and possible pathologic changes during aging and other disease conditions, such as AD, drug abuse, cardiovascular disorders, and cancers.

2.3 GRK2 Function

Although GRK2 is most abundant in the leukocytes and in the brain frontal cortex, the roles of GRK2 in cardiovascular system appear to have received most attention so far. For example, GRK2 was originally known as βARK1 (for β-adrenergic receptor kinase-1) [33], and its upregulation in the injured and stressed heart is believed to be responsible for βAR dysfunction in the heart failure (HF), which has led to actively pursued therapeutic strategies targeting GRK2 [34–37]. On the vascular side, GRK2 has been suggested to mediate hypertension [38–40], though downregulation of GRK2 by different approaches has led to opposite results in hypertension [41–43]. In addition, emerging evidence indicates that GRK2 upregulation may be associated with worsened hypoxic and ischemic brain damages [44, 45]. Therefore, a primary role of GRK2 in cardiovascular system health is indubitable.

Aside from the cardiovascular system, GRK2 in the leukocytes may be related to chemokine receptor regulation and inflammation [46, 47]. The very high levels of GRK2 in the brain frontal cortex might be indicative of an equally important function. This is not to overlook the evidence for GRK2's role in other brain functions related to drug addiction, reward, and even cholinergic neuronal function [26, 48–56].

2.4 GRK5 Function

As a GRK family member, the primary function of GRK5 is to desensitize activated GPCRs. Previous studies have shown that GRK5 regulates desensitization of many GPCRs, including ß-adrenergic receptor (ßAR), μ-opioid receptor (μ-OR), muscarinic receptors, and angiotensin II Receptor (AngIIR) [31, 57–68]. Nonetheless, increasing evidence indicates that GRK5 can also phosphorylate certain none-GPCR substrates (Table 1) and thus affect their functions. For example, phosphorylation of α-synuclein [69, 70] and tubulin [71] by GRK5 has been suggested to regulate their polymerization, and may therefore be related to neuronal function and possibly neurodegenerative disorders. Phosphorylation of p53 by GRK5 regulates p53 degradation [72], which implies a role of GRK5 in oncology. Whether the substrate is a GPCR or not, such GRK5 functions require its kinase activity.

Beyond the kinase-dependent function, GRK5 has also been suggested to have kinase-independent regulatory function. For example, GRK5 inhibits nuclear factor κB (NFκB) transcriptional activity by inducing nuclear accumulation of IκB alpha [73, 74]. GRK5 binds to Akt and negatively regulates vascular endothelial growth factor (VEGF) signaling [75]. Even more dramatically, GRK5 has been shown to contain a DNA-binding nuclear localization sequence, and may possess potential nuclear transcriptional regulatory function [76]. Therefore, it appears that GRK5 may have more divergent regulatory functions than just being a GPCR kinase.

3 GRK2 Dysfunction and Its Potential Pathogenic Impact on AD

Abnormal GRK2 levels were initially reported as a consequence of mild to moderate soluble Aß accumulation at prodromal stage of AD [65]. The change was described as twofold: (1) the total GRK2 protein level was increased in the CRND8 transgenic mice and so was the cytosolic GRK2 level; and (2) the plasma membrane associated monomeric GRK2 was decreased in the CRND8 mice even though high molecular weight GRK2 was increased. It seems Aß alters cellular behavior of GRK2: in Aß treated cells, GRK2 co-localizes with F-actin in the cytosol and the translocation from the cytosol to the membrane in response to GPCR stimuli is suppressed by the Aß treatment. Increased GRK2 was found in the cerebrovasculature, especially endothelial cells following

Table 1
GRK5 substrates

me	GPCR	Origin	Function	Reference
AngIIR	Yes	Mouse	AngIIR desensitization, and hypertension	[31, 57]
ßAR, ß1AR, ß2AR	Yes	Mouse	Desensitization of ßAR (G_i), ß1AR, and ß2AR, related to hypertension and heart failure	[57–61]
δ-OR	Yes	In vitro/cells	δ-OR desensitization and drug abuse	[62]
FSHR	Yes	In vitro/cells	FSHR desensitization and FSH signaling	[140]
hSPR	Yes	In vitro	hSPR desensitization	[141]
M2 muscarinic receptor	Yes	Mouse/airway smooth muscle/brain	M2 muscarinic receptor desensitization: asthma or pulmonary disease, and AD	[63–68]
PAR-1	Yes	Endothelial cells	PAR-1 desensitization	[142]
TSHR	Yes	Thyroid cells	TSHR desensitization	[86, 143]
α-synuclein	No	In vitro/cells/Lewy body	α-synuclein oligomer formation and aggregation in Parkinson's disease?	[69, 70]
HDAC	No	Cardiomyocyte/mouse	Myocardial hypertrophy	[144]
Hip	No	In vitro/cells	CXCR4 internalization	[145]
NFkB p105	No	Macrophages/mouse	LPS-induced inflammation/TLR4 signaling	[146, 147]
P53	No	Osteosarcoma cells	P53 degradation	[72]
PDGFRß	No	In vitro	PDGFRß desensitization	[84, 148]
Tubulin	No	In vitro/cells	Tubulin dimer assembling into microtubules	[71]

Abbreviations: *AngIIR* angiotensin II Receptor, *ßAR* ß-adrenergic receptor; *δ-OR* δ-opioid receptor, *FSHR* follicle-stimulating hormone receptor, *HDAC* histone deacetylase, *Hip* Hsp70 interacting protein, *hSPR* human substance P receptor, *PAR-1* thrombin receptor proteinase-activated receptor-1, *PDGFRß* platelet-derived growth factor receptor-ß, and *TSHR* thyrotropin receptor

experimental chronic brain hypoperfusion, as well as in select cells from human AD tissue, co-localizing with damaged cellular compartments, especially mitochondria and/or mitochondria-derived lysosomes or granular/vacuolar degenerative structures [77]. Such co-localization was also found with neurofibrillary tangles in AD brains in the same study. Another interesting finding is that the GRK2 levels in AD patients were reported to be elevated in peripheral lymphocytes in a manner correlated with the cognitive decline [78]. The pathogenic significance of the apparent abnormal levels of GRK2 in AD remains to be elucidated.

GRK2 overexpression may contribute to the cerebrovascular component of AD pathogenesis. AD pathology includes an apparent cerebrovascular component, ranging from cerebral hypoperfusion at functional level to the degeneration of the cerebrovasculature itself [79–82]. Increased vascular GRK2 expression was associated with attenuation of vasorelaxation and/or reduced cerebral blood flow, possibly, via inhibition of endothelial cell nitric oxide synthase, leading to reduced nitric oxide production or via reduced β-adrenergic-mediated cAMP accumulation, and ERK1/2 phosphorylation [38–40, 77, 83]. GRK2 upregulation could also worsen hypoxia and ischemic brain damages [44, 45]. Therefore, it is conceivable that the upregulated vascular GRK2 could compromise brain functions and accelerate AD pathogenesis by reducing local blood supply. Nevertheless, current evidence in this regard is mostly correlational. More stringent mechanistic studies remain to be performed.

4   GRK5 Deficiency and Its Pathological Consequences in AD

4.1   GRK5 Deficiency

Although dynamic regulation of the GRK5 expression remains to be systematically investigated, scattered reports have indicated that GRK5 downregulation may result from prolonged platelet-derived growth factor receptor-ß (PDGFRß) signaling, and treatments with gonadotropin-releasing hormone (GnRH), thyroid stimulating hormone (TSH), morphine, or lipopolysaccharide (LPS) [32, 84–87].

Even if the total GRK5 levels remain normal, the membrane or functional GRK5 deficiency could occur due to reduced membrane-associated GRK5 (mGRK5) levels [65, 88]. Given that desensitizing membrane-integrated GPCRs is the primary function of GRK, the kinase itself has to be physically associated with membrane to execute such a function. At physiological condition, GRK5 is primarily plasma membrane-associated by binding to phosphatidylinositol-4,5-bisphosphate (PIP2) and phosphoserine (PS), and is ready to act when GPCRs are activated by their agonists [19, 20]. In certain circumstances, however, the balance of the binding force for GRK5 between membrane (e.g., PIP2) and cytosol (e.g., Ca2+/Calmodulin) can be disrupted, which may cause translocation mGRK5 to cytosol [88]. For example, in cultured cells, Aß can cause rapid (within minutes) GRK5 membrane disassociation and lead to functional mGRK5 deficiency [65, 89, 90]. Therefore, GRK5 deficiency may be caused by either decreased grk5 gene expression or reduced membrane distribution of the GRK5 protein, or both.

4.2   Loss-of-Function in GRK5 Deficiency

As described above, emerging evidence indicates that GRK5 may have multiple regulatory roles, in addition to primarily functioning as a GPCR kinase. Previous studies have suggested that functional redundancy exists between the seven GRK members in phosphorylating different GPCR substrates. It was even suspected that there might be little or no specificity among the GRK members, mainly due the fact that seven or so GRK members are responsible for regulating hundreds to thousands of GPCRs [20, 88]. However, studies using GRK knockout (KO) mice have generated unambiguous and convincing results that illustrate selective loss-of-function for each particular GRK member in vivo. For example, the mice deficient in GRK2, 3, 5 and 6 display selectively impaired desensitization of adrenergic, odorant, muscarinic, and dopaminergic receptors, respectively [63, 91–93]. While recognizing the selective loss-of-function, many of the known functions of a GRK member are indeed not affected by the absence or deficiency of this GRK member, which on the other hand proves the redundancy or compensation between different GRK members. In the case of GRK5 deficiency, for example, the selective loss-of-function is evidenced only for muscarinic, but not for adrenergic or opioid receptors [63]. Nonetheless, many known GRK5 functions (i.e., those listed in Table 1) have not been specifically studied for their contribution to functional loss in relation to GRK5 deficiency. Therefore, it is possible that other functional loss caused by GRK5 deficiency, in additional to the impaired muscarinic receptor desensitization, remains to be discovered.

Interestingly, the impact of the GRK5 deficiency on muscarinic receptor desensitization is receptor-subtype selective. To date, five muscarinic acetylcholine (ACh) receptor subtypes have been identified, with M1, M3, and M5 receptors being $G_{q/11}$-coupled, and M2 and M4 receptors being $G_{i/o}$-coupled [94]. GRK5KO mice, when challenged with nonselective muscarinic agonists, display augmented hypothermia, hypoactivity, tremor, and salivation, as well as antinociceptive changes [63]. These behavioral changes are typical M2 and/or M4 receptor-mediated functions, according to the findings from muscarinic receptor subtype KO mice [94, 95]. Therefore, Gainetdinov et al initially speculated that GRK5 deficiency primarily affected the desensitization of M2 subtype of muscarinic receptors (M2R), based on the behavioral changes in the GRK5 KO (GRK5KO) mice [63]. It was later demonstrated that GRK5 deficiency led to reduced hippocampal ACh release that could be fully restored by blocking presynaptic M2/M4 autoreceptors [67]. Moreover, nonselective muscarinic agonist-induced internalization of muscarinic receptors was primarily impaired for M2R, partially for M4R, but not for M1R. This study provided the molecular evidence for the subtype-selective effect of GRK5 deficiency on the inhibitory G protein-coupled M2R and M4R, and revealed that the immediate pathophysiological consequence of GRK5 deficiency was the reduced ACh release (Fig. 1).

4.3 Pathologic Role of GRK5 Deficiency in AD

Beyond the reduced ACh release, GRK5 deficiency may have additional pathologic impact on AD pathogenesis. As mentioned earlier, GRK5 may have multiple functions that can be either

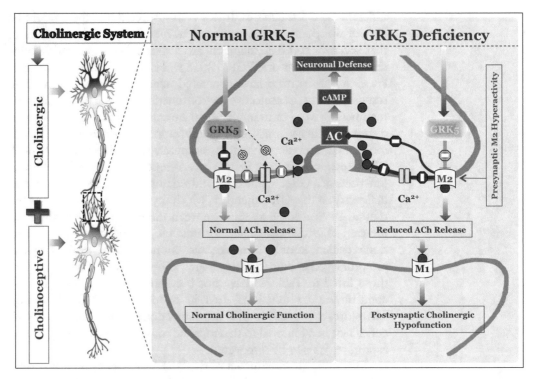

Fig. 1 Schematic diagram of molecular interactions between GRK5 and muscarinic receptors. The selective impact of GRK5 deficiency on presynaptic M2, but NOT postsynaptic M1, determines that its major impact is on the side of presynaptic cholinergic neurons, whereas its impact on the postsynaptic cholinoceptive neurons is limited to the indirect effects of the reduced ACh release. Presynaptically, GRK5 deficiency leads to hyperactive M2 autoreceptors, which may not only inhibit ACh release but also persistently suppress adenylyl cyclase (AC) activity. The latter may impair the intrinsic defense mechanisms and increase the cholinergic neuronal vulnerability to degeneration

kinase-dependent or independent [88]. Of note, the GRK5KO mouse was created by targeted deletion of exons 7 and 8 of the murine grk5 gene [63]. It was predicted that this mouse should produce a transcript encoding a peptide that contains 194 amino acid (a.a.). This speculative peptide should include the N-terminal a.a. 1–178 of the native GRK5 protein and an extra fragment of 16 novel residues. Given that the RH domain of GRK5 locates at a.a. 50-176, this means that the GRK5KO mice are only deficient in the kinase-dependent function of GRK5, while the kinase-independent or RH domain-dependent GRK5 function remains unaltered. In other words, the phenotypes revealed in the GRK5KO mice are irrelevant to the recently proposed RH domain-dependent GRK5 function [73, 74] or any other functions of GRK5 that are dependent upon the N-terminal of 1-178 a.a. In addition, compared to other AD mouse models, no genetic modifications were made to those commonly known AD-relevant genes, such as ßAPP, presenilins, tau, or apolipoprotein E. Therefore, the phenotypes of these mice are solely caused by the loss or lack of the GRK5 kinase activity.

The initial characterization of the GRK5KO mice revealed that the young mice exhibited mild spontaneous hypothermia as well as pronounced behavioral supersensitivity (i.e., hypothermia, hypoactivity, tremor, salivation, and antinociception) upon challenge with the nonselective muscarinic agonist oxotremorine [63]. The aged (18 months), unchallenged homozygous mice were found to display significant short-term (working) memory deficit, along with hypoalertness [66].

At pathological level, the most prominent change was the increased swollen axonal clusters (SACs) [66]. Interestingly, this hallmark pathologic change in GRK5KO mice primarily affected the hippocampus. In the advanced cases, it also affected the brain regions of the piriform cortex, amygdaloid and anterior olfactory nuclei, while most of other brain regions were free of such pathological structures. Normal GRK5 expression in the brain is relatively enriched in the limbic system [26], which coincidently overlaps with the subregions where the SACs occur. Besides, aged GRK5KO mice also displayed decreased synaptic proteins (SNAP-25, synaptotagmin, and growth-associated protein-43) and muscarinic receptors (M1R and M2R), as well as increased soluble Aß and tau phosphorylation levels in the hippocampus [66]. In addition, mild cognitive impairment (MCI) of aged mice positively correlated with the number of SACs and negatively correlated with the levels of M2R in the hippocampus. Although it remains unknown how GRK5 deficiency causes all these changes, these apparent correlations show that GRK5 deficiency can have detrimental effect on neuronal health.

It is worth noting that there were barely any observable senile plaques (SPs) or inflammatory changes, except for a few "micro" plaques captured under electronic microscope that showed fibrillar Aß-like structures and degenerating axonal components wrapped by reactive astrocytes. In particular, the lack of inflammation in this model was somewhat contrary to earlier expectations, given that the initial in vitro observation of Aß-induced GRK5 deficiency was performed in microglial cells [65]. One possible explanation is that the GRK5 deficiency can only act as an amplifier if there are GPCR ligands. However, there was lack of significant extracellular Aß fibrils and/or any other inflammatory initiators in the GRK5KO mice [66]. This speculation was tested later in a new transgenic line created by cross-breeding GRK5KO mice with Tg2576 mice that overexpress the Swedish mutant human ßAPP [96]. The produced heterozygous GRK5 deficient APP mice are referred to as GAP mice hereafter, although they have been previously referred to as GRK5KO/APPsw double mice [68, 97]. Studies in 18-month-old GAP mice revealed significantly exaggerated brain inflammatory changes, including microgliosis and astrogliosis, as compared to those in the age-matched Tg2576 (APPsw) mice [97]. Therefore, it seemed that the GRK5 deficiency indeed amplified the brain inflammation in aged GAP mice.

With respect to the detailed underlying mechanisms, however, it was initially speculated that GRK5 deficiency might lead to impaired desensitization of one or more GPCRs that are involved in the fibrillar Aß-triggered inflammatory reactions [88, 97]. The latter could include a score of GPCRs, such as formyl chemotactic receptor 2 (FPR2 or FPRL-1) [98, 99], C3aR and C5aR anaphylatoxin receptors [100], and CCR, CXCR, and CXCXR chemokine receptors [101]. In addition, another possible explanation was the increased Aß production itself [88]. The latest evidence indicated the latter explanation (the increased Aß rather than the impaired inflammatory GPCR desensitization) is likely to be truth. First, none of the aforementioned inflammatory GPCRs was affected by GRK5 deficiency. Second, not only soluble Aß production but also the fibrillar Aß burden (both plaque number and area) were significantly increased in GAP mice. Moreover, the increased Aß accumulation long preceded exaggerated inflammation in GAP mice [68]. Furthermore, there existed strong positive correlations between the fibrillar Aß burden and the gliosis in GAP mice [102]. Therefore, it becomes clear now that enhanced inflammation in GAP mice occurs only after and as a consequence of the increased fibrillar Aß deposits.

5   Mechanistic Links Between Molecular Events Driven by GRK2/5 Dysfunction

5.1 Cholinergic Dysfunction and ß-Amyloidogenesis

The pathologic impact of GRK5 deficiency in the GAP mice is dual: the increased Aß production along with the reduced ACh release [67]. Is there an internal relation between these two changes? In this regard, the latest study revealed that GRK5 deficiency altered ßAPP processing in favor of ß-amyloidogenic pathway, which was mediated by the impaired cholinergic activity [68].

In the GRK5KO mice the GRK5 deficiency was found to promote soluble Aß accumulation [66]. Perhaps, because that was murine Aß, it failed to cause significant fibrillar Aß deposit in GRK5KO mice. In GAP mice, however, the excessive Aß accumulation included not only the soluble form, but also the fibrils deposited in the plaques. Comparatively, the total Aß burden in GAP mice at 18 month old was roughly doubled than that in Tg2576 mice of the same age [68]. Therefore, both models confirmed that GRK5 deficiency promoted Aß accumulation. As for the relevant mechanism, it was revealed that there was an increase in secreted APPß fragment without change in the full length APP in GAP mice, indicating there was an increased ß-amyloidogenic APP processing in this animal model. In an acute experiment, the interstitial fluid (ISF) Aß in the hippocampus decreased in Tg2576 mice when the animals were challenged with novel object introduction (NOI) in the novel object recognition test. In contrast, this effect was lacking in GAP mice. Interestingly, this difference between the GAP and Tg2675 mice was completely corrected by selective M2 blockade, which appears to link the increased Aß production in GAP mice to a cholinergic dysfunction, or, more specifically, to the presynaptic M2 hyperactivity that we previously described [68, 88].

The impaired desensitization of M2R is so far the only functional loss demonstrated for the GRK5 deficiency [63, 67]. It is known that M1, M2 and M4, but not M3 and M5, are enriched in hippocampus, with M2/M4 being primarily presynaptic autoreceptors that negatively regulate ACh release in the hippocampal memory circuits [103, 104]. Therefore, once presynaptic M2R or M4R are activated, it is conceivable that the M2/M4 signaling will be prolonged, if GRK5 is deficient. This prolonged presynaptic M2/M4 autoreceptor signaling was referred to as presynaptic cholinergic hyperactivity [67, 68, 88]. The best-known effect of the presynaptic cholinergic hyperactivity is reduced ACh release [67], which in turn leads to postsynaptic cholinergic hypoactivity, including the postsynaptic M1 hypoactivity. In fact, postsynaptic cholinergic hypoactivity (reduced ACh) has been previously shown to promote the ß-amyloidogenic APP processing and Aß production [105–109]. Therefore, it is no surprise that blocking the presynaptic M2R and the prolonged M2 signaling completely restored the ability for GAP mice to downregulate the ISF Aß production.

Aside from the increased Aß accumulation and the subsequently exaggerated inflammation, another prominent pathologic change associated with GRK5 deficiency is the axonal defects and the reduced synaptic proteins and muscarinic receptors [66]. It remains to be established whether the observed axonal defects and synaptic degenerative changes are cholinergic and/or cholinoceptive selective. Emerging evidence suggests that these pathologic changes could result from the presynaptic cholinergic hyperactivity. For example, previous studies suggested that the signaling of M1, M3, and M5, but not M2 or M4, appears to be anti-apoptotic [110]. The M1 signaling was shown not only to inhibit ß-amyloidogenic APP processing but also to decrease tau phosphorylation in vitro [105, 111, 112]. Therefore, M1 signaling is generally characterized as "cholinergic protective." On the other hand, M1 and M2 are typical G_q and G_i-coupled receptors, respectively, and often mediate distinct or even opposing signals [113, 114]. The M2 signaling is known to reduce cAMP level [113, 114], and downregulate protein kinase A (PKA) activity, a vital signaling pathway for cell survival and apoptotic resistance [115–120]. Perhaps, more relevant to axonal defects and synaptic degeneration, PKA phosphorylates and inactivates glycogen synthase kinase 3 (GSK3) to facilitate glucose metabolism and cell/neurite growth [121–124]. In the case of M2 hyperactivity, PKA could be persistently inhibited. In this case, GSK3 will be released from their complex, and become dephosphorylated and activated. GSK3, especially GSK3ß, which is also known as tau protein kinase-1

(TPK1), is one main cause of tau hyperphosphorylation [125]. Tau hyperphosphorylation destabilizes microtubules and renders it more prone to aggregation [126, 127], which can contribute to axonal defects. Moreover, GSK3ß can also phosphorylate kinesin light chain (KLC), which leads to detachment of the kinesin motor from the cargo, thus preventing further transport of cargo and resulting in axonal swellings [126, 128, 129]. Therefore, if the M1 signaling is "cholinergic protective," then the M2 signaling appears to be "cholinergic destructive," at least, when it is prolonged. In the case of GRK5 deficiency, both presynaptic M2 hyperactivity (destructive) and postsynaptic M2 hypoactivity (less protective) would be detrimental to the cholinergic neuronal system (see Fig. 2 for schematic illustration of the hypothesis). Consistent with this hypothesis, GRK5 deficient neurons were found to be more vulnerable to spontaneous degeneration or neuronal death triggered by Aß [130]. Therefore, it remains interesting to see if the GRK5 deficiency in GAP mice promotes selective cholinergic neurodegeneration in the basal forebrain.

Importantly, aside from GRK5 deficiency, GRK2 upregulation caused by Aß may worsen the cholinergic dysfunction as well. In conditional GRK2KO from cholinergic neurons, the mice displayed cholinergic hypo-responsiveness to oxotremorine-M [53], which is the opposite of the muscarinic cholinergic super responsiveness observed in the GRK5KO mice [63].

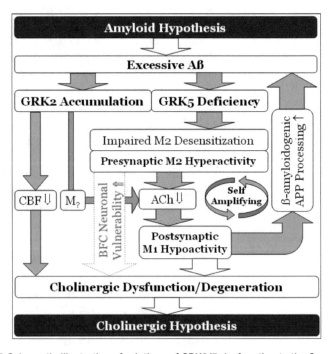

Fig. 2 Schematic illustration of relations of GRK2/5 dysfunction to the ß-amyloid and the cholinergic hypotheses. *BFC* basal forebrain cholinergic

Although the detailed underlying molecular mechanisms remain to be determined, the GRK2 upregulation by Aß, rather than compensating for the detrimental impact of GRK5 deficiency on cholinergic neurons, works with the GRK5 deficiency to compromise the cholinergic functions in AD.

5.2 GRK2/5 Dysfunction Links the Amyloid and Cholinergic Hypotheses Together

Despite various views on detailed causes and processes of AD, two major hypotheses have driven pharmaceutical research in AD in recent three decades: the amyloid hypothesis and the cholinergic hypothesis [131]. The cholinergic hypothesis states that the central cholinergic neuronal dysfunction is largely responsible for the cognitive decline in AD [5]. The amyloid hypothesis proposes that Aß is the central pathogenic molecule in AD [6]. Although the details of these two hypotheses may evolve over time with increasing insights into disease pathogenesis, the principal concepts of these distinct hypotheses appear to stand solidly [6, 131–137]. In addition, compelling evidence supports that cerebrovascular dysfunction and/or degeneration contributes to AD pathogenesis [79–82]. Compared to the amyloid and cholinergic hypotheses that focus on elucidating molecular events in neurons, the compromised cerebral blood and oxygen supplies provide poorer environment for vulnerable neurons to survive and may also slow down the waste clearance process that requires participation of circulating blood.

In brief, Aß is one of the main causes for GRK5 deficiency and GRK2 upregulation in AD [65]. In case of GRK5 deficiency, it selectively impairs desensitization of presynaptic M2/M4 autoreceptors, which leads to presynaptic inhibitory cholinergic receptors hyperactivity and the subsequent postsynaptic cholinergic hypoactivity. The latter, as the key component of the cholinergic hypothesis, further accelerates Aß production. Therefore, these studies directly connect Aß → GRK5 deficiency → cholinergic dysfunction → Aß into a self-promoting loop or vicious cycle. In this vicious cycle, Aß and cholinergic dysfunction each can serve as the cause and consequence, while GRK5 deficiency is the pivotal mediator (Fig. 2). Although the mechanisms are unclear, the GRK2 upregulation caused by Aß seems also to joins this process to make things worse [53]. This is in addition to the hostile cerebrovascular consequences imposed by the GRK2 upregulation [38–40, 44, 45, 77, 83]. Therefore, given the dominating importance of both amyloid and cholinergic hypotheses in AD, more efforts should be directed to studies of GRK2/5 dysfunction, which has been overlooked in the past.

It is worth noting that cholinergic dysfunction is a relatively broad term describing the deficiency of neurotransmitter ACh at cholinergic terminals. Cholinergic dysfunction in AD, according to the cholinergic hypothesis, is characterized by cholinergic hypofunction or a reduction of ACh, which may result from known changes in AD brains, such as reduced choline acetyltransferase (ChAT) and choline uptake, cholinergic neuronal and axonal abnormalities, and degeneration of cholinergic neurons [5, 135]. These pathological characteristics of AD observed in the postmortem brain tissues of AD patients are changes evident at very late stages of the disease. Such late stage changes may not necessarily reveal or reflect more causative alterations that occur early in the disease process. For example, activity of cholinergic markers, such as ChAT and acetylcholinesterase (AChE), do not decrease until relatively late in the disease process [138]. Since neither ChAT nor AChE is rate-limiting, changes in these markers do not necessarily reflect cholinergic function [139]. In fact, ChAT can be inhibited up to 90% with no measurable effects on ACh synthesis or release [132], while pharmacological and neurophysiological deficits in cholinergic response can exist without significant changes in ChAT activity during normal aging [139]. In support of the latter argument, it has been shown that cholinergic hypofunction (reduced ACh release) can exist in the absence of cholinergic structural degeneration in young GRK5KO mice [67], and the structural degenerative change only occurs in aged GRK5KO mice [66]. Therefore, it is possible that an early nonstructural cholinergic dysfunction precedes the structural cholinergic dysfunction/degeneration in AD [67].

While recognizing the importance of the GRK2/5 dysfunction in AD, many important questions remain to be addressed. Based on existing literature information and our own evidence, we present a hypothetical model that links GRK2/5 dysfunction to the amyloid and cholinergic hypotheses in AD (Fig. 2). This model attempts to integrate several most important hypotheses in AD into one unifying hypothesis, in the hope of encouraging additional investigations to ultimately improve our understanding of the disease pathogenesis.

6   Conclusion

As described, GRK2/5 dysfunction emerges to become a critical player in the AD pathogenesis, not only due to its close relation to Aß, but also because of their selective effects on cerebrovascular and cholinergic dysfunctions. As being proposed in the ß-amyloid cascade hypothesis, multiple molecular events subsequently resulting from the Aß accumulation lead to detrimental changes both inside and outside of neurons that eventually cause specific neurodegeneration and cognitive decline. The work on the GRK2/5 dysfunction unveils some of the mystery subsequent to Aß yet prior to cerebrovascular and cholinergic dysfunctions. This may in part shed a light on why AD is viewed as a neurodegenerative disorder featured with more profound cholinergic neurodegeneration. Future effort should address whether or not a selective cholinergic neuronal loss can be discovered in GAP mice and if blocking the presynaptic M2 hyperactivity abolishes the pathologic events driven by GRK5 deficiency.

Acknowledgment

This work was supported by grants to W.Z.S. from the Medical Research and Development Service, Department of Veterans Affairs, the Alzheimer's Association, and resources from the Midwest Biomedical Research Foundation.

References

1. Duyckaerts C, Delatour B, Potier MC (2009) Classification and basic pathology of Alzheimer disease. Acta Neuropathol 118(1):5–36

2. Nelson PT, Braak H, Markesbery WR (2009) Neuropathology and cognitive impairment in Alzheimer disease: a complex but coherent relationship. J Neuropathol Exp Neurol 68(1):1–14

3. Jellinger KA, Bancher C (1998) Neuropathology of Alzheimer's disease: a critical update. J Neural Transm Suppl 54:77–95

4. Mahler ME, Cummings JL (1990) Alzheimer disease and the dementia of Parkinson disease: comparative investigations. Alzheimer Dis Assoc Disord 4(3):133–149

5. Bartus RT, Dean RL 3rd, Beer B, Lippa AS (1982) The cholinergic hypothesis of geriatric memory dysfunction. Science 217(4558):408–414

6. Hardy J, Selkoe DJ (2002) The amyloid hypothesis of Alzheimer's disease: progress and problems on the road to therapeutics. Science 297(5580):353–356

7. Zatta PF (1995) Aluminum binds to the hyperphosphorylated tau in Alzheimer's disease: a hypothesis. Med Hypotheses 44(3):169–172

8. Hoyer S (2000) Brain glucose and energy metabolism abnormalities in sporadic Alzheimer disease. Causes and consequences: an update. Exp Gerontol 35(9-10):1363–1372

9. Aisen PS (1996) Inflammation and Alzheimer disease. Mol Chem Neuropathol 28(1-3):83–88

10. McGeer EG, McGeer PL (1999) Brain inflammation in Alzheimer disease and the therapeutic implications. Curr Pharm Des 5(10):821–836

11. Blennow K, Wallin A, Uhlemann C, Gottfries CG (1991) White-matter lesions on CT in Alzheimer patients: relation to clinical symptomatology and vascular factors. Acta Neurol Scand 83(3):187–193

12. Smith MA, Richey PL, Kalaria RN, Perry G (1996) Elastase is associated with the neurofibrillary pathology of Alzheimer disease: a putative link between proteolytic imbalance and oxidative stress. Restor Neurol Neurosci 9(4):213–217

13. Pappolla MA, Sos M, Omar RA, Sambamurti K (1996) The heat shock/oxidative stress connection. Relevance to Alzheimer disease. Mol Chem Neuropathol 28(1-3):21–34

14. Hoyer S (1998) Is sporadic Alzheimer disease the brain type of non-insulin dependent diabetes mellitus? A challenging hypothesis. J Neural Transm 105(4-5):415–422

15. Supnet C, Bezprozvanny I (2010) The dysregulation of intracellular calcium in Alzheimer disease. Cell Calcium 47(2):183–189

16. Sallese M, Mariggio S, Collodel G, Moretti E, Piomboni P, Baccetti B, De Blasi A (1997) G protein-coupled receptor kinase GRK4. Molecular analysis of the four isoforms and ultrastructural localization in spermatozoa and germinal cells. J Biol Chem 272(15):10188–10195

17. Virlon B, Firsov D, Cheval L, Reiter E, Troispoux C, Guillou F, Elalouf JM (1998) Rat G protein-coupled receptor kinase GRK4: identification, functional expression, and differential tissue distribution of two splice variants. Endocrinology 139(6):2784–2795

18. Sallese M, Salvatore L, D'Urbano E, Sala G, Storto M, Launey T, Nicoletti F, Knopfel T, De Blasi A (2000) The G-protein-coupled receptor kinase GRK4 mediates homologous desensitization of metabotropic glutamate receptor 1. FASEB J 14(15):2569–2580

19. Pitcher JA, Freedman NJ, Lefkowitz RJ (1998) G protein-coupled receptor kinases. Annu Rev Biochem 67:653–692

20. Kohout TA, Lefkowitz RJ (2003) Regulation of G protein-coupled receptor kinases and

arrestins during receptor desensitization. Mol Pharmacol 63(1):9–18

21. Ribas C, Penela P, Murga C, Salcedo A, Garcia-Hoz C, Jurado-Pueyo M, Aymerich I, Mayor F Jr (2007) The G protein-coupled receptor kinase (GRK) interactome: role of GRKs in GPCR regulation and signaling. Biochim Biophys Acta 1768(4):913–922

22. Reiter E, Lefkowitz RJ (2006) GRKs and beta-arrestins: roles in receptor silencing, trafficking and signaling. Trends Endocrinol Metab 17(4):159–165

23. Kunapuli P, Benovic JL (1993) Cloning and expression of GRK5: a member of the G protein-coupled receptor kinase family. Proc Natl Acad Sci U S A 90(12):5588–5592

24. Premont RT, Koch WJ, Inglese J, Lefkowitz RJ (1994) Identification, purification, and characterization of GRK5, a member of the family of G protein-coupled receptor kinases. J Biol Chem 269(9):6832–6841

25. Inglese J, Freedman NJ, Koch WJ, Lefkowitz RJ (1993) Structure and mechanism of the G protein-coupled receptor kinases. J Biol Chem 268(32):23735–23738

26. Erdtmann-Vourliotis M, Mayer P, Ammon S, Riechert U, Hollt V (2001) Distribution of G-protein-coupled receptor kinase (GRK) isoforms 2, 3, 5 and 6 mRNA in the rat brain. Brain Res Mol Brain Res 95(1-2):129–137

27. Wu CC, Tsai FM, Shyu RY, Tsai YM, Wang CH, Jiang SY (2011) G protein-coupled receptor kinase 5 mediates Tazarotene-induced gene 1-induced growth suppression of human colon cancer cells. BMC Cancer 11:175

28. Liu P, Wang X, Gao N, Zhu H, Dai X, Xu Y, Ma C, Huang L, Liu Y, Qin C (2010) G protein-coupled receptor kinase 5, overexpressed in the alpha-synuclein up-regulation model of Parkinson's disease, regulates bcl-2 expression. Brain Res 1307:134–141

29. Ahn MJ, Lee KH, Ahn JI, Yu DH, Lee HS, Choi JH, Jang JS, Bae JM, Lee YS (2004) The differential gene expression profiles between sensitive and resistant breast cancer cells to adriamycin by cDNA microarray. Cancer Res Treat 36(1):43–49

30. Penela P, Barradas M, Alvarez-Dolado M, Munoz A, Mayor F Jr (2001) Effect of hypothyroidism on G protein-coupled receptor kinase 2 expression levels in rat liver, lung, and heart. Endocrinology 142(3):987–991

31. Ishizaka N, Alexander RW, Laursen JB, Kai H, Fukui T, Oppermann M, Lefkowitz RJ, Lyons PR, Griendling KK (1997) G protein-coupled receptor kinase 5 in cultured vascular smooth muscle cells and rat aorta. Regulation by angiotensin II and hypertension. J Biol Chem 272(51):32482–32488

32. Fan J, Malik AB (2003) Toll-like receptor-4 (TLR4) signaling augments chemokine-induced neutrophil migration by modulating cell surface expression of chemokine receptors. Nat Med 9(3):315–321

33. Benovic JL, DeBlasi A, Stone WC, Caron MG, Lefkowitz RJ (1989) Beta-adrenergic receptor kinase: primary structure delineates a multigene family. Science 246(4927):235–240

34. Rengo G, Lymperopoulos A, Leosco D, Koch WJ (2011) GRK2 as a novel gene therapy target in heart failure. J Mol Cell Cardiol 50(5):785–792

35. Brinks H, Das A, Koch WJ (2011) A role for GRK2 in myocardial ischemic injury: indicators of a potential future therapy and diagnostic. Future Cardiol 7(4):547–556

36. Reinkober J, Tscheschner H, Pleger ST, Most P, Katus HA, Koch WJ, Raake PW (2012) Targeting GRK2 by gene therapy for heart failure: benefits above beta-blockade. Gene Ther 19(6):686–693

37. Cannavo A, Liccardo D, Koch WJ (2013) Targeting cardiac beta-adrenergic signaling via GRK2 inhibition for heart failure therapy. Front Physiol 4:264

38. Feldman RD (2002) Deactivation of vasodilator responses by GRK2 overexpression: a mechanism or the mechanism for hypertension? Mol Pharmacol 61(4):707–709

39. Liu S, Premont RT, Kontos CD, Zhu S, Rockey DC (2005) A crucial role for GRK2 in regulation of endothelial cell nitric oxide synthase function in portal hypertension. Nat Med 11(9):952–958

40. Semela D, Langer DA, Shah V (2006) GRK2 makes trouble: a no-NO in portal hypertension. Gastroenterology 130(3):1001–1003

41. Xing W, Li Y, Zhang H, Mi C, Hou Z, Quon MJ, Gao F (2013) Improvement of vascular insulin sensitivity by downregulation of GRK2 mediates exercise-induced alleviation of hypertension in spontaneously hypertensive rats. Am J Physiol 305(8):H1111–1119

42. Avendano MS, Lucas E, Jurado-Pueyo M, Martinez-Revelles S, Vila-Bedmar R, Mayor F Jr, Salaices M, Briones AM, Murga C (2014) Increased nitric oxide bioavailability in adult GRK2 hemizygous mice protects against angiotensin II-induced hypertension. Hypertension 63(2):369–375

43. Tutunea-Fatan E, Caetano FA, Gros R, Ferguson SS (2015) GRK2 targeted knockdown results in spontaneous hypertension, and altered vascular GPCR signaling. J Biol Chem 290(8):5141–5155

44. Nijboer CH, Kavelaars A, Vroon A, Groenendaal F, van Bel F, Heijnen CJ (2008) Low endogenous G-protein-coupled receptor kinase 2 sensitizes the immature brain to hypoxia-ischemia-induced gray and white matter damage. J Neurosci 28(13):3324–3332

45. Lombardi MS, van den Tweel E, Kavelaars A, Groenendaal F, van Bel F, Heijnen CJ (2004) Hypoxia/ischemia modulates G protein-coupled receptor kinase 2 and beta-arrestin-1 levels in the neonatal rat brain. Stroke 35(4):981–986

46. Penela P, Murga C, Ribas C, Salcedo A, Jurado-Pueyo M, Rivas V, Aymerich I, Mayor F Jr (2008) G protein-coupled receptor kinase 2 (GRK2) in migration and inflammation. Arch Physiol Biochem 114(3):195–200

47. Zhang C, Wang ZJ, Lok KH, Yin M (2012) beta-amyloid42 induces desensitization of CXC chemokine receptor-4 via formyl peptide receptor in neural stem/progenitor cells. Biol Pharm Bull 35(2):131–138

48. Ozaita A, Escriba PV, Ventayol P, Murga C, Mayor F Jr, Garcia-Sevilla JA (1998) Regulation of G protein-coupled receptor kinase 2 in brains of opiate-treated rats and human opiate addicts. J Neurochem 70(3):1249–1257

49. Bailey CP, Oldfield S, Llorente J, Caunt CJ, Teschemacher AG, Roberts L, McArdle CA, Smith FL, Dewey WL, Kelly E, Henderson G (2009) Involvement of PKC alpha and G-protein-coupled receptor kinase 2 in agonist-selective desensitization of mu-opioid receptors in mature brain neurons. Br J Pharmacol 158(1):157–164

50. Quillinan N, Lau EK, Virk M, von Zastrow M, Williams JT (2011) Recovery from mu-opioid receptor desensitization after chronic treatment with morphine and methadone. J Neurosci 31(12):4434–4443

51. Llorente J, Lowe JD, Sanderson HS, Tsisanova E, Kelly E, Henderson G, Bailey CP (2012) mu-Opioid receptor desensitization: homologous or heterologous? Eur J Neurosci 36(12):3636–3642

52. Doll C, Poll F, Peuker K, Loktev A, Gluck L, Schulz S (2012) Deciphering micro-opioid receptor phosphorylation and dephosphorylation in HEK293 cells. Br J Pharmacol 167(6):1259–1270

53. Daigle TL, Caron MG (2012) Elimination of GRK2 from cholinergic neurons reduces behavioral sensitivity to muscarinic receptor activation. J Neurosci 32(33):11461–11466

54. Alvaro-Bartolome M, Garcia-Sevilla JA (2013) Dysregulation of cannabinoid CB1 receptor and associated signaling networks in brains of cocaine addicts and cocaine-treated rodents. Neuroscience 247:294–308

55. Nimitvilai S, McElvain MA, Brodie MS (2013) Reversal of dopamine D2 agonist-induced inhibition of ventral tegmental area neurons by Gq-linked neurotransmitters is dependent on protein kinase C, G protein-coupled receptor kinase, and dynamin. J Pharmacol Exp Ther 344(1):253–263

56. Lowe JD, Sanderson HS, Cooke AE, Ostovar M, Tsisanova E, Withey SL, Chavkin C, Husbands SM, Kelly E, Henderson G, Bailey CP (2015) Role of G protein-coupled receptor kinases 2 and 3 in mu-opioid receptor desensitization and internalization. Mol Pharmacol 88(2):347–356

57. Keys JR, Zhou RH, Harris DM, Druckman CA, Eckhart AD (2005) Vascular smooth muscle overexpression of G protein-coupled receptor kinase 5 elevates blood pressure, which segregates with sex and is dependent on Gi-mediated signaling. Circulation 112(8):1145–1153

58. Rockman HA, Choi DJ, Rahman NU, Akhter SA, Lefkowitz RJ, Koch WJ (1996) Receptor-specific in vivo desensitization by the G protein-coupled receptor kinase-5 in transgenic mice. Proc Natl Acad Sci U S A 93(18):9954–9959

59. Cao TT, Deacon HW, Reczek D, Bretscher A, von Zastrow M (1999) A kinase-regulated PDZ-domain interaction controls endocytic sorting of the beta2-adrenergic receptor. Nature 401(6750):286–290

60. Iwata M, Yoshikawa T, Baba A, Anzai T, Nakamura I, Wainai Y, Takahashi T, Ogawa S (2001) Autoimmunity against the second extracellular loop of beta(1)-adrenergic receptors induces beta-adrenergic receptor desensitization and myocardial hypertrophy in vivo. Circ Res 88(6):578–586

61. Hu LA, Chen W, Premont RT, Cong M, Lefkowitz RJ (2002) G protein-coupled receptor kinase 5 regulates beta 1-adrenergic receptor association with PSD-95. J Biol Chem 277(2):1607–1613

62. Pei G, Kieffer BL, Lefkowitz RJ, Freedman NJ (1995) Agonist-dependent phosphorylation of the mouse delta-opioid receptor: involvement of G protein-coupled receptor kinases but not protein kinase C. Mol Pharmacol 48(2):173–177

63. Gainetdinov RR, Bohn LM, Walker JK, Laporte SA, Macrae AD, Caron MG, Lefkowitz RJ, Premont RT (1999) Muscarinic supersensitivity and impaired

receptor desensitization in G protein-coupled receptor kinase 5-deficient mice. Neuron 24(4):1029–1036

64. Walker JK, Gainetdinov RR, Feldman DS, McFawn PK, Caron MG, Lefkowitz RJ, Premont RT, Fisher JT (2004) G protein-coupled receptor kinase 5 regulates airway responses induced by muscarinic receptor activation. Am J Physiol Lung Cell Mol Physiol 286(2):L312–319

65. Suo Z, Wu M, Citron BA, Wong GT, Festoff BW (2004) Abnormality of G-protein-coupled receptor kinases at prodromal and early stages of Alzheimer's disease: an association with early beta-amyloid accumulation. J Neurosci 24(13):3444–3452

66. Suo Z, Cox AA, Bartelli N, Rasul I, Festoff BW, Premont RT, Arendash GW (2007) GRK5 deficiency leads to early Alzheimer-like pathology and working memory impairment. Neurobiol Aging 28(12):1873–1888

67. Liu J, Rasul I, Sun Y, Wu G, Li L, Premont RT, Suo WZ (2009) GRK5 deficiency leads to reduced hippocampal acetylcholine level via impaired presynaptic M2/M4 autoreceptor desensitization. J Biol Chem 284(29):19564–19571

68. Cheng S, Li L, He S, Liu J, Sun Y, He M, Grasing K, Premont RT, Suo WZ (2010) GRK5 deficiency accelerates {beta}-amyloid accumulation in Tg2576 mice via impaired cholinergic activity. J Biol Chem 285(53):41541–41548

69. Arawaka S, Wada M, Goto S, Karube H, Sakamoto M, Ren CH, Koyama S, Nagasawa H, Kimura H, Kawanami T, Kurita K, Tajima K, Daimon M, Baba M, Kido T, Saino S, Goto K, Asao H, Kitanaka C, Takashita E, Hongo S, Nakamura T, Kayama T, Suzuki Y, Kobayashi K, Katagiri T, Kurokawa K, Kurimura M, Toyoshima I, Niizato K, Tsuchiya K, Iwatsubo T, Muramatsu M, Matsumine H, Kato T (2006) The role of G-protein-coupled receptor kinase 5 in pathogenesis of sporadic Parkinson's disease. J Neurosci 26(36):9227–9238

70. Pronin AN, Morris AJ, Surguchov A, Benovic JL (2000) Synucleins are a novel class of substrates for G protein-coupled receptor kinases. J Biol Chem 275(34):26515–26522

71. Carman CV, Som T, Kim CM, Benovic JL (1998) Binding and phosphorylation of tubulin by G protein-coupled receptor kinases. J Biol Chem 273(32):20308–20316

72. Chen X, Zhu H, Yuan M, Fu J, Zhou Y, Ma L (2010) G-protein-coupled receptor kinase 5 phosphorylates p53 and inhibits DNA damage-induced apoptosis. J Biol Chem 285(17):12823–12830

73. Sorriento D, Ciccarelli M, Santulli G, Campanile A, Altobelli GG, Cimini V, Galasso G, Astone D, Piscione F, Pastore L, Trimarco B, Iaccarino G (2008) The G-protein-coupled receptor kinase 5 inhibits NFkappaB transcriptional activity by inducing nuclear accumulation of IkappaB alpha. Proc Natl Acad Sci U S A 105(46):17818–17823

74. Sorriento D, Campanile A, Santulli G, Leggiero E, Pastore L, Trimarco B, Iaccarino G (2009) A new synthetic protein, TAT-RH, inhibits tumor growth through the regulation of NFkappaB activity. Mol Cancer 8:97

75. Zhou RH, Pesant S, Cohn HI, Soltys S, Koch WJ, Eckhart AD (2009) Negative regulation of VEGF signaling in human coronary artery endothelial cells by G protein-coupled receptor kinase 5. Clin Transl Sci 2(1):57–61

76. Johnson LR, Scott MG, Pitcher JA (2004) G protein-coupled receptor kinase 5 contains a DNA-binding nuclear localization sequence. Mol Cell Biol 24(23):10169–10179

77. Obrenovich ME, Smith MA, Siedlak SL, Chen SG, de la Torre JC, Perry G, Aliev G (2006) Overexpression of GRK2 in Alzheimer disease and in a chronic hypoperfusion rat model is an early marker of brain mitochondrial lesions. Neurotox Res 10(1):43–56

78. Leosco D, Fortunato F, Rengo G, Iaccarino G, Sanzari E, Golino L, Zincarelli C, Canonico V, Marchese M, Koch WJ, Rengo F (2007) Lymphocyte G-protein-coupled receptor kinase-2 is upregulated in patients with Alzheimer's disease. Neurosci Lett 415(3):279–282

79. Zhu X, Smith MA, Honda K, Aliev G, Moreira PI, Nunomura A, Casadesus G, Harris PL, Siedlak SL, Perry G (2007) Vascular oxidative stress in Alzheimer disease. J Neurol Sci 257(1-2):240–246

80. Correia SC, Santos RX, Cardoso S, Carvalho C, Candeias E, Duarte AI, Placido AI, Santos MS, Moreira PI (2012) Alzheimer disease as a vascular disorder: where do mitochondria fit? Exp Gerontol 47(11):878–886

81. Diomedi M, Misaggi G (2013) Vascular contribution to Alzheimer disease: predictors of rapid progression. CNS Neurol Disord Drug Targets 12(4):532–537

82. Takeda S, Sato N, Morishita R (2014) Systemic inflammation, blood-brain barrier vulnerability and cognitive/non-cognitive symptoms in Alzheimer disease: relevance to pathogenesis and therapy. Front Aging Neurosci 6:171

83. Obrenovich ME, Morales LA, Cobb CJ, Shenk JC, Mendez GM, Fischbach K, Smith MA, Qasimov EK, Perry G, Aliev G (2009) Insights into cerebrovascular complications and Alzheimer disease through the selective loss of GRK2 regulation. J Cell Mol Med 13(5):853–865

84. Wu JH, Goswami R, Cai X, Exum ST, Huang X, Zhang L, Brian L, Premont RT, Peppel K, Freedman NJ (2006) Regulation of the platelet-derived growth factor receptor-beta by G protein-coupled receptor kinase-5 in vascular smooth muscle cells involves the phosphatase Shp2. J Biol Chem 281(49):37758–37772

85. Luo X, Ding L, Xu J, Williams RS, Chegini N (2005) Leiomyoma and myometrial gene expression profiles and their responses to gonadotropin-releasing hormone analog therapy. Endocrinology 146(3):1074–1096

86. Nagayama Y, Tanaka K, Namba H, Yamashita S, Niwa M (1996) Expression and regulation of G protein-coupled receptor kinase 5 and beta-arrestin-1 in rat thyroid FRTL5 cells. Thyroid 6(6):627–631

87. Fan X, Zhang J, Zhang X, Yue W, Ma L (2002) Acute and chronic morphine treatments and morphine withdrawal differentially regulate GRK2 and GRK5 gene expression in rat brain. Neuropharmacology 43(5):809–816

88. Suo WZ, Li L (2010) Dysfunction of G protein-coupled receptor kinases in Alzheimer's disease. ScientificWorldJournal 10:1667–1678

89. Pitcher JA, Fredericks ZL, Stone WC, Premont RT, Stoffel RH, Koch WJ, Lefkowitz RJ (1996) Phosphatidylinositol 4,5-bisphosphate (PIP2)-enhanced G protein-coupled receptor kinase (GRK) activity. Location, structure, and regulation of the PIP2 binding site distinguishes the GRK subfamilies. J Biol Chem 271(40):24907–24913

90. Pronin AN, Satpaev DK, Slepak VZ, Benovic JL (1997) Regulation of G protein-coupled receptor kinases by calmodulin and localization of the calmodulin binding domain. J Biol Chem 272(29):18273–18280

91. Jaber M, Koch WJ, Rockman H, Smith B, Bond RA, Sulik KK, Ross J Jr, Lefkowitz RJ, Caron MG, Giros B (1996) Essential role of beta-adrenergic receptor kinase 1 in cardiac development and function. Proc Natl Acad Sci U S A 93(23):12974–12979

92. Peppel K, Boekhoff I, McDonald P, Breer H, Caron MG, Lefkowitz RJ (1997) G protein-coupled receptor kinase 3 (GRK3) gene disruption leads to loss of odorant receptor desensitization. J Biol Chem 272(41):25425–25428

93. Gainetdinov RR, Bohn LM, Sotnikova TD, Cyr M, Laakso A, Macrae AD, Torres GE, Kim KM, Lefkowitz RJ, Caron MG, Premont RT (2003) Dopaminergic supersensitivity in g protein-coupled receptor kinase 6-deficient mice. Neuron 38(2):291–303

94. Matsui M, Yamada S, Oki T, Manabe T, Taketo MM, Ehlert FJ (2004) Functional analysis of muscarinic acetylcholine receptors using knockout mice. Life Sci 75(25):2971–2981

95. Wess J (2004) Muscarinic acetylcholine receptor knockout mice: novel phenotypes and clinical implications. Annu Rev Pharmacol Toxicol 44:423–450

96. Hsiao K, Chapman P, Nilsen S, Eckman C, Harigaya Y, Younkin S, Yang F, Cole G (1996) Correlative memory deficits, Abeta elevation, and amyloid plaques in transgenic mice. Science 274(5284):99–102

97. Li L, Liu J, Suo WZ (2008) GRK5 deficiency exaggerates inflammatory changes in TgAPPsw mice. J Neuroinflammation 5:24

98. Le Y, Gong W, Tiffany HL, Tumanov A, Nedospasov S, Shen W, Dunlop NM, Gao JL, Murphy PM, Oppenheim JJ, Wang JM (2001) Amyloid (beta)42 activates a G-protein-coupled chemoattractant receptor, FPR-like-1. J Neurosci 21(2):RC123

99. Yazawa H, Yu ZX, Le Takeda Y, Gong W, Ferrans VJ, Oppenheim JJ, Li CC, Wang JM (2001) Beta amyloid peptide (Abeta42) is internalized via the G-protein-coupled receptor FPRL1 and forms fibrillar aggregates in macrophages. FASEB J 15(13):2454–2462

100. Langkabel P, Zwirner J, Oppermann M (1999) Ligand-induced phosphorylation of anaphylatoxin receptors C3aR and C5aR is mediated by "G protein-coupled receptor kinases. Eur J Immunol 29(9):3035–3046

101. Streit WJ, Conde JR, Harrison JK (2001) Chemokines and Alzheimer's disease. Neurobiol Aging 22(6):909–913

102. Suo WZ (2013) Accelerating Alzheimer's pathogenesis by GRK5 deficiency via cholinergic dysfunction. Adv Alzheimers Dis 2:148–160

103. Levey AI (1996) Muscarinic acetylcholine receptor expression in memory circuits: implications for treatment of Alzheimer disease. Proc Natl Acad Sci U S A 93(24):13541–13546

104. Zhang W, Basile AS, Gomeza J, Volpicelli LA, Levey AI, Wess J (2002) Characterization of central inhibitory muscarinic autoreceptors

by the use of muscarinic acetylcholine receptor knock-out mice. J Neurosci 22(5):1709–1717

105. Rossner S, Ueberham U, Schliebs R, Perez-Polo JR, Bigl V (1998) The regulation of amyloid precursor protein metabolism by cholinergic mechanisms and neurotrophin receptor signaling. Prog Neurobiol 56(5):541–569

106. DeLapp N, Wu S, Belagaje R, Johnstone E, Little S, Shannon H, Bymaster F, Calligaro D, Mitch C, Whitesitt C, Ward J, Sheardown M, Fink-Jensen A, Jeppesen L, Thomsen C, Sauerberg P (1998) Effects of the M1 agonist xanomeline on processing of human beta-amyloid precursor protein (FAD, Swedish mutant) transfected into Chinese hamster ovary-m1 cells. Biochem Biophys Res Commun 244(1):156–160

107. Lin L, Georgievska B, Mattsson A, Isacson O (1999) Cognitive changes and modified processing of amyloid precursor protein in the cortical and hippocampal system after cholinergic synapse loss and muscarinic receptor activation. Proc Natl Acad Sci U S A 96(21):12108–12113

108. Fisher A, Pittel Z, Haring R, Bar-Ner N, Kliger-Spatz M, Natan N, Egozi I, Sonego H, Marcovitch I, Brandeis R (2003) M1 muscarinic agonists can modulate some of the hallmarks in Alzheimer's disease: implications in future therapy. J Mol Neurosci 20(3):349–356

109. Liskowsky W, Schliebs R (2006) Muscarinic acetylcholine receptor inhibition in transgenic Alzheimer-like Tg2576 mice by scopolamine favours the amyloidogenic route of processing of amyloid precursor protein. Int J Dev Neurosci 24(2-3):149–156

110. Budd DC, McDonald J, Emsley N, Cain K, Tobin AB (2003) The C-terminal tail of the M3-muscarinic receptor possesses anti-apoptotic properties. J Biol Chem 278(21):19565–19573

111. Postina R (2008) A closer look at alpha-secretase. Curr Alzheimer Res 5(2):179–186

112. Sadot E, Gurwitz D, Barg J, Behar L, Ginzburg I, Fisher A (1996) Activation of m1 muscarinic acetylcholine receptor regulates tau phosphorylation in transfected PC12 cells. J Neurochem 66(2):877–880

113. Pemberton KE, Hill-Eubanks LJ, Jones SV (2000) Modulation of low-threshold T-type calcium channels by the five muscarinic receptor subtypes in NIH 3 T3 cells. Pflugers Arch 440(3):452–461

114. Crespo P, Xu N, Simonds WF, Gutkind JS (1994) Ras-dependent activation of MAP kinase pathway mediated by G-protein beta gamma subunits. Nature 369(6479):418–420

115. Kim SS, Choi JM, Kim JW, Ham DS, Ghil SH, Kim MK, Kim-Kwon Y, Hong SY, Ahn SC, Kim SU, Lee YD, Suh-Kim H (2005) cAMP induces neuronal differentiation of mesenchymal stem cells via activation of extracellular signal-regulated kinase/MAPK. Neuroreport 16(12):1357–1361

116. Kiermayer S, Biondi RM, Imig J, Plotz G, Haupenthal J, Zeuzem S, Piiper A (2005) Epac activation converts cAMP from a proliferative into a differentiation signal in PC12 cells. Mol Biol Cell 16(12):5639–5648

117. Malbon CC, Tao J, Wang HY (2004) AKAPs (A-kinase anchoring proteins) and molecules that compose their G-protein-coupled receptor signalling complexes. Biochem J 379(Pt 1):1–9

118. Tasken K, Aandahl EM (2004) Localized effects of cAMP mediated by distinct routes of protein kinase A. Physiol Rev 84(1):137–167

119. Dumaz N, Marais R (2005) Integrating signals between cAMP and the RAS/RAF/MEK/ERK signalling pathways. Based on the anniversary prize of the Gesellschaft fur Biochemie und Molekularbiologie Lecture delivered on 5 July 2003 at the Special FEBS Meeting in Brussels. FEBS J 272(14):3491–3504

120. Chin PC, Majdzadeh N, D'Mello SR (2005) Inhibition of GSK3beta is a common event in neuroprotection by different survival factors. Brain Res Mol Brain Res 137(1-2):193–201

121. Fang X, Yu SX, Lu Y, Bast RC Jr, Woodgett JR, Mills GB (2000) Phosphorylation and inactivation of glycogen synthase kinase 3 by protein kinase A. Proc Natl Acad Sci U S A 97(22):11960–11965

122. Buller CL, Loberg RD, Fan MH, Zhu Q, Park JL, Vesely E, Inoki K, Guan KL, Brosius FC 3rd (2008) A GSK-3/TSC2/mTOR pathway regulates glucose uptake and GLUT1 glucose transporter expression. Am J Physiol Cell Physiol 295(3):C836–843

123. Zhao Y, Altman BJ, Coloff JL, Herman CE, Jacobs SR, Wieman HL, Wofford JA, Dimascio LN, Ilkayeva O, Kelekar A, Reya T, Rathmell JC (2007) Glycogen synthase kinase 3alpha and 3beta mediate a glucose-sensitive antiapoptotic signaling pathway to stabilize Mcl-1. Mol Cell Biol 27(12):4328–4339

124. Hur EM, Zhou FQ (2010) GSK3 signalling in neural development. Nat Rev 11(8):539–551

125. Imahori K, Uchida T (1997) Physiology and pathology of tau protein kinases in relation to Alzheimer's disease. J Biochem (Tokyo) 121(2):179–188

126. Roy S, Zhang B, Lee VM, Trojanowski JQ (2005) Axonal transport defects: a common theme in neurodegenerative diseases. Acta Neuropathol 109(1):5–13

127. Trojanowski JQ, Lee VM (1995) Phosphorylation of paired helical filament tau in Alzheimer's disease neurofibrillary lesions: focusing on phosphatases. FASEB J 9(15):1570–1576

128. Morfini G, Szebenyi G, Elluru R, Ratner N, Brady ST (2002) Glycogen synthase kinase 3 phosphorylates kinesin light chains and negatively regulates kinesin-based motility. EMBO J 21(3):281–293

129. Stokin GB, Lillo C, Falzone TL, Brusch RG, Rockenstein E, Mount SL, Raman R, Davies P, Masliah E, Williams DS, Goldstein LS (2005) Axonopathy and transport deficits early in the pathogenesis of Alzheimer's disease. Science 307(5713):1282–1288

130. Suo WZ, Cheng S, He M (2012) Accelerating Alzheimer's pathogenesis by GRK5 deficiency via cholinergic dysfunction. Alzheimers Dement 2:646

131. Thathiah A, De Strooper B (2009) G protein-coupled receptors, cholinergic dysfunction, and Abeta toxicity in Alzheimer's disease. Sci Signal 2(93):re8

132. Bartus RT, Dean RL, Pontecorvo MJ, Flicker C (1985) The cholinergic hypothesis: a historical overview, current perspective, and future directions. Ann N Y Acad Sci 444:332–358

133. Woolf NJ (1996) The critical role of cholinergic basal forebrain neurons in morphological change and memory encoding: a hypothesis. Neurobiol Learn Mem 66(3):258–266

134. Ladner CJ, Lee JM (1998) Pharmacological drug treatment of Alzheimer disease: the cholinergic hypothesis revisited. J Neuropathol Exp Neurol 57(8):719–731

135. Fisher A (2008) Cholinergic treatments with emphasis on m1 muscarinic agonists as potential disease-modifying agents for Alzheimer's disease. Neurotherapeutics 5(3):433–442

136. Small DH, Cappai R (2006) Alois Alzheimer and Alzheimer's disease: a centennial perspective. J Neurochem 99(3):708–710

137. De Strooper B, Vassar R, Golde T (2010) The secretases: enzymes with therapeutic potential in Alzheimer disease. Nat Rev Neurol 6(2):99–107

138. Davis KL, Mohs RC, Marin D, Purohit DP, Perl DP, Lantz M, Austin G, Haroutunian V (1999) Cholinergic markers in elderly patients with early signs of Alzheimer disease. JAMA 281(15):1401–1406

139. Bartus RT, Emerich DF (1999) Cholinergic markers in Alzheimer disease. JAMA 282(23):2208–2209

140. Kara E, Crepieux P, Gauthier C, Martinat N, Piketty V, Guillou F, Reiter E (2006) A phosphorylation cluster of five serine and threonine residues in the C-terminus of the follicle-stimulating hormone receptor is important for desensitization but not for beta-arrestin-mediated ERK activation. Mol Endocrinol 20(11):3014–3026

141. Warabi K, Richardson MD, Barry WT, Yamaguchi K, Roush ED, Nishimura K, Kwatra MM (2002) Human substance P receptor undergoes agonist-dependent phosphorylation by G protein-coupled receptor kinase 5 in vitro. FEBS Lett 521(1-3):140–144

142. Tiruppathi C, Yan W, Sandoval R, Naqvi T, Pronin AN, Benovic JL, Malik AB (2000) G protein-coupled receptor kinase-5 regulates thrombin-activated signaling in endothelial cells. Proc Natl Acad Sci U S A 97(13):7440–7445

143. Nagayama Y, Tanaka K, Hara T, Namba H, Yamashita S, Taniyama K, Niwa M (1996) Involvement of G protein-coupled receptor kinase 5 in homologous desensitization of the thyrotropin receptor. J Biol Chem 271(17):10143–10148

144. Martini JS, Raake P, Vinge LE, DeGeorge BR Jr, Chuprun JK, Harris DM, Gao E, Eckhart AD, Pitcher JA, Koch WJ (2008) Uncovering G protein-coupled receptor kinase-5 as a histone deacetylase kinase in the nucleus of cardiomyocytes. Proc Natl Acad Sci U S A 105(34):12457–12462

145. Barker BL, Benovic JL (2011) G protein-coupled receptor kinase 5 phosphorylation of hip regulates internalization of the chemokine receptor CXCR4. Biochemistry 50(32):6933–6941

146. Parameswaran N, Pao CS, Leonhard KS, Kang DS, Kratz M, Ley SC, Benovic JL (2006) Arrestin-2 and G protein-coupled receptor kinase 5 interact with NFkappaB1 p105 and negatively regulate lipopolysaccharide-stimulated ERK1/2 activation in macrophages. J Biol Chem 281(45):34159–34170

147. Patial S, Shahi S, Saini Y, Lee T, Packiriswamy N, Appledorn DM, Lapres JJ, Amalfitano A, Parameswaran N (2011) G-protein coupled receptor kinase 5 mediates lipopolysaccharide-induced NFkappaB activation in primary macrophages and modulates inflammation in vivo in mice. J Cell Physiol 226(5):1323–1333

148. Cai X, Wu JH, Exum ST, Oppermann M, Premont RT, Shenoy SK, Freedman NJ (2009) Reciprocal regulation of the platelet-derived growth factor receptor-beta and G protein-coupled receptor kinase 5 by cross-phosphorylation: effects on catalysis. Mol Pharmacol 75(3):626–636

Chapter 11

Regulation of Dopamine-Dependent Behaviors by G Protein-Coupled Receptor Kinases

Eugenia V. Gurevich, Raul R. Gainetdinov, and Vsevolod V. Gurevich

Abstract

Neurotransmitter dopamine exerts its effects via five subtypes of dopamine receptors, D1 through D5, all of which belong to the superfamily of G protein-coupled receptors (GPCRs). Agonist-activated GPCRs are selectively phosphorylated by GRKs, whereupon arrestin proteins bind active phosphoreceptors, blocking further G protein activation, facilitating GPCR internalization via coated pits, and initiating G protein-independent round of signaling. GRKs are rate limiting in this process. Four non-visual GRK subtypes are ubiquitously expressed and present in virtually every neuron expressing dopamine receptors. Here we describe the effects of individual GRKs on the dopamine receptor signaling and trafficking in cultured cells, as well as in in vivo models of dopamine-mediated signaling: response to psychostimulants and L-DOPA-induced dyskinesia, a debilitating side effect of L-DOPA replacement therapy in Parkinson's disease. The in vivo findings demonstrate differential effects of GRK subtypes on signaling of individual dopamine receptors in the brain. Effect of GRK isoform on psychostimulant-induced behavior is not only dependent on the dopamine receptor but also on the neuronal type in which the isoform operates, as evidenced by the cell-selective GRK deletions. In addition, certain behavioral effects of GRK3 do not require its kinase activity, and are apparently mediated by the ability of its RGS-like domain to bind α-subunits of $G_{q/11}$ and suppress their signaling. Thus, in vivo dopamine signaling in the brain serves as a powerful model for unraveling biological actions of different GRK subtypes.

Key words Dopamine, Dopamine receptors, GPCRs, GRKs, Psychostimulants, Parkinson's disease, L-DOPA, Dyskinesia, G proteins

1 Introduction

The parameters of signaling via dopamine (DA) receptors, as of most G protein-coupled receptors (GPCRs), are defined to a significant extent by a conserved desensitization mechanism [1]. An active DA receptor is phosphorylated by one or more of GPCR kinases (GRKs), whereupon arrestin proteins, which specifically recognize active phospho-receptors [2], bind them and block further G protein activation via competition for overlapping binding sites on the receptor [3]. Furthermore, arrestin binding initiates receptor internalization [4]. This mechanism ensures appropriate

Vsevolod V. Gurevich et al. (eds.), *G Protein-Coupled Receptor Kinases*, Methods in Pharmacology and Toxicology, DOI 10.1007/978-1-4939-3798-1_11, © Springer Science+Business Media New York 2016

length and intensity of G protein activation by GPCRs preventing their overactivity. Arrestin binding to the receptor also initiates another round of signaling independent of G proteins, via scaffolding of signaling proteins by arrestins [5]. GPCR signaling is strictly controlled by this process, and the rate and extent of desensitization depend on the availability of GRKs [6–16]. Since most GPCRs require phosphorylation by GRKs for high-affinity arrestin binding [4], GRKs promote arrestin-dependent signaling, in addition to initiating GPCR desensitization towards G proteins [17, 18]. Most mammals express seven GRKs, four of which, GRK2, GRK3, GRK5, and GRK6, are fairly ubiquitous and collectively target hundreds of GPCR subtypes [19].

DA receptors belong to the superfamily of GPCRs, first identified by the similarity of sequence and overall topology of β2-adrenergic receptor and rhodopsin [20]. Mammals have five DA receptor subtypes, which were cloned in 1988–91, essentially in the order of their decreasing abundance in the brain: D2 [21], which has two splice variants [22, 23], D1 [24–26], D3 [27], D4 [28], and last D5 [29]. Thus, the first question that needs to be asked is whether any GRK preferentially targets particular dopamine receptors, and if so, which receptors are regulated by which GRK(s).

The question consists of two parts: first, which GRK isoforms are capable of phosphorylating which DA receptor subtypes and with what efficacy and, second, which isoforms phosphorylate which DA receptors in vivo. These two topics are related but not identical. The performance of the GRK isoforms in the living tissue will depend not only on their biochemical specificity but also on the relative expression and subcellular distribution. For example, if one isoform is considerably more abundant than the other, the second will likely have little chance of regulating a particular receptor, because the more abundant isoform will always get there first. Similarly, if a GRK isoform is localized in a subcellular compartment away from the receptor in question, it has little chance to regulate it, even if it is capable of phosphorylating it in simpler biochemical or cell culture experiments. Therefore, biochemical competence is necessary but not sufficient to conclude that a GRK plays a role in regulating a particular DA receptor in vivo.

2 GRK Interaction with Dopamine Receptors

2.1 Dopamine Receptor Subtypes and GRK Isoforms

Even in its simplest biochemical form, the question which dopamine receptor is phosphorylated by which GRK isoform turned out to be nontrivial. The first study used the rat D1 (called D1A at the time to distinguish it from another Gs-coupled dopamine subtype, D5) heterologously expressed in HEK293 cells with GRK2, GRK3, and GRK5 [30]. Co-expression of all of these GRKs increased D1 phosphorylation to a similar extent. All three GRKs preferentially phosphorylated serines in the D1. However, functional consequences of phosphorylation (the effects on cAMP production) were shown to be quite different: while all GRKs shifted dopamine dose–response curve to the right (to higher dopamine concentrations), GRK2/3 did not affect maximum response, whereas GRK5 reduced it by ~40 % [30]. Next study addressed the issue of sites in the D1 receptor targeted not by GRKs, but by cAMP-activated PKA, and the effect of removal of these sites by mutagenesis on desensitization of D1-mediated activation of adenylyl cyclase [31]. Among four potential PKA phosphorylation sites, Thr268 was identified as the most important. Interestingly, the removal of PKA sites slowed down the loss of responsiveness to dopamine, but did not affect the rate of receptor internalization [31]. Thus, the authors concluded that PKA phosphorylation likely affects the D1 coupling to Gs, but not endocytosis, apparently mediated by GRK phosphorylation and subsequent arrestin binding [31].

Both D2 and D3 receptors couple to Gi subfamily of G proteins. The study of their regulation suggested that while the D2 undergoes rapid GRK phosphorylation and arrestin binding, which leads to its internalization, the D3 receptor is relatively resistant to this regulation [10]. GRK2, GRK3, and both non-visual arrestins were shown to play a role in phosphorylation and internalization of the D2 receptor [10]. Interestingly, the exchange of intracellular loops i2 and i3 between the D2 and D3 reversed this phenotype, indicating that these elements (rather than the C-terminus phosphorylated by GRKs in rhodopsin and β2-adrenergic receptor), determine their susceptibility to GRK/arrestin-mediated regulation [10].

An interesting model for the role of GRK-mediated phosphorylation of the D1 receptor in arrestin binding was proposed based on the extensive mutagenesis that included progressive truncation of the C-terminus and elimination of putative phosphorylation sites in the i3 [32]. Full deletion of the C-terminus with all Ser/Thr residues in it completely blocked the D1 phosphorylation, but did not preclude desensitization, arrestin recruitment, or endocytosis. In contrast, elimination of putative phosphorylation sites from the i3 reduced phosphorylation and significantly impaired desensitization and arrestin recruitment [32]. The data are consistent with the idea that the phosphorylation of the D1 C-terminus and i3 serves to unmask arrestin binding site. Thus, in the D1 lacking the C-terminus no unmasking is necessary, so that arrestin binds without phosphorylation [32]. Interestingly, a similar mechanism, where phosphorylation of certain elements serves to get them out of the way to promote arrestin access to the active receptor, was earlier proposed for the M2 muscarinic [33] and later for δ-opioid [34] receptors.

Another unconventional mode of regulation by GRK2/3 was described in case of the D3, which in part acts as a presynaptic autoreceptor [17]. The D3 receptor phosphorylation by GRK2/3 was shown to disrupt the D3 interaction with filamin, which appears to ensure the D3 localization in filamin-rich lipid rafts, where its cognate G protein is localized. Arrestin-3 was also found to be localized near the D3 via direct interactions with filamin [17]. Thus, the D3 receptor phosphorylation by GRK2/3 desensitizes the D3 by breaking its association with filamin, and therefore localization in G protein-rich subcellular compartments, whereas the interaction of GRK-phosphorylated the D3 with arrestin might play only a secondary role [17].

2.2 Selectivity of GRKs for Active GPCRs

GRKs are widely believed to selectively phosphorylate only active GPCRs (reviewed in ref. 19). This notion received strong support by the elucidation of the molecular mechanism of rhodopsin kinase (GRK1) activation [35]. This study showed that GRK1 physically binds light-activated rhodopsin, and that this interaction increases its enzymatic activity [35]. This mechanism explained why GRKs selectively phosphorylate active GPCRs. Interestingly, the D1 receptor was the first GPCR where this assumption was shown not to be universally correct [36]. It was shown that α isoform of GRK4 (but not the other three splice variants of this GRK) constitutively phosphorylates the D1 at two sites in the C-terminus, Thr428 and Ser431. This phosphorylation reduces the D1 responsiveness and facilitates the D1 receptor elimination from plasma membrane, and both effects are abolished by the elimination of these two sites in T428V+S431A mutant [36]. This finding showed that at least some GPCRs can be directly regulated by the complement of GRKs expressed in the same cell [36]. Importantly, two splice variants of the same GRK, GRK4α and GRK4γ, were shown to phosphorylate a different dopamine receptor subtype, the D3, in a strictly activation-dependent manner [37]. Elimination of GRK4 by RNAi in that case leads to the abolition of ERK1/2 activation and mitogenic response to dopamine [37], suggesting that these responses are mediated by arrestins associated with the phosphorylated D3.

GRK2 and GRK3, but not other GRKs, were shown to phosphorylate the agonist-activated D2 receptor, targeting eight Ser/Thr residues in its i3 [38]. Interestingly, mutational elimination of all these GRK targets, while predictably prevented the D2 phosphorylation, did not affect receptor association with arrestin-3 or internalization [38]. This finding suggests that, similar to the D1 [32], phosphorylation of the D2 by GRKs is not required to create arrestin-3 (beta-arrestin 2) binding site, but, more likely, acts to allow arrestin access to a site created by receptor activation [38]. Importantly, upon internalization, unphosphorylated D2 was mostly degraded, whereas phosphorylated WT D2 was recycled. Thus, in case of the D2, phosphorylation by GRKs appears to primarily regulate post-endocytic trafficking [38]. Another study of the D2 receptor also concluded that agonist-induced GRK phosphorylation of the D2, as well as its arrestin-dependent internalization (which has both phosphorylation-dependent and -independent components) plays a greater role in receptor resensitization than in desensitization [39].

Recent systematic analysis of the phosphorylation of six different GPCRs, including two dopamine receptors, by four ubiquitously expressed receptor kinases, GRK2, GRK3, GRK5, and GRK6, has showed that there is no universal rule regarding the dependence of receptor phosphorylation on the receptor activation [40]. In most cases GRK2/3 are selective for active GPCRs, whereas GRK5 and GRK6, which belong to the GRK4 subfamily [41], phosphorylate both active and inactive GPCRs [40]. The D1 showed higher dependence on activation than many other GPCRs: in contrast to GRK4α, which phosphorylated both active and inactive form of the D1 [36], the other members of the GRK4 subfamily, GRKs 5 and 6, and well as GRKs 2 and 3 tested in this study preferentially phosphorylated agonist-activated D1 [40]. The situation with the D2 receptor was somewhat different: it was phosphorylated in activation-dependent manner by GRK2/3, and not phosphorylated at all by GRK5/6 [40].

Three classes of proteins preferentially bind ligand-activated GPCRs: G proteins [42, 43], GRKs [35, 44, 45], and arrestins [46, 47]. So far, the evidence is consistent with the idea that all three classes engage the cavity between GPCR helices that opens on the cytoplasmic side upon receptor activation [48, 49]. Apparently G proteins [50], arrestins [51], and GRKs [52, 53] insert an amphipathic α-helix into this cavity. The findings that certain synthetic ligands can bias signaling towards G proteins or arrestins (see [54] and references therein) suggests that the binding of different agonists to the same GPCR can produce distinct conformational changes that lead to preferential engagement of G proteins or GRKs/arrestins. Structural differences between Gs-associated β2-adrenergic receptor [49] and arrestin-1-associated rhodopsin [51] are consistent with this idea, although to determine whether these differences reflect the difference in receptor or its interaction partner, we need more structures of GPCR complexes with G proteins and arrestins.

3   DA Receptor Signaling and the Actions of Psychostimulant Drugs

Studying the role of GRKs in behaviors induced by drugs targeting DA receptors would be the way to address the question of the in vivo regulation of the DA receptors by GRK isoforms. Experiments in living animals bypass the problems associated with heterologous expression of receptors and GRKs and allow for assessing specificity of GRK isoforms derived from the cell-specific expression and/or subcellular localization rather than from biochemical specificity. These studies have demonstrated that GRKs play important roles in the DA-dependent behavior and suggests that GRK could be viable therapeutic targets for pathological conditions associated with abnormal dopaminergic signaling.

3.1 Effects of Psychostimulants on the DA Neurotransmission

Psychostimulant drugs such as cocaine and amphetamine produce multiple physiological and psychological effects in humans including an increase in blood pressure, heart rate and respiration, increased stimulation, confidence, euphoria and exhilaration, reduced fatigue and appetite, and improved performance in simple cognitive and motor tasks [55]. In rodents, administration of psychostimulant drugs causes a sharp elevation in the locomotor activity. Psychostimulants elevate synaptic concentration of monoamines (serotonin, norepinephrine, DA) by blocking their transporters and/or inducing non-vesicular release. Their action at the mesolimbic dopaminergic system is thought to be primarily responsible for their physiological and behavioral effects. Psychostimulants enhance the DA concentration in the nucleus accumbens, the key structure in the brain reward system that receives massive projections from dopaminergic neurons in the ventral tegmental area [56, 57]. Robust increases in extracellular dopamine levels caused by psychostimulants result in the enhanced stimulation of dopamine receptors, which, in its turn, leads to the elevated locomotor activity.

The dopaminergic projections terminate on the output neurons in the striatum, including the nucleus accumbens (Fig. 1). Based on the structure these neurons project to, they are classified into the striatonigral (projecting to the substantia nigra reticulata) and striatopallidal (projecting to the globus pallidus external) neurons. The D1 and D2 receptors are the main subtypes expressed by the output neurons in the striatum and nucleus accumbens. In the caudate–putamen region (Fig. 1), the D1 and D2 subtypes are segregated: the D1 receptor is expressed predominantly on striatonigral, and the D2 — on the striatopallidal neurons with little overlap [58–65]. In the nucleus accumbens, the concentration of the D1 and D2 receptors is lower than in the caudate–putamen, and the degree of co-expression higher [64–66]. The third DA receptor subtype expressed in the nucleus accumbens is the D3 receptor, which is particularly abundant in the shell region and is largely co-expressed with the D1 receptor [67, 68]. Cholinergic interneurons, which exert powerful influence over the striatal output neurons [69–71], bear the dopamine D2 and D5 receptors [64, 72–74]. As the major receptor subtypes in the nucleus accumbens, D1 and D2 dopamine receptors play a critical role in mediating the locomotion-stimulating effects of psychostimulants [75, 76]. Since GRKs can regulate dopamine receptors in vitro (reviewed in refs. 77, 78), several studies have focused on evaluation of the role of

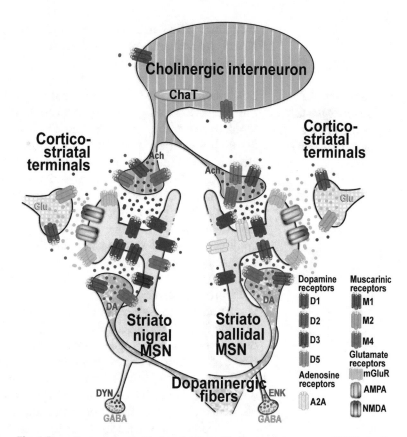

Fig. 1 Receptors expressed in the striatum. Medium spiny neurons (MSN) are the most abundant cell type in the striatum. MSNs are GABAergic output neurons subdivided based on their projections into striatonigral (projecting to the substantia nigra reticulata) and striatopallidal (projecting to the globus pallidus external). MSNs receive heavy glutamatergic corticostriatal projections terminating on the heads of spines. Corticostriatal terminals express D2 dopamine and M3 muscarinic presynaptic receptors regulating the release of glutamate. The action of glutamate is mediated by ionotropic glutamate AMPA and NMDA receptors located on spine synapses and by metabotropic glutamate receptor located on the periphery of the synapses. The metabotropic glutamate receptors of the Group I (mGluRI and mGluRV) are found on both types of MSNs. Striatonigral MSNs can be identified by dynorphin expression. They selectively express Gs/olf-coupled D1 receptors. The Gi/o-coupled D3 dopamine receptors also seem to be predominantly co-expressed in the rat with the D1 receptor on the striatonigral neurons, whereas in the human striatum there is high level of co-expression with the D2 receptor. Striatopallidal MSNs are identified by enkephalin expression. They express selectively Gi/o-coupled D2 dopamine and Gs-coupled A2A adenosine receptors. Both types of MSN express M1 muscarinic receptors, whereas M4 are mostly expressed on striatonigral MSNs. Dopaminergic fibers come from substantia nigra. Their activity is regulated by presynaptic D2 and M4 receptors, both of which couple to Gi/o. Cholinergic interneurons that are the source of acetylcholine in the striatum express D2 and M4 receptors, as well as D5, which, similar to D1, couples to Gs/olf and stimulates cAMP production

individual GRKs in regulating dopamine receptor responsiveness in vivo by assessing behavioral sensitivity to cocaine and amphetamine in GRK mutant mice.

3.2 Role of GRK2 Isoform in Regulating Behavioral Effects of Psychostimulants

It is known that GRK2 is ubiquitously expressed in various areas of the brain, including primary dopaminergic areas [79], and can regulate dopamine D1, D2, and D3 receptors in vitro [10, 30, 80–83]. Alterations in GRK2 expression in the striatum following chronic cocaine were also documented [84]. Since mice with global GRK2 deficiency are not viable due to embryonic lethality caused by cardiac hypoplasia [85], hemizygous GRK2+/- mice were initially used to explore the role of GRK2 in dopamine receptor functions [77]. While locomotor effects of psychostimulant amphetamine and nonselective D1/D2 dopamine agonist apomorphine, were not altered in hemizygous GRK2+/- mice, cocaine treatment at certain doses caused significant enhancement of locomotor activity suggesting that even partial GRK2 deficiency is sufficient to cause certain alterations in dopamine receptors sensitivity [77]. However, the fact that this enhancement was observed only in very narrow range of doses indicated quite complex regulation of populations of dopamine receptors by this GRK that might be different in various cellular populations. Recent studies with mice with cell-specific deletion of GRK2 in various groups of striatal neurons have indeed demonstrated an intricate and strictly organized role of GRK2 in the control of dopaminergic responses and action of psychostimulants. Several strains of GRK2 deficient mice with Cre-lox system-mediated conditional transgenic deletion of this kinase under control of specific cellular promoters have been developed [86, 87].

The mice lacking GRK2 specifically in cholinergic interneurons (ChATcreGrk2f/f mice), D1-dopamine expressing striatal output synaptic neurons (D1RcreGrk2f/f mice), DAT-expressing presynaptic dopaminergic neurons (DATcreGrk2f/f mice), D2 dopamine receptor-expressing presynaptic dopaminergic neurons as well as striatal output neurons (D2RcreGrk2f/f mice) and adenosine A2A receptor-expressing striatal output neurons (A2AcreGrk2f/f mice) (Fig. 1) were tested for basal and cocaine-induced locomotor activity [86, 87]. Earlier work with mice lacking specific GRKs globally has revealed a very modest phenotype in unchallenged animals, suggesting that global lack of GRK kinases has little impact on dopamine-related physiological processes under basal conditions [14, 16]. Similarly, no overt alterations in spontaneous locomotor activity were observed in drug-naive mice lacking GRK2 in either cholinergic [86] or D1R-expressing neurons [87]. At the same time, the selective deletion of GRK2 in D2 dopamine receptor-expressing neurons and DAT-expressing dopaminergic neurons, but not postsynaptic A2AR-expressing striatopallidal MSNs resulted in increased spontaneous locomotor activity.

These data strongly suggest that the hyperactivity phenotype of D2RcreGrk2f/f mice is caused by the loss of GRK2 specifically in dopaminergic neurons.

Interestingly, while cocaine-mediated effects remained intact following deletion of GRK2 from A2AR-expressing striatopallidal MSNs or cholinergic neurons [86] the deletion of GRK2 in D1R- and D2R-expressing neurons caused opposite effects on acute cocaine-induced locomotion. Particularly, mice lacking GRK2 in D1 dopamine receptor-containing neurons showed enhanced locomotor response to cocaine, while mice lacking GRK2 in D2 dopamine receptor containing neurons showed less activity following cocaine. Taking into account the fact that mice with GRK2 deficiency in dopaminergic neurons were also markedly less sensitive to the acute effects of cocaine, these results suggest that the reduced sensitivity of D2RcreGrk2f/f mice to cocaine is primarily caused by altered regulation of D2 dopamine autoreceptors due to loss of GRK2 function in dopaminergic neurons.

Sensitization to the locomotion-stimulating effects of cocaine was also tested in all these strains, and only mice with deficiency of GRK2 in D2R-expressing neurons showed reduced chronic cocaine sensitization response. These results indicate that not only GRK2 function in D2R-expressing neurons in the striatal cells but also in other brain areas such as the medial prefrontal cortex [88] might be required for the full expression of behavioral sensitization to cocaine. Further indication of specific role of GRK2 in the regulation of presynaptic D2 dopamine autoreceptors was obtained in studies involving Fast Scan Cyclic Voltammetry. Particularly, GRK2 deficiency in D2R-expressing neurons caused a significant reduction in striatal DA release directly demonstrating that GRK2 deficiency in D2R-expressing neurons leads to overactivity of presynaptic D2 autoreceptors, which results in the persistent suppression of evoked DA release from striatal DA terminals. Enhanced D2 autoreceptor activity may thus be due to impaired GRK2-mediated desensitization of these presynaptic receptors. Interestingly, although GRK2 is expressed at a relatively higher level in cholinergic interneurons as compared to striatal output neurons [89], selective knockout of GRK2 in this neuronal subtype has no effect on the cocaine-induced psychomotor activation, behavioral sensitization to psychostimulants, or conditioned place preference [86] suggesting little role for GRK2 in these neurons in regulating dopaminergic responses.

3.3 Role of Other GRK Isoforms in Regulating Behavioral Effects of Psychostimulants

It should be noted, that the direct assessment of the potential role of GRK3, GRK4 and GRK5 in the regulation of dopamine receptors in mice with global deletion of these GRKs revealed essentially normal responses to several dopaminergic drugs including cocaine and amphetamine, indicating that regulation of dopamine receptors is not significantly affected by deletion of these GRKs [16].

However, the absence of GRK6 has also been reported to strongly enhance striatal D2 dopamine receptor activity [14], but in contrast to the present findings, this work implicated postsynaptic D2 dopamine receptors as the principal physiological target of GRK6. GRK6 seems to be one of the most prominent GRKs in the striatum and other dopaminergic brain areas [90]. Particularly, high expression of GRK6 protein was found in the dopamine-receptive GABAergic medium spiny neurons as well as in cholinergic interneurons in the striatum [14]. In vivo assessment of dopaminergic function in mice lacking GRK6 revealed significantly enhanced responsiveness to primarily dopaminergic psychostimulant drugs and direct dopamine agonists [14, 91]. An increased coupling of striatal D2-like dopamine receptors to G proteins and higher proportion of high-affinity D2 receptors was also documented in these mutants [14, 92]. These observations have indicated that postsynaptic D2 dopamine receptors are direct physiological targets for GRK6-mediated regulation. Thus, while it is now evident that multiple GRKs can regulate DA receptors in vivo, regulation of D2 dopamine receptors by GRK2- and GRK6 seems to be functionally the most important. The two kinases demonstrate strict neuronal specificity of this regulation: GRK2 and GRK6 regulate distinct populations of the D2 receptors, i.e., the receptors localized on dopaminergic presynaptic neurons and on postsynaptic striatal output neurons, respectively. Role of GRK2 in the regulation of D1 dopamine receptors is also noteworthy. Taken together, it appears that GRKs (particularly, GRK2 and GRK6) play an important role in the control of the functions of dopamine receptors and the central dopaminergic system in general and, thus, may represent promising novel therapeutic targets for DA-related pathologies.

4   DA Receptor Signaling in Parkinson's Disease

4.1 Dopamine Receptors in Parkinson's Disease and L-DOPA-induced Dyskinesia

The striatum receives dense dopaminergic innervation, and striatal neurons express high levels of DA receptors. DA released by midbrain dopaminergic neurons regulates the striatal output and plays an essential role in movement control. Loss of dopaminergic neurons and depletion of DA in the striatum in Parkinson's disease (PD) leads to the dysfunction of the striatal circuits and motor deficits. The action of DA in the striatum is mediated by DA receptors, with the D1 and D2 subtypes being the most prominent (Fig. 1).

PD is a neurodegenerative disorder primarily caused by the degeneration of nigral dopaminergic neurons that provide dopamine (DA) to the striatum. DA depletion in rodents with neurotoxin 6-hydroxydopamine (6-OHDA) produces movement defects reminiscent of akinesia in PD and is often used as a model of

PD. Most of what is known regarding signaling alterations in striatal neurons in PD comes from studies utilizing this model. Nonhuman primates treated with the neurotoxin 1-methyl-4-phenyl-1,2,3,6-tetrahydropyridine (MPTP) to deplete dopaminergic neurons faithfully reproduce PD symptoms and, thus, the model is considered the "golden standard" of the animal models of PD. However, it is impractical for molecular studies and is used for such studies considerably less often than hemiparkinsonian rodents. Loss of striatal DA in PD causes complex alterations in cellular signaling: numerous pathways in the DA-depleted striatum show strikingly exaggerated responses to stimulation by dopaminergic drugs [60, 93–95] linked to supersensitivity of D1 [96, 97] and D2 [98, 99] receptors. The mechanisms that maintain the aberrant receptor responses remain poorly understood.

The best symptomatic therapeutic agent is the DA precursor L-3,4-dihydroxyphenylalanine (L-DOPA), which is very effective initially in reversing akinesia in PD patients. However, long-term treatment leads to L-DOPA-induced motor complications, including dyskinesia (LID), or involuntary aimless movements [100–102]. Surprisingly, the pathophysiology of LID, despite decades of research, is still poorly understood. The reason for this is that mechanisms of signaling alterations triggered by loss of DA and subsequent L-DOPA treatment remain obscure. In 6-OHDA-lesioned rodents, treatment with L-DOPA induces rotations, the frequency of which increases with repeated administration of the drug (this process is referred to as behavioral sensitization to L-DOPA), and abnormal involuntary movements (AIMs), which also become more prominent with the chronic treatment. The chronic treatment with L-DOPA desensitizes some supersensitive signaling responses, in parallel with the reversal of DA depletion-induced akinesia. E.g., chronic L-DOPA suppresses supersensitivity of the ERK pathway caused by loss of DA [93, 103–106]. Chronic L-DOPA treatment is also known to augment lesion-induced supersensitivity of select pathways and/or further deregulate their activity [93, 106, 107]. These signaling alterations correlate with progressively increasing frequency of L-DOPA-induced rotations [67, 93, 108, 109] and of abnormal involuntary movements (AIMs) [108, 110–113]. The exaggerated signaling via the striatal D1 [96, 107, 112], D2 [99], and D3 [67, 93, 114] receptors has been implicated in LID in rodents and primates.

Because both dyskinetic and antiparkinsonian actions of L-DOPA are mediated by signaling through DA receptors, the molecular mechanisms of these effects are likely intertwined. Since dopaminergic signaling is required for proper movement control, the clinical challenge is to suppress signaling responsible for LID while preserving enough dopaminergic activity to support the antiparkinsonian action of the drug. Previous attempts to dissociate the detrimental and beneficial effect of the drug with pharmacological or molecular tools that inhibit the former while preserving the latter have been only moderately successful [99, 114]. To successfully manage LID, molecular mechanisms regulating signaling via DA receptors under normal and pathological conditions must be unraveled to enable selective targeting of those specifically responsible for LID. Exaggerated signaling via DA receptors implicated in LID suggests that that normalization of this excessive signaling may be beneficial. The challenge is to reduce the signaling in a way that alleviates LID while preserving the antiparkinsonian activity of the drug, which is also mediated by DA receptors.

4.2 Effect of DA Depletion and L-DOPA on the GRK Expression

Five GRK isoforms are expressed in the brain [79, 89, 103, 115, 116]. Striatal neurons express four GRK isoforms, GRKs 2, 3, 5, and 6 at various levels In the rat striatum, GRK6 is expressed at the highest level followed by GRK2 [109], whereas in the monkey and human brain GRK5 is expressed at the highest level followed by GRK2 in most striatal subdivisions [103, 116].

A simple way how the loss of DA and/or L-DOPA treatment can influence the signaling via GPCRs is by modulating the availability of GRKs (Fig. 2a, b). In rats with unilateral DA depletion the concentration of GRK6 and GRK3 isoforms in the dopamine-depleted motor striatum is reduced, and L-DOPA fails to alter the GRK expression [108, 109]. This can contribute to faulty receptor desensitization and enhanced signaling. Although the degree of reduction in case of GRK6 is not large (25–40%), it could be quite functionally significant in view of the demand created by huge surge of DA produced from L-DOPA. Furthermore, hemizygous GRK6 knockout mice expressing approximately 50% of GRK6 display full phenotype when treated with psychostimulant drugs [14], suggesting that the concentration of GRK6 is critically important for the normal functioning of the DA receptors, particularly in the conditions of the dopaminergic overload. The GRK3 was the only other GRK isoform consistently reduced across striatal regions by the DA depletion in the hemiparkinsonian rat, with chronic L-DOPA having no effect [109, 117]. In contrast, GRK2, the major isoform in the rat striatum and the closest relative of GRK3, is unchanged by the loss of DA and upregulated by chronic L-DOPA treatment [109, 117].

In parkinsonian monkeys, loss of DA leads to the upregulation of several GRKs [103], which may temper dopaminergic signaling upon initial L-DOPA administration and ensure a therapeutic response to the drug. However, chronic L-DOPA treatment suppresses the GRK expression [103]. The elevated membrane expression and reduced internalization of D1 receptors in the striatum of dyskinetic monkeys [118] has been demonstrated, suggesting that LID is associated with deficits in the D1 receptor desensitization and trafficking. Additionally, we found a strong tendency to a

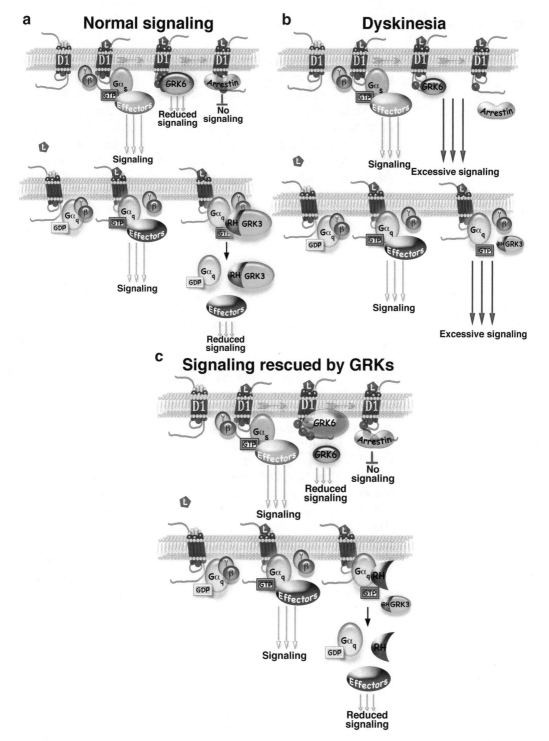

Fig. 2 Signaling abnormalities associated with dyskinesia and their correction by GRKs. (**a**) In the normal striatum, GRK6 controls GPCR signaling via receptor phosphorylation followed by arrestin binding, whereas GRK3
regulates the signaling of Gq/11-coupled GPCRs by sequestering active GTP-liganded Gαq/11. (**b**) Dopamine
depletion and/or subsequent pulsatile stimulation in the course of I-DOPA therapy may cause a reduction in the
expression of GRK6 and/or GRK3 in the striatum. Alternatively the amount of available GRKs becomes insufficient due to increased demand at the peak of the stimulation. In either case, this leads to uncontrolled excessive
signaling (sensitization to dopamine) and ultimately to I-DOPA-induced dyskinesia. (**c**) The delivery of exogenous
GRK6, which increases total availability of GRK6, and the expression of wild type GRK3 or its isolated RGS
homology domain (RH, shown) restores normal signaling regulation, thereby alleviating dyskinesia

decrease in the concentration of GRK2 and GRK5 in the striatal regions in human patients with PD at post mortem [116], which points to possible loss of GRKs following long-term L-DOPA use.

Thus, reduced GRK availability caused by either the loss of DA or by subsequent chronic treatment with L-DOPA likely contributes to the exaggerated dopaminergic signaling in the dyskinetic brain (Fig. 2b). Alternatively, defective desensitization and resulting receptor supersensitivity could be due to insufficient GRK availability in relation to the demand imposed by the DA surges in the course of L-DOPA therapy, even if the GRK concentration is not reduced, as compared to the normal striatum. Collectively, these results suggest that increasing the capacity of the desensitization machinery in the parkinsonian striatum may ameliorate LID.

4.3 Effect of the GRK Manipulation on LID and Antiparkinsonian Effect of L-DOPA

Based on the hypothesis that the GPCR desensitization machinery is defective in LID, whether due to reduced concentration of specific GRK isoforms or insufficient GRK availability relative to the demand, we set out to examine the effect of enhancing the capacity of the system on LID. The only feasible way to enhance the function of GRKs was to increase their concentration in the brain. Therefore, we chose to overexpress GRK6 in the DA-depleted striatum in hemiparkinsonian rats using the lentivirus-mediated gene transfer. GRK6 was chosen for these experiments, because, as described above, it was reported to be the primary GRK isoform [14, 77] regulating the signaling via DA receptors in vivo.

We found that lentivirus-mediated overexpression of GRK6 in the motor striatum in hemiparkinsonian rats suppressed L-DOPA-induced contralateral rotations and ameliorated abnormal involuntary movements (AIMs), suggesting that increased GRK availability alleviates LID [108] (Fig. 2c). Using lentivirus-mediated miRNA knockdown approach, we demonstrated that reduced availability of GRK6 promoted rotational behavior and increased AIMs scores, in agreement with our finding [109] that dopamine depletion reduces the expression of GRK6 and L-DOPA treatment does not reverse this reduction. We found that, although both GRK6A and GRK6B splice variants are reduced by the DA depletion, GRK6A is most affected by the lesion. The loss of GRK6 in the lesioned hemisphere suggests a link between lower GRK6 availability and dyskinesia. MiRNA-mediated GRK6 knockdown exacerbated the decrease in the GRK6 expression in the lesioned hemisphere and aggravated the behavioral consequences of DA depletion and L-DOPA treatment, supporting the role of low GRK6 in dyskinesia. The lesion reduced the GRK6 concentration by approximately 40%, and lentiviral knockdown further reduced it by 36–40%, whereas overexpression doubled GRK6 concentration. These numbers are in a good agreement with the work by Gainetdinov et al. [14], who found in GRK6 hemizygous mice (with ~50% reduction in the GRK6 concentration) a behavioral phenotype close to that of knockout animals. Thus, even a modest modulation of GRK6 concentration seems to have critical impact on dopaminergic signaling and dopamine-dependent behavior. These data underscore an important functional role of GRK6 in signaling mechanisms underlying dyskinesia (Fig. 2b).

Nonhuman primates lesioned with dopaminergic toxin 1-methyl-4-phenyl-1,2,3,6-tetrahydropyridine (MPTP) are considered a "golden standard" animal model of PD, since they faithfully reproduce the PD symptoms seen in human patients and develop dyskinesia upon chronic treatment with L-DOPA. We have examined the effect of upregulation of GRK6 in the striatum of parkinsonian monkeys on the manifestation of LID. The monkeys lesioned with MPTP and treated with L-DOPA until they developed LID were given injections into the motor putamen of the lentivirus encoding human GRK6. Upon recovery, the animals were tested for LID, as well as for the antiparkinsonian effect of L-DOPA. We found that elevating the concentration of GRK6 leads to significant amelioration of LID with complete preservation of the therapeutic potential of L-DOPA. Furthermore, the therapeutic effect was even extended in duration in animals expressing GRK6, as compared with control monkeys. In the clinical setting, patients with severe LID are often prescribed reduced dose of L-DOPA to help control LID. This comes at the expense of the anti-akinetic effect of the drug. We reproduced the situation in the parkinsonian monkeys by treating them with half the regular dose of L-DOPA and testing for both therapeutic and LID-inducing effects. To our surprise, we found that in GRK6-expressing monkeys half the L-DOPA dose was just as effective therapeutically as the full dose in control animals, but without inducing LID. In contrast, in control animal LID was reduced, albeit to a lower extent than in the GRK6 expressing monkeys, but so was the therapeutic effect of L-DOPA [108].

Therefore, our data demonstrate that promoting GPCR desensitization in the DA-depleted striatum via virus-mediated overexpression of GRK6 attenuates LID in both primate and rodent models. GRK6 suppresses LID in dyskinetic monkeys without compromising the antiparkinsonian effects of L-DOPA. In fact, GRK6 prolongs the antiparkinsonian effect, especially at the lower L-DOPA dose. The duration of the antiparkinsonian effect of the half-dose in GRK6-expressing animals was even slightly longer than that of the full L-DOPA dose in controls. Importantly, the additional time afforded by GRK6 was LID-free. In the rodent model, GRK6 consistently reduced the rotation frequency and the appearance of AIMs. The inhibition of the rotations and AIMs in rats by GRK6 parallels its potent anti-dyskinetic activity in the primate model of PD, suggesting an overlap between the molecular mechanisms underlying LID in primates and dyskinetic behaviors in rodents. Collectively, these data demonstrate that increased availability of GRK6 helps to control LID without sacrificing the antiparkinsonian benefits of L-DOPA.

A distinguishing feature of the GRKs is the presence, in addition to the kinase domain, of the RGS homology (RH) domain [119]. The RGS proteins are known to be critical regulators of GPCR signaling playing important roles in a variety of physiological and pathological processes [120]. The kinase domain of all GRKs is inserted within in a loop within the RH domain structure, which is a very unusual feature for multi-domain proteins [19, 121]. The RH domain of GRKs was originally identified *in silico* [119] but later shown to be functionally active in cultured cells [122–127]. In contrast to "conventional" RGS proteins, many of which accelerate GTP hydrolysis by G proteins [120], the RH of GRKs possess almost no GTPase accelerating activity but binds and sequesters active $G\alpha q/11$, thereby reducing the signaling via $Gq/11$-coupled GPCRs [123–126] (Fig. 2a). Thus, GRK2/3 can suppress GPCR signaling by two independent mechanisms: receptor phosphorylation and scavenging active $G\alpha q/11$. While the latter mechanism was demonstrated in cultured cells [122–126, 128, 129], it was never shown to operate in vivo.

Since GRK3 is downregulated in the lesioned striatum of the hemiparkinsonian rat, we tested whether overexpression of GRK3 would inhibit L-DOPA-induced rotations and AIMs and found that to be the case [117]. If the action of GRK3 is mediated by receptor phosphorylation, it could be due to facilitated receptor desensitization or enhanced arrestin-mediated signaling upon arrestin binding to phosphorylated receptors [17, 18]. However, in contrast to GRK6 that acted via receptor phosphorylation, the action of GRK3 was phosphorylation-independent, since kinase-dead mutant GRK3 retained full activity, which effectively ruled out both phosphorylation-dependent desensitization and arrestin-dependent signaling [117]. The GRK3 construct with inactivated RH domain but with other domains functionally intact (GRK3-RHD) did not affect L-DOPA-induced rotations, demonstrating that functional RH domain is required for the anti-LID activity of GRK3, whereas other domains do not make a measurable contribution. We also found that isolated RH domain lacking other domains recapitulated the effect of full-length GRK3, further supporting the conclusion that RH domain is sufficient for the GRK3 action. Moreover, in the context of similar subcellular localization of full-length GRK3 and its separated RH domain, the finding that both show the same anti-LID activity strongly suggests that full-length GRK3 exerts its effect in this paradigm via its RH domain. Taken together, these experiments provided definitive proof that the functional RH domain is necessary and sufficient for the anti-LID activity of GRK3 [117] (Fig. 2c).

The fact that GRK6 was proven to act exclusively via phosphorylation is not surprising. Although all GRKs possess the RH domain, only the RH domains of GRK2 and GRK3 seem to be capable of binding $G\alpha q/11$ [123]. The structure of GRK6 revealed that its RH domain has a shorter α5 helix than that of GRKs2/3 [121] and lacks structural elements known to be required for binding to Gαq/11 [122, 125, 126].

4.4 Receptors Mediating Effects of GRK on LID

GRK6 likely alters DA-dependent behavior by facilitating desensitization of DA receptors. Previous work with mice has demonstrated that behavioral supersensitivity to psychostimulants caused by GRK6 knockout is due to modified signaling through the D2 but not the D1 receptor [14]. However, dopamine depletion and subsequent development of LID in the course of L-DOPA treatment precipitates multiple dramatic changes in the striatal signaling pathways [97, 130]. Although both receptor subtypes are involved in LID, the D1 receptor seems to play a particularly important role [96, 118, 131]. Furthermore, deletion of the D1 receptor, but not the D2 receptor, abrogates both L-DOPA-induced rotations and AIMs [132], proving that only the D1 receptor is indispensable for LID. Thus, we expected that the dyskinetic action of GRK6 might require it to act on the D1 or both major DA receptor subtypes. We found that GRK6 reduced LID caused by selective D1 and D2 agonists in parkinsonian monkeys, indicating that signaling via both receptor subtypes was altered. In this respect, the effect of GRK6 is qualitatively different from our previous results with RGS9-2 [99], which only affected D2 receptors coupled to its target Gαi/o, but not D1 receptors coupled to Gαs [120]. In hemiparkinsonian rats, GRK6 promoted the D1 receptor internalization and suppressed the L-DOPA-induced upregulation of prodynorphin and of the D3 receptor attributed to the enhanced D1 receptor signaling [67]. Similarly, GRK6 reduced the prodynorphin expression in dyskinetic monkeys. Although we did not detect any increase in D2 receptor internalization, GRK6 reduced the upregulation of preproenkephalin mRNA expressed in D2 receptor-bearing neurons [60, 61, 133].

These findings should be interpreted with some caution, however, since some of the effects, behavioral as well as molecular, could be indirect occurring at the circuitry level. Earlier studies with selective D1 and D2 agonists demonstrated functional cooperation between the receptor systems. Synergism between the D1 and D2 receptors, i.e., a phenomenon when concomitant administration of a D1 and a D2 agonist produces much stronger behavioral and molecular effects than either drug alone. Such synergism as well as cross-priming effect (priming is an enhancement of a response to subsequent as compared to previous administrations of a drug; D1 and D2 agonists can prime for each other) seriously complicate understanding the relative role of these receptor subtypes in LID using pharmacological approaches (reviewed in refs. 134, 135). The mechanisms of either phenomenon remain unknown but likely indirect, involving interactions at the level of the neural circuitry, with the important role played by glutamate release [136–138]. Quite likely, GRK6 altered the D1 receptor desensitization directly, since we detected altered D1 receptor trafficking [108]. In contrast, the effect on the behavior produced by the D2 agonists is more likely indirect involving circuitry mechanisms, first, because there was no change in the D2 receptor trafficking, and, second, because GRK6 did not appear to be able to phosphorylate the D2 receptor, as demonstrated by in-cell phosphorylation experiments [38, 40]. Further experiments with neuron-selective modulation of the GRK6 activity are required to settle this issue.

In animals treated with selective D1 or D2/D3 agonists, GRK6 not only suppressed LID, but also shortened the overall duration of their effects, including the antiparkinsonian activity, and this effect was particularly obvious when the D1 agonist was used. This is consistent with faster receptor desensitization due to increased GRK6 availability. Conversely, in GRK6-expressing animals L-DOPA-induced antiparkinsonian effect lasted longer than in control monkeys. Due to high selectivity of GRKs for active receptors [139], we expected the anti-LID effect of GRK6 to be coupled with the preservation of the antiparkinsonian activity. The receptor must be activated, allowing the signal to go through, before it is desensitized by GRK-mediated phosphorylation. Apparently, this initial signaling is sufficient for the antiparkinsonian effect but not for LID. Although we have shown that GRK6 is able to phosphorylate many GPCRs in the inactive state, it shows high preference for the active D1 receptor over its inactive form [40]. Unique effects of L-DOPA might arise from its simultaneous action at both D1 and D2 receptors. The presence of GRK6 is likely to shift the balance in favor of D2-like receptors, since it may not promote their desensitization directly, and they generally do not desensitize as readily as D1 receptors [10, 30]. This conclusion is consistent with our finding that in monkeys GRK6 had only a modest effect on the duration of D2-mediated effects, whereas it substantially shortened that of the D1 agonist. Such rebalancing of the activity of D1 and D2 receptors and, consequently, of the direct and indirect pathways, might contribute to extended antiparkinsonian benefits.

GRK6 likely modulated DA-dependent behavior by facilitating desensitization of DA receptors. Previous work with GRK6 knockout mice has demonstrated that GRK6 is the key isoform regulating the signaling via the DA receptors [14]. Our results supported that conclusion although emphasizing the role of the D1 receptor regulation by GRK6 rather than that of the D2 receptor [108]. With GRK3, the situation is different. The canonical signaling of either the D1 or the D2 receptor does not involve Gq/11. The notion that D1R can couple to Gq, as an alternative to Gs/olf, persists [66, 140–152], although it is disputed [153–155]. Recent reports have shown that the striatal D1 receptors on the striatonigral neurons and D5 receptors on cholinergic interneurons couple to Gq in vivo [156, 157]. D1R/D2R heterodimers were reported to couple to Gq [63, 66] However, dimer formation requires the D1/D2 receptor co-expression in the same neuron, and only a limited proportion (5–7%) of neurons in the dorsal striatum co-express both receptors [64–66, 147, 158–160], although the proportion is higher in the nucleus accumbens [66, 147, 159]. Furthermore, the existence of the D1/D2R dimers has recently been called into question [153]. Therefore, the question whether the D1 receptor can engage the Gq signaling directly remains unresolved, and the origin of the Gq/11 signaling in LID affected by GRK3 is unclear.

Since RH directly binds active $G\alpha q/11$, its action does not depend on GRK3 biding to a particular receptor. GRK3 could sequester via it RH domain active $G\alpha q/11$ generated by activation of a number of non-DA Gq/11-coupled receptors expressed in striatal neurons. For example, active $G\alpha q/11$ could be generated by Group I mGluRs indirectly activated by L-DOPA. mGluR1 and, particularly, mGluR5 is highly expressed in medium spiny striatal neurons and interneurons [161–164]. Studies showing that drugs targeting these receptors modulate L-DOPA-induced behaviors and LID [165, 166] support the involvement of these receptors in the action of L-DOPA. Other Gq-coupled receptors could also contribute, including 5-HT2A receptors expressed by medium spiny striatal neurons [167]. Antagonists of these receptors reduce LID, suggesting a role in L-DOPA action, although it is unclear whether the mechanism is presynaptic or postsynaptic [168]. A major Gq-coupled receptor expressed by both types of medium spiny striatal neurons, but not by interneurons, is the M1 muscarinic receptor [169, 170]. Anticholinergic drugs targeting this receptor are used to treat stiffness and tremor in PD [170], but so far there is no evidence of its involvement in LID.

4.5 Signaling Mechanisms Affected by GRKs in the Parkinsonian Brain

We hypothesized that the origin of multiple signaling abnormalities in the DA-depleted striatum is inadequate desensitization of DA receptors that is either not normalized or further deregulated by subsequent chronic L-DOPA treatment. Defective receptor desensitization may partially stem from reduced expression of GRK isoforms in the DA depleted striatum that is not normalized by L-DOPA [109]. GRK6 affects desensitization of the DA receptors directly via conventional phosphorylation-arrestin binding mechanisms, whereas GRK3 acts via its RH domain facilitating inactivation of active $G\alpha q/11$, i.e., in a manner similar to other RGS proteins. Signaling abnormalities could then be propagated throughout the signaling network. The corollary of this hypothesis is that elevated expression of GRKs should rescue desensitization of DA receptors, thus ameliorating abnormal signaling via multiple pathways and improving behavior.

Several signaling pathways that are not normally activated by DA (or L-DOPA) show strong activation by L-DOPA or other dopaminergic agonists following DA depletion. The MAP kinase ERK is the best-studied pathway in the context of DA depletion and LID mechanisms. The supersensitivity of the ERK pathway to dopaminergic stimulation following DA depletion has been reported by many laboratories, and elevated ERK activity has been linked to LID development [60, 93, 94, 103, 106, 171, 172]. However, the exact role of the ERK deregulation in the LID development is still unclear. Moreover, chronic treatment with L-DOPA required for LID development desensitizes the ERK response, making it more likely that high ERK activity is associated with priming rather than with LID per se [60, 93, 103, 106]. Since priming is an important component of LID pathophysiology, reducing the ERK hyperactivity may have an anti-LID effect. Successful attempt has been made to ameliorate LID by controlling the activity of the neuron-specific ERK1/2 activator Ras-GRF1 factor [173]. We have demonstrated that expression of GRK6 in the lesioned striatum significantly suppressed ERK1/2 activation in response to L-DOPA challenge. We also found, in agreement with previous reports [93, 103–106], that chronic L-DOPA treatment reduced the degree of ERK supersensitivity to L-DOPA. The effect of GRK6 was strong in drug-naïve animals but diminished with chronic L-DOPA treatment. In fact, GRK6 brought down the ERK1/2 response in drug-naïve animals to the level of the desensitized ERK1/2 response in chronically L-DOPA-treated animals.

In contrast to ERK, the role of the p38 pathway in general has not previously attracted attention in connection to LID, although evidence exists as to the role of the p38 pathway in neuronal death in PD [174]. We detected elevated basal activity of p38 kinase in the lesioned striatum and found that p38, similarly to ERK1/2, was rendered supersensitive to L-DOPA challenge by DA depletion. In saline-treated animals, elevated level of phospho-p38 in the lesioned striatum was reflective of the increased p38 expression, since phospho-p38 to total p38 ratio was unchanged. In L-DOPA-treated animals, the ratio was elevated to a comparable degree in saline- and L-DOPA challenged rats, suggesting increased basal activity of the p38 pathway in the course of chronic L-DOPA treatment that was not further increased by the acute challenge. Thus, elevated p38 activity may be associated not only with peak-dose LID, as is the case with ERK1/2, but with the dyskinetic state itself. In contrast to ERK, chronic L-DOPA did not significantly desensitize the p38 response to L-DOPA challenge. The overexpression of GRK6 reduced the degree of the p38 supersensitivity across experimental groups, also reducing the basal activity in the L-DOPA-treated rats, but the effect was most noticeable in drug-naïve L-DOPA-challenged animals.

We have reported that loss of DA in the striatum resulted in a sustained elevation of the responsiveness of the Akt pathway to dopaminergic stimulation, which was not desensitized by chronic L-DOPA [93]. The hyperphosphorylation of Akt at the main activating residue Thr[308] in response to L-DOPA challenge in both drug-naïve and L-DOPA-treated rats is ameliorated by overexpression of GRK6, similarly to the effect seen on ERK1/2 and p38 activation. Therefore, our data demonstrate that by overexpressing GRK6, which presumably facilitated desensitization of DA receptors in the lesioned striatum, it was possible to partially normalize signaling via at least three pathways, ERK, p38, and Akt, all of which became supersensitive to DA upon DA depletion.

Enhanced ERK response to DA stimulation in the DA-depleted striatum has been linked to the D1 receptor supersensitivity [60, 94, 175, 176]. The elevated GRK6 likely reduced the ERK activation by L-DOPA via facilitation of the D1 receptor desensitization and normalization of the D1 intracellular trafficking and regulation [108]. The supersensitivity of the p38 or Akt pathways has not yet been attributed to a specific receptor. However, it is reasonable to conclude that they are also normalized via improved receptor desensitization. GRKs are believed to have rather broad receptor specificity, although detailed information for individual GRK isoforms is lacking (for review see [19]). GRK6 has been shown to preferentially regulate the D2 receptor in vivo [14]. Our previous data demonstrated that in the conditions of DA depletion GRK6 effectively modulates the signaling and trafficking of the supersensitive D1 receptor [108]. There is no information whether GRK6 regulates other GPCRs expressed by striatal neurons that are involved in the movement control and/or LID, such as adenosine A1 [177] and A2A [178, 179], serotonin 5-HT1A [180–184] and 5-HT1B [184, 185], or opioid [186–188] receptors in vitro or in vivo.

Chronic L-DOPA treatment appeared to diminish the normalizing effect of GRK6 on signaling, most obviously in case of ERK [95]. This was a somewhat unexpected finding. It seems that GRK6 suppressed acute signaling effects of L-DOPA, thus alleviating peak-dose LID, but not the long-term L-DOPA effects that predispose the animals to LID. This conclusion is consistent with the fact that overexpression of GRK6 diminished locomotor sensitization to L-DOPA, but does not abolish it. Sensitization still occurs, albeit at a reduced rate. The reduction is possibly due to weakened priming effect of every dose of L-DOPA. Chronic L-DOPA has no further effect on the GRK6 concentration reduced by DA depletion [95, 108, 109]. Therefore, GRK6 overexpression should be expected to normalize signaling even following chronic L-DOPA treatment, which was only partially the case. It is conceivable that overexpressed GRK6 facilitates acute desensitization of DA receptors, whereas upon chronic L-DOPA additional factors are introduced, which are either not under GRK6 control or affected by GRK6 in a different manner.

Reduced potency of every dose of the drug may be the cause of lower accumulation of transcription factor ΔFosB in the lesioned striatum of GRK6-overexpressing rats observed in this study. ΔFosB has been shown to directly contribute to the development of LID [189–191]. A lower level of ΔFosB in GRK6-overexpressing rats is consistent with the reduced rate of behavioral sensitization and LID in these animals. We also showed that the increase of ΔFosB concentration in the lesioned striatum occurs in the nuclear fraction, and this accumulation is blunted by GRK6. Weakened priming effect of every single L-DOPA dose accumulated over the course of the chronic treatment eventually may result in reduced gene expression associated with LID. We found that overexpressed GRK6 also reduced the degree of upregulation of dynorphin and enkephalin mRNA and the increase in the D3 DA receptor concentration [108]. These molecular changes are well-known markers of LID [134, 135], although their causal connection with LID development has never been convincingly demonstrated.

In case of GRK3, we detected no significant alterations in the MAP kinase or Akt signaling upon overexpression of full-length GRK3 or isolated RH domain. However, GRK3 and RH diminished accumulation of ΔFosB [117]. Interestingly, the effect of GRK3 on the accumulation of ΔFosB, the transcription factor implicated in LID development [189, 192], is phosphorylation-independent and is mediated via the RH domain of GRK3 [117]. Since the RH of GRK3 is only capable of interacting with Gαq/11 [123], these data for the first time implicate Gq-mediated signaling in the L-DOPA-induced ΔFosB accumulation. Gq-mediated signaling could affect ΔFosB accumulation via modulation of the protein kinase C [193] or calcium/calmodulin-dependent protein kinase II (CaMKII) activity [194].

These data show that modulation of the function of GRK6 and GRK3 impact the signaling network affected by the loss of DA and L-DOPA treatment. GRKs 6 and 3 affect different segments of the network mediated by second messengers cAMP and diacylglycerol/calcium, respectively. The signaling affected by the two GRK isoforms seems to converge at the level of the transcription factor ΔFosB and, presumably, downstream regulation of the gene expression.

4.6 Conclusions

Taken together, these in vitro studies and studies in transgenic mice with focus on assessing the effects of DA-targeting psychostimulant drugs and of L-DOPA in the models of PD and LID have convincingly demonstrated critical roles of select GRK isoforms in regulating the DA receptor signaling. Particularly, the roles of GRK2, GRK3 and GRK6 seem to be most critical in the regulation of both the D1-like and D2-like DA receptors. DA receptors, the same as other GPCRs, are known to have two modes of signaling—G protein-dependent and arrestin-dependent [195]. The role of GRKs in regulating the arrestin-dependent signaling remains essentially unexplored. It would be interesting to determine whether specific GRK are specifically connected with one versus another mode of the DA receptor signaling or the same GRK-mediated phosphorylation process equally promotes both events.

Further understanding of the specifics of such regulation should be critical for elucidating the pathological mechanisms of dopamine-related conditions. The addiction to psychostimulants remains quite high, and the illicit use of some psychostimulant drugs such as amphetamines is on the rise worldwide [196]. Furthermore, currently there is no viable strategy for treatment of the psychostimulant addiction or prevention of relapse of drug use. There is little doubt that GRKs, as the key regulators of the DA receptor signaling, play an essential role in neurological adaptations underlying the transition from persistent drug use to addiction. GRKs could impact addiction processes, for example, via modulation of ΔFosB accumulation involved in the cocaine-induced neuroplasticity [197] or by affecting the arrestin recruitment to DA receptors and arrestin-dependent signaling known to play a role in the psychostimulant action [198–200]

Clear understanding of the signaling regulation could be particularly important for LID, which remains an unmet medical need in the management of PD severely affecting the efficacy of treatment and the patients' quality of life. Advanced degeneration of dopaminergic innervation observed shortly after diagnosis of PD [201] makes the improvement of existing symptomatic therapies, in addition to the development of neuroprotective therapies, critical. In recent years, investigations have uncovered numerous signaling alterations associated with LID [reviewed in refs. 111, 134, 202]. Reduced supersensitivity of the ERK pathway and reduced accumulation of ΔFosB have been shown to lead to amelioration of LID [173, 189, 190]. However, the role of most signaling pathways deregulated by loss of DA and/or chronic L-DOPA in LID simply has not been explored. Furthermore, many signaling pathways that operate in the striatum have never been investigated in connection with PD or LID. A good example of this is the involvement in LID of the Gq/11-mediated signaling we discovered in connection with the GRK3 function that has never been suspected before. Thus, the sheer number of signaling pathways potentially involved in LID makes an informed choice of proper targets for anti-LID therapy difficult. It might be necessary to normalize most of them to achieve sustained anti-LID benefits, and it is unclear how to accomplish that. The root cause of signaling changes following DA depletion and chronic L-DOPA treatment seems to be abnormal signaling via DA receptors. Managing signaling at the receptor level may be a more effective way of normalizing multiple pathways and bringing about anti-LID benefits than targeting each pathway separately. As shown above, facilitation of receptor desensitization via GRK-dependent mechanisms leads to improvement in the function of multiple signaling pathways, amelioration of molecular abnormalities associated with LID, together with reduction of LID at the behavioral level. The results give further support to the notion that GRK6 and GRK3 are attractive targets for anti-LID therapy that may offer multiple therapeutic benefits unattainable by directly targeting signaling pathways.

References

1. Carman CV, Benovic JL (1998) G-protein-coupled receptors: turn-ons and turn-offs. Curr Opin Neurobiol 8:335–344

2. Gurevich VV, Gurevich EV (2004) The molecular acrobatics of arrestin activation. Trends Pharmacol Sci 25(2):105–111

3. Gurevich VV, Gurevich EV (2006) The structural basis of arrestin-mediated regulation of G-protein-coupled receptors. Pharmacol Ther 110(3):465–502

4. Gurevich EV, Gurevich VV (2006) Arrestins: ubiquitous regulators of cellular signaling pathways. Genome Biol 7(9):236

5. Gurevich VV, Gurevich EV (2014) Overview of different mechanisms of arrestin-mediated signaling. Curr Protoc Pharmacol 67(2.10):1–9

6. Willets JM, Parent JL, Benovic JL, Kelly E (1999) Selective reduction in A2 adenosine receptor desensitization following antisense-induced suppression of G protein-coupled receptor kinase 2 expression. J Neurochem 73:1781–1789

7. Bohn LM, Gainetdinov RR, Sotnikova TD, Medvedev IO, Lefkowitz RJ, Dykstra LA, Caron MG (2003) Enhanced rewarding properties of morphine, but not cocaine, in beta(arrestin)-2 knock-out mice. J Neurosci 23(32):10265–10273

8. Bohn LM, Lefkowitz RJ, Gainetdinov RR, Peppel K, Caron MG, Lin FT (1999) Enhanced morphine analgesia in mice lacking beta-arrestin2. Science 286:2495–2498

9. Pan L, Gurevich EV, Gurevich VV (2003) The nature of the arrestin x receptor complex determines the ultimate fate of the internalized receptor. J Biol Chem 278:11623–11632

10. Kim KM, Valenzano KJ, Robinson SR, Yao WD, Barak LS, Caron MG (2001) Differential regulation of the dopamine D2 and D3 receptors by G protein-coupled receptor kinases and beta-arrestins. J Biol Chem 276:37409–37414

11. Xu J, Dodd RL, Makino CL, Simon MI, Baylor DA, Chen J (1997) Prolonged photoresponses in transgenic mouse rods lacking arrestin. Nature 389(6650):505–509

12. Menard L, Ferguson SS, Zhang J, Lin FT, Lefkowitz RJ, Caron MG, Barak LS (1997) Synergistic regulation of beta2-adrenergic receptor sequestration: intracellular complement of beta-adrenergic receptor kinase and beta-arrestin determine kinetics of internalization. Mol Pharmacol 51:800–808

13. Iaccarino G, Rockman HA, Shotwell KF, Tomhave ED, Koch WJ (1998) Myocardial overexpression of GRK3 in transgenic mice: evidence for in vivo selectivity of GRKs. Am J Physiol 275:1298–1306

14. Gainetdinov RR, Bohn LM, Sotnikova TD, Cyr M, Laakso A, Macrae AD, Torres GE, Kim KM, Lefkowitz RJ, Caron MG, Premont RT (2003) Dopaminergic supersensitivity in G protein-coupled receptor kinase 6-deficient mice. Neuron 38:291–303

15. Willets JM, Nash MS, Challiss RA, Nahorski SR (2004) Imaging of muscarinic acetylcholine receptor signaling in hippocampal neurons: evidence for phosphorylation-dependent and -independent regulation by G-protein-coupled receptor kinases. J Neurosci 24(17):4157–4162

16. Gainetdinov RR, Bohn LM, Walker JK, Laporte SA, Macrae AD, Caron MG, Lefkowitz RJ, Premont RT (1999) Muscarinic supersensitivity and impaired receptor desensitization in G protein-coupled receptor kinase 5-deficient mice. Neuron 24(4):1029–1036

17. Kim J, Ahn S, Ren XR, Whalen EJ, Reiter E, Wei H, Lefkowitz RJ (2005) Functional antagonism of different G protein-coupled receptor kinases for beta-arrestin-mediated angiotensin II receptor signaling. Proc Natl Acad Sci U S A 102:142–1447

18. Ren XR, Reiter E, Ahn S, Kim J, Chen W, Lefkowitz RJ (2005) Different G protein-coupled receptor kinases govern G protein and beta-arrestin-mediated signaling of V2 vasopressin receptor. Proc Natl Acad Sci U S A 102:1448–1453

19. Gurevich EV, Tesmer JJ, Mushegian A, Gurevich VV (2012) G protein-coupled receptor

kinases: more than just kinases and not only for GPCRs. Pharmacol Ther 133:40–69

20. Dixon RA, Kobilka BK, Strader DJ, Benovic JL, Dohlman HG, Frielle T, Bolanowski MA, Bennett CD, Rands E, Diehl RE, Mumford RA, Slater EE, Sigal IS, Caron MG, Lefkowitz RJ, Strader CD (1986) Cloning of the gene and cDNA for mammalian beta-adrenergic receptor and homology with rhodopsin. Nature 321:75–79

21. Bunzow JR, Van Tol HH, Grandy DK, Albert P, Salon J, Christie M, Machida CA, Neve KA, Civelli O (1988) Cloning and expression of a rat D2 dopamine receptor cDNA. Nature 336(6201):783–787

22. Dal Toso R, Sommer B, Ewert M, Herb A, Pritchett DB, Bach A, Shivers BD, Seeburg PH (1989) The dopamine D2 receptor: two molecular forms generated by alternative splicing. EMBO J 8(13):4025–4034

23. Monsma FJ Jr, McVittie LD, Gerfen CR, Mahan LC, Sibley DR (1989) Multiple D2 dopamine receptors produced by alternative RNA splicing. Nature 342(6252):926–929

24. Dearry A, Gingrich JA, Falardeau P, Fremeau RT Jr, Bates MD, Caron MG (1990) Molecular cloning and expression of the gene for a human D1 dopamine receptor. Nature 347(6288):72–76

25. Monsma FJ Jr, Mahan LC, McVittie LD, Gerfen CR, Sibley DR (1990) Molecular cloning and expression of a D1 dopamine receptor linked to adenylyl cyclase activation. Proc Natl Acad Sci U S A 87(17):6723–6727

26. Sunahara RK, Niznik HB, Weiner DM, Stormann TM, Brann MR, Kennedy JL, Gelernter JE, Rozmahel R, Yang YL, Israel Y, Seeman P, O'Dowd BF (1990) Human dopamine D1 receptor encoded by an intronless gene on chromosome 5. Nature 347(6288):80–83

27. Giros B, Martres MP, Sokoloff P, Schwartz JC (1990) Gene cloning of human dopaminergic D3 receptor and identification of its chromosome. C R Acad Sci III 311(13):501–508

28. Van Tol HH, Bunzow JR, Guan HC, Sunahara RK, Seeman P, Niznik HB, Civelli O (1991) Cloning of the gene for a human dopamine D4 receptor with high affinity for the antipsychotic clozapine. Nature 350(6319):610–614

29. Sunahara RK, Guan HC, O'Dowd BF, Seeman P, Laurier LG, Ng G, George SR, Torchia J, Van Tol HH, Niznik HB (1991) Cloning of the gene for a human dopamine D5 receptor with higher affinity for dopamine than D1. Nature 350(6319):614–619

30. Tiberi M, Nash S, Bertrand L, Lefkowitz RJ, Caron MG (1996) Differential regulation of dopamine D1A receptor responsiveness by various G protein-coupled receptor kinases. J Biol Chem 271(7):3771–3778

31. Jiang D, Sibley DR (1999) Regulation of D(1) dopamine receptors with mutations of protein kinase phosphorylation sites: attenuation of the rate of agonist-induced desensitization. Mol Pharmacol 56(4):675–683

32. Kim OJ, Gardner BR, Williams DB, Marinec PS, Cabrera DM, Peters JD, Mak CC, Kim KM, Sibley DR (2004) The role of phosphorylation in D1 dopamine receptor desensitization: evidence for a novel mechanism of arrestin association. J Biol Chem 279:7999–8010

33. Pals-Rylaarsdam R, Gurevich VV, Lee KB, Ptasienski J, Benovic JL, Hosey MM (1997) Internalization of the m2 muscarinic acetylcholine receptor: arrestin-independent and -dependent pathways. J Biol Chem 272:23682–23689

34. Whistler JL, Tsao P, von Zastrow M (2001) A phosphorylation-regulated brake mechanism controls the initial endocytosis of opioid receptors but is not required for post-endocytic sorting to lysosomes. J Biol Chem 276:34331–34338

35. Palczewski K, Buczylko J, Kaplan MW, Polans AS, Crabb JW (1991) Mechanism of rhodopsin kinase activation. J Biol Chem 266:12949–12955

36. Rankin ML, Marinec PS, Cabrera DM, Wang Z, Jose PA, Sibley DR (2006) The D1 dopamine receptor is constitutively phosphorylated by G protein-coupled receptor kinase 4. Mol Pharmacol 69(3):759–769

37. Villar VA, Jones JE, Armando I, Palmes-Saloma C, Yu P, Pascua AM, Keever L, Arnaldo FB, Wang Z, Luo Y, Felder RA, Jose PA (2009) G protein-coupled receptor kinase 4 (GRK4) regulates the phosphorylation and function of the dopamine D3 receptor. J Biol Chem 284(32):21425–21434

38. Namkung Y, Dipace C, Javitch JA, Sibley DR (2009) G protein-coupled receptor kinase-mediated phosphorylation regulates post-endocytic trafficking of the D2 dopamine receptor. J Biol Chem 284(22):15038–15051

39. Cho D, Zheng M, Min C, Ma L, Kurose H, Park JH, Kim KM (2010) Agonist-induced endocytosis and receptor phosphorylation mediate resensitization of dopamine D(2) receptors. Mol Endocrinol 24(3):574–586

40. Li L, Homan KT, Vishnivetskiy SA, Manglik A, Tesmer JJ, Gurevich VV, Gurevich EV (2015) G Protein-coupled receptor kinases of the GRK4 protein subfamily phosphorylate inactive

G Protein-coupled Receptors (GPCRs). J Biol Chem 290(17):10775–10790

41. Mushegian A, Gurevich VV, Gurevich EV (2012) The origin and evolution of G protein-coupled receptor kinases. PLoS One 7(3):e33806

42. De Lean A, Stadel JM, Lefkowitz RJ (1980) A ternary complex model explains the agonist-specific binding properties of the adenylate cyclase-coupled beta-adrenergic receptor. J Biol Chem 255(15):7108–7117

43. Samama P, Cotecchia S, Costa T, Lefkowitz RJ (1993) A mutation-induced activated state of the beta 2-adrenergic receptor. Extending the ternary complex model. J Biol Chem 268(7):4625–4636

44. Benovic JL, Strasser RH, Caron MG, Lefkowitz RJ (1986) Beta-adrenergic receptor kinase: identification of a novel protein kinase that phosphorylates the agonist-occupied form of the receptor. Proc Natl Acad Sci U S A 83(9):2797–2801

45. Benovic JL, Mayor FJ, Somers RL, Caron MG, Lefkowitz RJ (1986) Light-dependent phosphorylation of rhodopsin by beta-adrenergic receptor kinase. Nature 321(6073):869–872

46. Gurevich VV, Benovic JL (1993) Visual arrestin interaction with rhodopsin: sequential multisite binding ensures strict selectivity towards light-activated phosphorylated rhodopsin. J Biol Chem 268:11628–11638

47. Gurevich VV, Pals-Rylaarsdam R, Benovic JL, Hosey MM, Onorato JJ (1997) Agonist-receptor-arrestin, an alternative ternary complex with high agonist affinity. J Biol Chem 272:28849–28852

48. Farrens DL, Altenbach C, Yang K, Hubbell WL, Khorana HG (1996) Requirement of rigid-body motion of transmembrane helices for light activation of rhodopsin. Science 274:768–770

49. Rasmussen SG, DeVree BT, Zou Y, Kruse AC, Chung KY, Kobilka TS, Thian FS, Chae PS, Pardon E, Calinski D, Mathiesen JM, Shah ST, Lyons JA, Caffrey M, Gellman SH, Steyaert J, Skiniotis G, Weis WI, Sunahara RK, Kobilka BK (2011) Crystal structure of the β2 adrenergic receptor-Gs protein complex. Nature 477:549–555

50. Rasmussen SG, Choi HJ, Fung JJ, Pardon E, Casarosa P, Chae PS, Devree BT, Rosenbaum DM, Thian FS, Kobilka TS, Schnapp A, Konetzki I, Sunahara RK, Gellman SH, Pautsch A, Steyaert J, Weis WI, Kobilka BK (2011) Structure of a nanobody-stabilized active state of the β(2) adrenoceptor. Nature 469:175–180

51. Kang Y, Zhou XE, Gao X, He Y, Liu W, Ishchenko A, Barty A, White TA, Yefanov O, Han GW, Xu Q, de Waal PW, Ke J, Tan MHE, Zhang C, Moeller A, West GM, Van Eps N, Caro LN, Vishnivetskiy SA, Lee RJ, Suino-Powell KM, Gu X, Pal K, Ma J, Zhi X, Boutet S, Williams GJ, Messerschmidt M, Gati C, Zatsepin NA, Wang D, James D, Basu S, Roy-Chowdhuty S, Conrad S, Coe J, Liu H, Lisova S, Kupitz C, Grotjohann I, Fromme R, Jiang Y, Tan M, Yang H, Li J, Wang M, Zheng Z, Li D, Zhao Y, Standfuss J, Diederichs K, Dong Y, Potter CS, Carragher B, Caffrey M, Jiang H, Chapman HN, Spence JCH, Fromme P, Weierstall U, Ernst OP, Katritch V, Gurevich VV, Griffin PR, Hubbell WL, Stevens RC, Cherezov V, Melcher K, Xu HE (2015) Crystal structure of rhodopsin bound to arrestin determined by femtosecond X-ray laser. Nature 523:561–567.

52. Pao CS, Barker BL, Benovic JL (2009) Role of the amino terminus of G protein-coupled receptor kinase 2 in receptor phosphorylation. Biochemistry 48(30):7325–7333

53. Beautrait A, Michalski KR, Lopez TS, Mannix KM, McDonald DJ, Cutter AR, Medina CB, Hebert AM, Francis CJ, Bouvier M, Tesmer JJ, Sterne-Marr R (2014) Mapping the putative G protein-coupled receptor (GPCR) docking site on GPCR kinase 2: insights from intact cell phosphorylation and recruitment assays. J Biol Chem 289(36):25262–25275

54. Strachan RT, Sun JP, Rominger DH, Violin JD, Ahn S, Rojas Bie Thomsen A, Zhu X, Kleist A, Costa T, Lefkowitz RJ (2014) Divergent transducer-specific molecular efficacies generate biased agonism at a G protein-coupled receptor (GPCR). J Biol Chem 289(20):14211–14224

55. Nestler EJ (2005) The neurobiology of cocaine addiction. Sci Pract Perspect 3:4–10

56. Thomas MJ, Kalivas PW, Shaham Y (2008) Neuroplasticity in the mesolimbic dopamine system and cocaine addiction. Br J Pharmacol 154:327–342

57. Feltenstein MW, See RE (2008) The neurocircuitry of addiction: an overview. Br J Pharmacol 154:261–274

58. Gerfen CR, Keefe KA, Gauda EB (1995) D1 and D2 dopamine receptor function in the striatum: coactivation of D1- and D2-dopamine receptors on separate populations of neurons results in potentiated immediate early gene response in D1-containing neurons. J Neurosci 15:8167–8176

59. Gerfen CR, McGinty JF, Young WS (1991) Dopamine differentially regulates dynorphin, substance P, and enkephalin expression in striatal neurons: in situ hybridization histochemical analysis. J Neurosci 11:1016–1031

60. Gerfen CR, Miyachi S, Paletzki R, Brown P (2002) D1 dopamine receptor supersensitivity in the dopamine-depleted striatum results from a switch in the regulation of ERK1/2 kinase. J Neurosci 22:5042–5054

61. Le Moine C, Bloch B (1995) D1 and D2 dopamine receptor gene expression in the rat striatum: sensitive cRNA probes demonstrate prominent segregation of D1 and D2 mRNAs in distinct neuronal populations of the dorsal and ventral striatum. J Comp Neurol 355:418–426

62. Rashid AJ, O'Dowd BF, Verma V, George SR (2007) Neuronal Gq/11-coupled dopamine receptors: an uncharted role for dopamine. Trends Pharmacol Sci 28:551–555

63. Rashid AJ, So CH, Kong MM, Furtak T, El-Ghundi M, Cheng R, O'Dowd BF, George SR (2007) D1-D2 dopamine receptor heterooligomers with unique pharmacology are coupled to rapid activation of Gq/11 in the striatum. Proc Natl Acad Sci U S A 104:654–659

64. Bertran-Gonzalez J, Bosch C, Maroteaux M, Matamales M, Hervé D, Valjent E, Girault JA (2008) Opposing patterns of signaling activation in dopamine D1 and D2 receptor-expressing striatal neurons in response to cocaine and haloperidol. J Neurosci 28:5671–5685

65. Matamales M, Bertran-Gonzalez J, Salomon L, Degos B, Deniau JM, Valjent E, Hervé D, Girault JA (2009) Striatal medium-sized spiny neurons: identification by nuclear staining and study of neuronal subpopulations in BAC transgenic mice. PLoS One 4:e4770

66. Lee SP, So CH, Rashid AJ, Varghese G, Cheng R, Lanca AJ, O'Dowd BF, George SR (2004) Dopamine D1 and D2 receptor co-activation generates a novel phospholipase C-mediated calcium signal. J Biol Chem 279:35671–35678

67. Bordet R, Ridray S, Carboni C, Diaz J, Sokoloff P, Schwartz JC (1997) Induction of dopamine D3 receptor expression as a mechanism of behavioral sensitization to levodopa. Proc Natl Acad Sci U S A 94:3363–3367

68. Bordet R, Ridray S, Schwartz JC, Sokoloff P (2000) Involvement of the direct striatonigral pathway in levodopa-induced sensitization in 6-hydroxydopamine-lesioned rats. Eur J Neurosci 12:2117–2123

69. Ding J, Guzman JN, Tkatch T, Chen S, Goldberg JA, Ebert PJ, Levitt P, Wilson CJ, Hamm HE, Surmeier DJ (2006) RGS4-dependent attenuation of M4 autoreceptor function in striatal cholinergic interneurons following dopamine depletion. Nat Neurosci 9:832–842

70. Ding Y, Won L, Britt JP, Lim SA, McGehee DS, Kang UJ (2011) Enhanced striatal cholinergic neuronal activity mediates L-DOPA-induced dyskinesia in parkinsonian mice. Proc Natl Acad Sci U S A 108:840–845

71. Wang Z, Kai L, Day M, Ronesi J, Yin HH, Ding J, Tkatch T, Lovinger DM, Surmeier DJ (2006) Dopaminergic control of corticostriatal long-term synaptic depression in medium spiny neurons is mediated by cholinergic interneurons. Neuron 50:443–452

72. Ciliax BJ, Nash N, Heilman C, Sunahara R, Hartney A, Tiberi M, Rye DB, Caron MG, Niznik HB, Levey AI (2000) Dopamine D_5 receptor immunolocalization in rat and monkey brain. Synapse 37:125–145

73. Khan ZU, Gutiérrez A, Martín R, Peñafiel A, Rivera A, de la Calle A (2000) Dopamine D5 receptors of rat and human brain. Neuroscience 100:689–699

74. Berlanga ML, Simpson TK, Alcantara AA (2005) Dopamine D5 receptor localization on cholinergic neurons of the rat forebrain and diencephalon: a potential neuroanatomical substrate involved in mediating dopaminergic influences on acetylcholine release. J Comp Neurol 492:34–49

75. Laakso A, Mohn AR, Gainetdinov RR, Caron MG (2002) Experimental genetic approaches to addiction. Neuron 36:213–228

76. Koob GF (1992) Drugs of abuse: anatomy, pharmacology and function of reward pathways. Trends Pharmacol Sci 13:177–184

77. Gainetdinov RR, Premont RT, Bohn LM, Lefkowitz RJ, Caron MG (2004) Desensitization of G protein-coupled receptors and neuronal functions. Annu Rev Neurosci 27:107–144

78. Premont RT, Gainetdinov RR (2007) Physiological roles of G protein-coupled receptor kinases and arrestins. Annu Rev Physiol 69:511–534

79. Arriza JL, Dawson TM, Simerly RB, Martin LJ, Caron MG, Snyder SH, Lefkowitz RJ (1992) The G-protein-coupled receptor kinases bARK1 and bARK2 are widely distributed at synapses in rat brain. J Neurosci 12:4045–4055

80. Iwata K, Ito K, Fukuzaki A, Inaki K, Haga T (1999) Dynamin and rab5 regulate GRK2-dependent internalization of dopamine D2 receptors. Eur J Biochem 263(2):596–602

81. Kabbani N, Negyessy L, Lin R, Goldman-Rakic P, Levenson R (2002) Interaction with neuronal calcium sensor NCS-1 mediates desensitization of the D2 dopamine receptor. J Neurosci 22(19):8476–8486

82. Banday AA, Fazili FR, Lokhandwala MF (2007) Insulin causes renal dopamine D1 receptor desensitization via GRK2-mediated receptor phosphorylation involving phosphatidylinositol 3-kinase and protein kinase C. Am J Physiol Renal Physiol 293(3):F877–F884

83. Sedaghat K, Nantel MF, Ginsberg S, Lalonde V, Tiberi M (2006) Molecular characterization of dopamine D2 receptor isoforms tagged with green fluorescent protein. Mol Biotechnol 34(1):1–14

84. Schroeder JA, McCafferty MR, Unterwald EM (2009) Regulation of dynamin 2 and G protein-coupled receptor kinase 2 in rat nucleus accumbens during acute and repeated cocaine administration. Synapse 63(10):863–870

85. Jaber M, Koch WJ, Rockman H, Smith B, Bond RA, Sulik KK, Ross J Jr, Lefkowitz RJ, Caron MG, Giros B (1996) Essential role of beta-adrenergic receptor kinase 1 in cardiac development and function. Proc Natl Acad Sci U S A 93(23):12974–12979

86. Daigle TL, Caron MG (2012) Elimination of GRK2 from cholinergic neurons reduces behavioral sensitivity to muscarinic receptor activation. J Neurosci 32:11461–11466

87. Daigle TL, Ferris MJ, Gainetdinov RR, Sotnikova TD, Urs NM, Jones SR, Caron MG (2014) Selective deletion of GRK2 alters psychostimulant-induced behaviors and dopamine neurotransmission. Neuropsychopharmacology 10:2450–2462

88. Beyer CE, Steketee JD (2002) Cocaine sensitization: modulation by dopamine D2 receptors. Cereb Cortex 12:526–535

89. Bychkov E, Zurkovsky L, Garret M, Ahmed MR, Gurevich EV (2013) Distinct cellular and subcellular distribution of G protein-coupled receptor kinase and arrestin isoforms in the striatum. PLoS One 7:e48912

90. Erdtmann-Vourliotis M, Mayer P, Ammon S, Riechert U, Hollt V (2001) Distribution of G-protein-coupled receptor kinase (GRK) isoforms 2, 3, 5 and 6 mRNA in the rat brain. Brain Res Mol Brain Res 95(1-2):129–137

91. Raehal KM, Schmid CL, Medvedev IO, Gainetdinov RR, Premont RT, Bohn LM (2009) Morphine-induced physiological and behavioral responses in mice lacking G protein-coupled receptor kinase 6. Drug Alcohol Depend 104(3):187–196

92. Seeman P, Weinshenker D, Quirion R, Srivastava LK, Bhardwaj SK, Grandy DK, Premont RT, Sotnikova TD, Boksa P, El-Ghundi M, O'Dowd BF, George SR, Perreault ML, Mannisto PT, Robinson S, Palmiter RD, Tallerico T (2005) Dopamine supersensitivity correlates with D2High states, implying many paths to psychosis. Proc Natl Acad Sci U S A 102(9):3513–3518

93. Bychkov E, Ahmed MR, Dalby KN, Gurevich EV (2007) Dopamine depletion and subsequent treatment with L-DOPA, but not the long-lived dopamine agonist pergolide, enhances activity of the Akt pathway in the rat striatum. J Neurochem 102:699–711

94. Santini E, Valjent E, Usiello A, Carta M, Borgkvist A, Girault J-A, Herve D, Greengard P, Fisone G (2007) Critical Involvement of cAMP/DARPP-32 and extracellular signal-regulated protein kinase signaling in L-DOPA-induced dyskinesia. J Neurosci 27:6995–7005

95. Ahmed MR, Bychkov E, Kook S, Zurkovsky L, Dalby KN, Gurevich EV (2015) Overexpression of GRK6 rescues L-DOPA-induced signaling abnormalities in the dopamine-depleted striatum of hemiparkinsonian rats. Exp Neurol 266:42–54

96. Aubert I, Guigoni HK, Li Q, Dovero S, Barthe N, Bioulac BH, Gross CE, Fisone G, Bloch B, Bezard E (2005) Increased D1 dopamine receptor signaling in levodopa-induced dyskinesia. Ann Neurol 57:17–26

97. Guigoni C, Aubert I, Li Q, Gurevich VV, Benovic JL, Ferry S, Mach U, Stark H, Leriche L, Hakansson K, Bioulac BH, Gross CE, Sokoloff P, Fisone G, Gurevich EV, Bloch B, Bezard E (2005) Pathogenesis of levodopa-induced dyskinesia: focus on D1 and D3 dopamine receptors. Parkinsonism Relat Disord 11(Suppl 1):S25–S29

98. Kovoor A, Seyffarth P, Ebert J, Barghshoon S, Chen C-K, Schwarz S, Axelrod JD, Cheyette BNR, Simon MI, Lester HA, Schwarz J (2005) D2 dopamine receptors colocalize regulator of G-protein signaling 9-2 (RGS9-2) via the RGS9 DEP domain, and RGS9 knock-out mice develop dyskinesias associated with dopamine pathways. J Neurosci 25:2157–2165

99. Gold SJ, Hoang CV, Potts BW, Porras G, Pioli E, Kim KW, Nadjar A, Qin C, LaHoste GJ, Li Q, Bioulac BH, Waugh JL, Gurevich E, Neve RL, Bezard E (2007) RGS9 2 negatively modulates l-3,4-dihydroxyphenylalanine-Induced dyskinesia in experimental Parkinson's disease. J Neurosci 27:14338–14348

100. Fahn S (2008) How do you treat motor complications in Parkinson's disease: medicine, surgery, or both? Ann Neurol 64(Suppl 2):S56–S64

101. Stocchi F, Nordera G, Marsden CD (1997) Strategies for treating patients with advanced

Parkinson's disease with disastrous fluctuations and dyskinesias. Clin Neuropharmacol 20:95–115

102. Cotzias GC, Papavasiliou PS, Gellene R (1969) Modification of Parkinsonism by chronic treatment with L-dopa. N Engl J Med 280(7):337–345

103. Bezard E, Gross CE, Qin L, Gurevich VV, Benovic JL, Gurevich EV (2005) L-DOPA reverses the MPTP-induced elevation of the arrestin2 and GRK6 expression and enhanced ERK activation in monkey brain. Neurobiol Dis 18:323–335

104. Brown A, Deutch AY, Colbran RJ (2005) Dopamine depletion alters phosphorylation of striatal proteins in a model of Parkinsonism. Eur J Neurosci 22:247–256

105. Kim DS, Palmiter RD, Cummins A, Gerfen CR (2006) Reversal of supersensitive striatal dopamine D1 receptor signaling and extracellular signal-regulated kinase activity in dopamine-deficient mice. Neuroscience 137:1381–1388

106. Santini E, Sgambato-Faure V, Li Q, Savasta M, Dovero S, Fisone G, Bezard E (2010) Distinct changes in cAMP and extracellular signal-regulated protein kinase signalling in L-DOPA-induced dyskinesia. PLoS One 5:e12322

107. Sgambato-Faure V, Buggia V, Gilbert F, Levesque D, Benabid AL, Berger F (2005) Coordinated and spatial upregulation of arc in striatonigral neurons correlates with L-dopa-induced behavioral sensitization in dyskinetic rats. J Neuropathol Exp Neurol 64:936–947

108. Ahmed MR, Berthet A, Bychkov E, Porras G, Li Q, Bioulac BH, Carl YT, Bloch B, Kook S, Aubert I, Dovero S, Doudnikoff E, Gurevich VV, Gurevich EV, Bezard E (2010) Lentiviral overexpression of GRK6 alleviates L-dopa-induced dyskinesia in experimental Parkinson's disease. Sci Transl Med 2:28ra28

109. Ahmed MR, Bychkov E, Gurevich VV, Benovic JL, Gurevich EV (2007) Altered expression and subcellular distribution of GRK subtypes in the dopamine-depleted rat basal ganglia is not normalized by l-DOPA treatment. J Neurochem 104:1622–1636

110. Cenci MA, Lundblad M (2007) Ratings of L-DOPA-induced dyskinesia in the unilateral 6-OHDA lesion model of Parkinson's disease in rats and mice. Curr Protoc Neurosci 9 (Unit 9.25)

111. Cenci MA, Konradi C (2010) Maladaptive striatal plasticity in L-DOPA-induced dyskinesia. Prog Brain Res 183:209–233

112. Cenci MA, Lee CS, Björklund A (1998) L-DOPA-induced dyskinesia in the rat is associated with striatal overexpression of prodynorphin- and glutamic acid decarboxylase mRNA. Eur J Neurosci 10:2694–2706

113. Cenci MA (2007) Dopamine dysregulation of movement control in L-DOPA-induced dyskinesia. Trends Neurosci 30:236–243

114. Bezard E, Ferry S, Mach U, Stark H, Leriche L, Boraud T, Gross CE, Sokoloff P (2003) Attenuation of levodopa-induced dyskinesia by normalizing dopamine D3 receptor function. Nat Med 9(6):762–767

115. Gurevich EV, Benovic JL, Gurevich VV (2004) Arrestin2 expression selectively increases during neural differentiation. J Neurochem 91(6):1404–1416

116. Bychkov E, Gurevich VV, Joyce JN, Benovic JL, Gurevich EV (2008) Arrestins and two receptor kinases are upregulated in Parkinson's disease with dementia. Neurobiol Aging 29:379–396

117. Ahmed MR, Bychkov E, Li L, Gurevich VV, Gurevich EV (2015) GRK3 suppresses L-DOPA-induced dyskinesia in the rat model of Parkinson's disease via its RGS homology domain. Sci Rep 5:10920

118. Guigoni C, Doudnikoff E, Li Q, Bloch B, Bezard E (2007) Altered D1 dopamine receptor trafficking in Parkinsonian and dyskinetic non-human primates. Neurobiol Dis 26(2):452

119. Siderovski DP, Hessel A, Chung S, Mak TW, Tyers M (1996) A new family of regulators of G-protein-coupled receptors? Curr Biol 6:211–212

120. Hollinger S, Hepler JR (2002) Cellular regulation of RGS proteins: modulators and integrators of G protein signaling. Pharmacol Rev 54:527–559

121. Lodowski DT, Tesmer VM, Benovic JL, Tesmer JJ (2006) The structure of G protein-coupled receptor kinase (GRK)-6 defines a second lineage of GRKs. J Biol Chem 281:16785–16793

122. Day PW, Wedegaertner PB, Benovic JL (2004) Analysis of G-protein-coupled receptor kinase RGS homology domains. Methods Enzymol 390:295–310

123. Carman CV, Parent JL, Day PW, Pronin AN, Sternweis PM, Wedegaertner PB, Gilman AG, Benovic JL, Kozasa T (1999) Selective regulation of Galpha(q/11) by an RGS domain in the G protein-coupled receptor kinase, GRK2. J Biol Chem 274:34483–34492

124. Day PW, Carman CV, Sterne-Marr R, Benovic JL, Wedegaertner PB (2003) Differential interaction of GRK2 with members of the Ga$_q$ family. Biochemistry 42:9176–9184

125. Sterne-Marr R, Dhami GK, Tesmer JJ, Ferguson SS (2004) Characterization of GRK2 RH domain-dependent regulation of GPCR coupling to heterotrimeric G proteins. Methods Enzymol 390:310–336

126. Sterne-Marr R, Tesmer JJ, Day PW, Stracquatanio RP, Cilente JA, O'Connor KE, Pronin AN, Benovic JL, Wedegaertner PB (2003) G protein-coupled receptor Kinase 2/G alpha/11 interaction. A novel surface on a regulator of G protein signaling homology domain for binding G alpha subunits. J Biol Chem 278:6050–6058

127. Usui I, Imamura T, Satoh H, Huang J, Babendure JL, Hupfeld CJ, Olefsky JM (2004) GRK2 is an endogenous protein inhibitor of the insulin signaling pathway for glucose transport stimulation. EMBO J 23:2821–2829

128. Dhami GK, Dale LB, Anborgh PH, O'Connor-Halligan KE, Sterne-Marr R, Ferguson SS (2004) G Protein-coupled receptor kinase 2 regulator of G protein signaling homology domain binds to both metabotropic glutamate receptor 1a and Galphaq to attenuate signaling. J Biol Chem 279:16614–16620

129. Dhami GK, Anborgh PH, Dale LB, Sterne-Marr R, Ferguson SSG (2002) Phosphorylation-independent regulation of metabotropic glutamate receptor signaling by G protein-coupled receptor kinase 2. J Biol Chem 277(28):25266–25272

130. Bezard E, Brotchie JM, Gross CE (2001) Pathophysiology of levodopa-induced dyskinesia: potential for new therapies. Nat Rev Neurosci 2:577–588

131. Berthet A, Porras G, Doudnikoff E, Stark H, Cador M, Bezard E, Bloch B (2009) Pharmacological analysis demonstrates dramatic alteration of D1 dopamine receptor neuronal distribution in the rat analog of L-DOPA-induced dyskinesia. J Neurosci 29:4829–4835

132. Darmopil S, Martín AB, De Diego IR, Ares S, Moratalla R (2009) Genetic inactivation of dopamine D1 but not D2 receptors inhibits L-DOPA-induced dyskinesia and histone activation. Biol Psychiatry 66:603–613

133. Morissette M, Grondin R, Goulet M, Bédard PJ, Di Paolo T (1999) Differential regulation of striatal preproenkephalin and preprotachykinin mRNA levels in MPTP-lesioned monkeys chronically treated with dopamine D1 or D2 agonists. J Neurochem 72:682–692

134. Gurevich EV, Gurevich VV (2008) Dopamine receptors and the treatment of Parkinson's disease. In: Neve KA (ed) Dopamine receptors, 2nd edn. Humana, Portland, OR, pp 525–584

135. Bastide MF, Meissner WG, Picconi B, Fasano S, Fernagut PO, Feyder M, Francardo V, Alcacer C, Ding Y, Brambilla R, Fisone G, Joe Stoessl A, Bourdenx M, Engeln M, Navailles S, De Deurwaerdère P, Ko WK, Simola N, Morelli M, Groc L, Rodriguez MC, Gurevich EV, Quik Morari M, Mellone M, Gardoni F, Tronci E, Guehl D, Tison F, Crossman AR, Kang UJ, Steece-Collier K, Fox S, Carta M, Angela-Cenci M, Bézard E (2015) Pathophysiology of L-dopa-induced motor and non-motor complications in Parkinson's disease. Prog Neurobiol 132:96–168

136. Paul ML, Currie RW, Robertson HA (1995) Priming of a D1 dopamine receptor behavioural response is dissociated from striatal immediate-early gene activity. Neuroscience 66:347–359

137. Paul ML, Graybiel AM, David JC, Robertson HA (1992) D1-like and D2-like dopamine receptors synergistically activate rotation and c-fos expression in the dopamine-depleted striatum in a rat model of Parkinson's disease. J Neurosci 12:3729–3742

138. Pollack AE, Strauss JB (1999) Time dependence and role of N-methyl-D-aspartate glutamate receptors in the priming of D2-mediated rotational behavior and striatal Fos expression in 6-hydroxydopamine lesioned rats. Brain Res 827:160–168

139. Moore CA, Milano SK, Benovic JL (2007) Regulation of receptor trafficking by GRKs and arrestins. Annu Rev Physiol 69:451–482

140. Banday AA, Lokhandwala MF (2007) Oxidative stress reduces renal dopamine D1 receptor-Gq/11alpha G protein-phospholipase C signaling involving G protein-coupled receptor kinase 2. Am J Physiol Ren Physiol 293:F306–F315

141. Felder CC, Blecher M, Jose PA (1989) Dopamine-1-mediated stimulation of phospholipase C activity in rat renal cortical membranes. J Biol Chem 264:8739–8745

142. Felder CC, Jose PA, Axelrod J (1989) The dopamine-1 agonist, SKF 82526, stimulates phospholipase-C activity independent of adenylate cyclase. J Pharmacol Exp Ther 248:171–175

143. Liu J, Wang F, Huang C, Long LH, Wu WN, Cai F, Wang JH, Ma LQ, Chen JG (2009)

Activation of phosphatidylinositol-linked novel D1 dopamine receptor contributes to the calcium mobilization in cultured rat prefrontal cortical astrocytes. Cell Mol Neurobiol 29:317–328

144. Liu J, Wang W, Wang F, Cai F, Hu ZL, Yang YJ, Chen J, Chen JG (2009) Phosphatidylinositol-linked novel D(1) dopamine receptor facilitates long-term depression in rat hippocampal CA1 synapses. Neuropharmacology 57:164–171

145. Mizuno K, Kurokawa K, Ohkuma S (2012) Dopamine D1 receptors regulate type 1 inositol 1,4,5-trisphosphate receptor expression via both AP-1- and NFATc4-mediated transcriptional processes. J Neurochem 122:702–713

146. Pacheco MA, Jope RS (1997) Comparison of [3H]phosphatidylinositol and [3H]phosphatidylinositol 4,5- bisphosphate hydrolysis in postmortem human brain membranes and characterization of stimulation by dopamine D1 receptors. J Neurochem 69:639–644

147. Perreault ML, Hasbi A, O'Dowd BF, George SR (2014) Heteromeric dopamine receptor signaling complexes: emerging neurobiology and disease relevance. Neuropsychopharmacology 39:156–168

148. Undie AS, Friedman E (1990) Stimulation of a dopamine D1 receptor enhances inositol phosphates formation in rat brain. J Pharmacol Exp Ther 253:987–992

149. Undie AS, Friedman E (1992) Selective dopaminergic mechanism of dopamine and SKF38393 stimulation of inositol phosphate formation in rat brain. Eur J Pharmacol 226:297–302

150. Undie AS, Friedman E (1994) Inhibition of dopamine agonist-induced phosphoinositide hydrolysis by concomitant stimulation of cyclic AMP formation in brain slices. J Neurochem 63:222–230

151. Yu Y, Wang JR, Sun PH, Guo Y, Zhang ZJ, Jin GZ, Zhen X (2008) Neuroprotective effects of atypical D1 receptor agonist SKF83959 are mediated via D1 receptor-dependent inhibition of glycogen synthase kinase-3 beta and a receptor-independent anti-oxidative action. J Neurochem 104:946–956

152. Zhang X, Zhou Z, Wang D, Li A, Yin Y, Gu X, Ding F, Zhen X, Zhou J (2009) Activation of phosphatidylinositol-linked D1-like receptor modulates FGF-2 expression in astrocytes via IP3-dependent Ca2+ signaling. J Neurosci 29:7766–7775

153. Frederick AL, Yano H, Trifilieff P, Vishwasrao HD, Biezonski D, Mészáros J, Urizar E, Sibley DR, Kellendonk C, Sonntag KC, Graham DL, Colbran RJ, Stanwood GD, Javitch JA (2015) Evidence against dopamine D1/D2 receptor heteromers. Mol Psychiatry 20(11):1373–85

154. Lee SM, Kant A, Blake D, Murthy V, Boyd K, Wyrick SJ, Mailman RB (2014) SKF-83959 is not a highly-biased functionally selective D1 dopamine receptor ligand with activity at phospholipase C. Neuropharmacology 86:145–154

155. Lee SM, Yang Y, Mailman RB (2014) Dopamine D1 receptor signaling: does GαQ-phospholipase C actually play a role? J Pharmacol Exp Ther 351:9–17

156. Medvedev IO, Ramsey AJ, Masoud ST, Bermejo MK, Urs N, Sotnikova TD, Beaulieu JM, Gainetdinov RR, Salahpour A (2013) D1 dopamine receptor coupling to PLCβ regulates forward locomotion in mice. J Neurosci 33:18125–18133

157. Sahu A, Tyeryar KR, Vongtau HO, Sibley DR, Undieh AS (2009) D5 dopamine receptors are required for dopaminergic activation of phospholipase C. Mol Pharmacol 75:447–453

158. Aubert I, Ghorayeb I, Normand E, Bloch B (2000) Phenotypical characterization of the neurons expressing the D1 and D2 dopamine receptors in the monkey striatum. J Comp Neurol 418:22–32

159. Perreault ML, Hasbi A, Alijaniaram M, Fan T, Varghese G, Fletcher PJ, Seeman P, O'Dowd BF, George SR (2010) The dopamine D1-D2 receptor heteromer localizes in dynorphin/enkephalin neurons: increased high affinity state following amphetamine and in schizophrenia. J Biol Chem 285:36625–36634

160. Surmeier DJ, Song WJ, Yan Z (1996) Coordinated expression of dopamine receptors in neostriatal medium spiny neurons. J Neurosci 16:6579–6591

161. Testa CM, Standaert DG, Landwehrmeyer GB, Penney JBJ, Young AB (1995) Differential expression of mGluR5 metabotropic glutamate receptor mRNA by rat striatal neurons. J Comp Neurol 354:241–252

162. Testa CM, Friberg IK, Weiss SW, Standaert DG (1998) Immunohistochemical localization of metabotropic glutamate receptors mGluR1a and mGluR2/3 in the rat basal ganglia. J Comp Neurol 390:5–19

163. Paquet M, Smith Y (2003) Group I metabotropic glutamate receptors in the monkey striatum: subsynaptic association with glutamatergic and dopaminergic afferents. J Neurosci 23:7659–7669

164. Smith Y, Charara A, Hanson JE, Paquet M, Levey AI (2000) GABA(B) and group I metabotropic glutamate receptors in the stria-

topallidal complex in primates. J Anat 196:555–576

165. Mela F, Marti M, Dekundy A, Danysz W, Morari M, Cenci MA (2007) Antagonism of metabotropic glutamate receptor type 5 attenuates l-DOPA-induced dyskinesia and its molecular and neurochemical correlates in a rat model of Parkinson's disease. J Neurochem 101:483–497

166. Rylander D, Recchia A, Mela F, Dekundy A, Danysz W, Cenci MA (2009) Pharmacological modulation of glutamate transmission in a rat model of L-DOPA-induced dyskinesia: effects on motor behavior and striatal nuclear signaling. J Pharmacol Exp Ther 330:227–235

167. Bubser M, Backstrom JR, Sanders-Bush E, Roth BL, Deutch AY (2001) Distribution of serotonin 5-HT2A receptors in afferents of the rat striatum. Synapse 39:297–304

168. Huot P, Fox SH, Newman-Tancredi A, Brotchie JM (2011) Anatomically selective serotonergic type 1A and serotonergic type 2A therapies for Parkinson's disease: an approach to reducing dyskinesia without exacerbating parkinsonism? J Pharmacol Exp Ther 339:2–8

169. Calabresi P, Centonze D, Gubellini P, Pisani A, Bernardi G (2000) Acetylcholine-mediated modulation of striatal function. Trends Neurosci 23:120–126

170. Pisani A, Bernardi G, Ding J, Surmeier DJ (2007) Re-emergence of striatal cholinergic interneurons in movement disorders. Trends Neurosci 30:545–553

171. Santini E, Feyder M, Gangarossa G, Bateup HS, Greengard P, Fisone G (2012) Dopamine- and cAMP-regulated phospho-protein of 32-kDa (DARPP-32)-dependent activation of extracellular signal-regulated kinase (ERK) and mammalian target of rapamycin complex 1 (mTORC1) signaling in experimental parkinsonism. J Biol Chem 287:27806–27812

172. Alcacer C, Santini E, Valjent E, Gaven F, Girault JA, Hervé D (2012) Gα(olf) mutation allows parsing the role of cAMP-dependent and extracellular signal-regulated kinase-dependent signaling in L-3,4-dihydroxyphenylalanine-induced dyskinesia. J Neurosci 32:5900–5910

173. Fasano S, Bezard E, D'Antoni A, Francardo V, Indrigo M, Qin L, Doveró S, Cerovic M, Cenci MA, Brambilla R (2010) Inhibition of Ras-guanine nucleotide-releasing factor 1 (Ras-GRF1) signaling in the striatum reverts motor symptoms associated with L-dopa-induced dyskinesia. Proc Natl Acad Sci U S A 107:21824–21829

174. Akerboom J, Chen TW, Wardill TJ, Tian L, Marvin JS, Mutlu S, Calderón NC, Esposti F, Borghuis BG, Sun XR, Gordus A, Orger MB, Portugues R, Engert F, Macklin JJ, Filosa A, Aggarwal A, Kerr RA, Takagi R, Kracun S, Shigetomi E, Khakh BS, Baier H, Lagnado L, Wang SS, Bargmann CI, Kimmel BE, Jayaraman V, Svoboda K, Kim DS, Schreiter ER, Looger LL (2012) Optimization of a GCaMP calcium indicator for neural activity imaging. J Neurosci 32:13819–13840

175. Santini E, Alcacer C, Cacciatore S, Heiman M, Hervé D, Greengard P, Girault JA, Valjent E, Fisone G (2009) L-DOPA activates ERK signaling and phosphorylates histone H3 in the striatonigral medium spiny neurons of hemiparkinsonian mice. J Neurochem 108:621–633

176. Westin JE, Vercammen L, Strome EM, Konradi C, Cenci MA (2007) Spatiotemporal pattern of striatal ERK1/2 phosphorylation in a rat model of L-DOPA-induced dyskinesia and the role of dopamine D1 receptors. Biol Psychiatry 62:800–810

177. Xiao K, McClatchy DB, Shukla AK, Zhao Y, Chen M, Shenoy SK, Yates JR 3rd, Lefkowitz RJ (2007) Functional specialization of beta-arrestin interactions revealed by proteomic analysis. Proc Natl Acad Sci U S A 104(29):12011–12016

178. Armentero MT, Pinna A, Ferré S, Lanciego JL, Müller CE, Franco R (2011) Past, present and future of A(2A) adenosine receptor antagonists in the therapy of Parkinson's disease. Pharmacol Ther 132:280–299

179. Fredduzzi S, Moratalla R, Monopoli A, Cuellar B, Xu K, Ongini E, Impagnatiello F, Schwarzschild MA, Chen JF (2002) Persistent behavioral sensitization to chronic L-DOPA requires A2A adenosine receptors. J Neurosci 22:1054–1062

180. Bibbiani F, Oh JD, Chase TN (2001) Serotonin 5-HT1A agonist improves motor complications in rodent and primate Parkinsonian models. Neurology 57:1829–1834

181. Dupre KB, Eskow KL, Barnum CJ, Bishop C (2008) Striatal 5-HT1A receptor stimulation reduces D1 receptor-induced dyskinesia and improves movement in the hemiparkinsonian rat. Neuropharmacology 55:1321–1328

182. Dupre KB, Ostock CY, Eskow Jaunarajs KL, Button T, Savage LM, Wolf W, Bishop C (2011) Local modulation of striatal glutamate efflux by serotonin 1A receptor stimulation in dyskinetic, hemiparkinsonian rat. Exp Neurol 229:288–299

183. Dupre KB, Ostock CY, George JA, Eskow Jaunarajs KL, Hueston CM, Bishop C (2013) Effects of 5-HT receptor stimulation on D1 receptor agonist-induced striatonigral activity and dyskinesia in hemiparkinsonian rats. ACS Chem Neurosci 4:747–760

184. Iderberg H, Rylander D, Bimpisidis Z, Cenci MA (2013) Modulating mGluR5 and 5-HT1A/1B receptors to treat l-DOPA-induced dyskinesia: effects of combined treatment and possible mechanisms of action. Exp Neurol 250:116–124

185. Zhang X, Andren PE, Greengard P, Svenningsson P (2008) Evidence for a role of the 5-HT1B receptor and its adaptor protein, p11, in l-DOPA treatment of an animal model of Parkinsonism. Proc Natl Acad Sci U S A 105:2163–2168

186. Chen L, Togasaki DM, Langston JW, Di Monte DA, Quik M (2005) Enhanced striatal opioid receptor-mediated G-protein activation in L-DOPA-treated dyskinetic monkeys. Neuroscience 132:409–420

187. Cox H, Togasaki DM, Chen L, Langston JW, Di Monte DA, Quik M (2007) The selective kappa-opioid receptor agonist U50,488 reduces L-dopa-induced dyskinesias but worsens Parkinsonism in MPTP-treated primates. Exp Neurol 205:101–107

188. Henrya B, Foxb SH, Crossmanb AR, Brotchieb JM (2001) μ- and δ-opioid receptor antagonists reduce levodopa-induced dyskinesia in the MPTP-lesioned primate model of Parkinson's disease. Exp Neurol 171:139–146

189. Cao X, Yasuda T, Uthayathas S, Watts RL, Mouradian MM, Mochizuki H, Papa SM (2010) Striatal overexpression of DeltaFosB reproduces chronic levodopa-induced involuntary movements. J Neurosci 30:7335–7343

190. Berton O, Guigoni C, Li Q, Bioulac BH, Aubert I, Gross CE, Dileone RJ, Nestler EJ, Bezard E (2009) Striatal overexpression of DeltaJunD resets L-DOPA-induced dyskinesia in a primate model of Parkinson disease. Biol Psychiatry 66:554–561

191. Engeln M, Bastide MF, Toulmé E, Dehay B, Bourdenx M, Doudnikoff E, Li Q, Gross CE, Boué-Grabot E, Pisani A, Bezard E, Fernagut PO (2016) Selective inactivation of striatal FosB/ΔFosB-expressing neurons alleviates l-dopa-induced dyskinesia. Biol Psychiatry 79(5):354–61

192. Cenci MA (2002) Transcription factors involved in the pathogenesis of L-DOPA-induced dyskinesia in a rat model of Parkinson's disease. Amino Acids 23:105–109

193. Ding WQ, Larsson C, Alling C (1998) Stimulation of muscarinic receptors induces expression of individual Fos and Jun genes through different transduction pathways. J Neurochem 70:1722–1729

194. Robison AJ, Vialou V, Mazei-Robison M, Feng J, Kourrich S, Collins M, Wee S, Koob G, Turecki G, Neve R, Thomas M, Nestler EJ (2013) Behavioral and structural responses to chronic cocaine require a feedforward loop involving ΔFosB and calcium/calmodulin-dependent protein kinase II in the nucleus accumbens shell. J Neurosci 33:4295–4307

195. Beaulieu JM, Espinoza S, Gainetdinov RR (2015) Dopamine receptors – IUPHAR Review 13. Br J Pharmacol 172:1–23

196. United Nations Office on Drugs and Crime (2014) World drug report 2014. United Nations Office on Drugs and Crime, Vienna

197. Robison AJ, Nestler EJ (2011) Transcriptional and epigenetic mechanisms of addiction. Nat Rev Neurosci 12:623–637

198. Beaulieu J-M, Tirotta E, Sotnikova TD, Masri B, Salahpour A, Gainetdinov RR, Borrelli E, Caron MG (2007) Regulation of Akt signaling by D2 and D3 dopamine receptors in vivo. J Neurosci 27(4):881–885

199. Beaulieu JM, Gainetdinov RR, Caron MG (2007) The Akt-GSK-3 signaling cascade in the actions of dopamine. Trends Pharmacol Sci 28:166–172

200. Beaulieu JM, Sotnikova TD, Marion S, Lefkowitz RJ, Gainetdinov RR, Caron MG (2005) An Akt/beta-arrestin 2/PP2A signaling complex mediates dopaminergic neurotransmission and behavior. Cell 122:261–273

201. Kordower JH, Olanow CW, Dodiya HB, Chu Y, Beach TG, Adler CH, Halliday GM, Bartus RT (2013) Disease duration and the integrity of the nigrostriatal system in Parkinson's disease. Brain 136:2419–2431

202. Murer MG, Moratalla R (2011) Striatal signaling in l-DOPA-induced dyskinesia: common mechanisms with drug abuse and long term memory involving D1 dopamine receptor stimulation. Front Neuroanat 5:51

Chapter 12

G-Protein-Coupled Receptors and Their Kinases in Cardiac Regulation

Alessandro Cannavo, Claudio de Lucia, and Walter J. Koch

Abstract

The superfamily of G-protein-coupled receptors (GPCRs), or seven transmembrane-spanning receptors (7TMRs), represents the largest family of membrane proteins that transduce cell signals via heterotrimeric G proteins from neurohormones, ions, and sensory stimuli to regulate virtually every aspect of mammalian physiology. In the normal and diseased heart, it is apparent that major players include the β-adrenergic receptors (βARs) and the angiotensin II type 1 receptors (AT$_1$Rs). Their crucial role is reflected by the fact that, currently, they represent the direct targets of different approved cardiovascular drugs used in clinical practice. However, other "minor" receptors and their signaling pathways have been identified for roles that they exert on cardiac pathophysiology. GPCRs can, individually or collectively, regulate cardiac growth and function, including processes such as heart rate, contractility, and blood pressure, in response to catecholamines and other neurohormones. For these reasons, GPCRs are dynamically regulated to prevent overstimulation that could lead to cardiac diseases like heart failure (HF). This dampening process, known as desensitization, is initiated through GPCR phosphorylation by second-messenger kinases like protein kinase A (PKA) and PKC or the GPCR kinases (GRKs). PKA and PKC initiate heterologous desensitization, while GRKs initiate homologous desensitization, phosphorylating only agonist-occupied GPCRs. This GPCR regulation by GRKs induces recruitment and binding of β-arrestins that displace bound G proteins, therefore uncoupling receptors from their downstream signaling effectors. This process continues through β-arrestin-dependent internalization of receptors, that lead either to their degradation and downregulation or recycling (resensitization) to the membrane. Moreover, β-arrestin recruitment to GRK-phosphorylated receptors has been shown to lead to intracellular signaling, a process called G protein-dependent and independent signaling. Given their central role in cardiac physiology and in pathology, GPCRs are critical therapeutic targets in cardiac diseases and GRKs are emerging as innovative targets.

Key words Cardiac function, G-protein-coupled receptor kinase, Heart failure

1 Introduction

GPCRs are nodal regulators of most aspects of cardiovascular biology. Over the past decades, different reports have revealed much about the signaling properties of the GPCRs [1]. Examples of GPCRs with well-recognized roles in cardiovascular physiology include the β-adrenergic receptors (βARs) that control cardiac contractility [2] and the angiotensin II (Ang II) type 1 receptors

Vsevolod V. Gurevich et al. (eds.), *G Protein-Coupled Receptor Kinases*, Methods in Pharmacology and Toxicology, DOI 10.1007/978-1-4939-3798-1_12, © Springer Science+Business Media New York 2016

(AT$_1$Rs) that are prominent receptors implicated in cardiac growth [3]. Much effort has focused on identification of the multiple ways in which GPCRs like the βARs and AT$_1$Rs regulate cardiac function, and also how those molecules take part in cardiac pathology. Importantly, great work has also been done in uncovering mechanisms by which GPCR signaling is regulated and led to the discovery of GPCR kinases (GRKs) [4, 5] and β-arrestins [6]. Thus, given that cardiac GPCRs and their signaling pathways represent nodal regulators of the cardiac function, there is an enormous potential for development of novel therapies targeting these receptors in cardiac diseases like heart failure (HF), either directly (e.g. GPCR blockers) or via their signaling regulating molecules (e.g. GRK inhibitors). Below, we discuss some of the major GPCR systems involved in cardiac health and disease and the role GRKs play in HF pathogenesis.

2   G-Protein-Coupled Receptors Involved in the Control of Heart Function

2.1   β-Adrenergic Receptors (βARs)

The adrenergic receptor (AR) function is modulated by the endogenous catecholamine hormones epinephrine and norepinephrine [2]. In the heart, βARs, comprise approximately 90% of the total cardiac ARs, with the α$_1$ARs, accounting for the remaining 10% [7]. Consistent with their expression and role in the heart, βARs are one of the most important molecular targets in the cardiovascular system. Three βAR subtypes (β$_1$AR, β$_2$AR, and β$_3$AR) have been identified in cardiac tissue [8], and among these β$_1$AR and β$_2$AR represent 80 and 20% of the expressed βARs, respectively [9]. In general, acute activation of cardiac βARs leads to activation of stimulatory G (G$_s$) protein inducing the subsequent activation of adenylyl cyclase (AC), which catalyzes the production of cAMP that, in turn, activates PKA [8]. This kinase activates different Ca^{2+} handling proteins and some myofilament components exerting important effects on cardiac contractility [10]. Importantly, chronic activation of βARs appears to be an important culprit in HF development, at least in part, by the induction of over-desensitization caused by increased sympatholytic nervous system activity and elevated catecholamines [11].

The effects on cardiac cell fate exerted by the three βAR isoforms are dependent on their distinct G protein coupling. While β$_1$AR and β$_3$AR are coupled with G$_s$, activation of cardiac β$_2$AR also can activate G inhibitory (G$_i$)-dependent signaling pathways [12]. G$_i$ concurrent activation spatially compartmentalizes β$_2$AR/G$_s$-mediated cAMP signaling, functionally inhibits AC activity, and stimulates novel mitogen-activated protein kinase (MAPK) pathways in the heart through Gα and βγ subunits. Importantly, several studies have demonstrated that β$_1$AR activation leads to cardiac apoptosis, whereas β$_2$AR activation leads to both pro-apoptotic and pro-survival signals [13]. In particular β_2ARs, but not β_1ARs, activate a G_i-$G\beta\gamma$-PI3K-Akt cell survival signaling pathway, and the inhibition of this pathway promotes pro-death signaling [13]. For its part, the β_3AR seems to play a role in cardiac metabolism, cardioprotection, and contractility [14]. Little is known about these mechanisms, but it has been proposed that β_3AR expression, which is lower in the healthy myocardium, is increased in HF animal models and in HF patients [15, 16] and, in limited studies, by treatment with β_1AR blockers [17, 18]. Moreover, a role for nitric oxide (NO) and cGMP has been recently proposed as a mechanism of β_3AR-mediated cardioprotection in animal models of cardiac pressure overload, neurohormone-induced hypertrophy, myocardial ischemia/reperfusion injury, and acute myocardial infarction [19]. Therefore, increased β_3AR signaling apparent after β_1AR blockade helps to explain why such treatment is beneficial in HF.

2.2 αARs

Whereas the role and the function of βARs are well studied, less is known about cardiac αARs. In myocytes, all α_1ARs (α_{1A}, α_{1B}, and α_{1D}) are expressed [7], however, no expression has been demonstrated for the α_2AR [20]. All three α_1ARs couple to the $G_{q/11}$ ($G\alpha_q$) family of G proteins and involve activation of phospholipase Cβ1 (PLCβ1) at the plasma membrane [7]. Activation of PLCβ1 leads to phosphatidylinositol (PI) cleavage, and to increased inositol trisphosphate (IP$_3$) and diacylglycerol (DAG). Following interaction of IP$_3$ with the IP$_3$ receptor, Ca^{2+} is released from intracellular stores. DAG is involved in activation of PKC and related signaling [7].

Regarding the functional role of α_1ARs in the heart, different reports from the last decade indicate that α_1ARs, following chronic activation, can induce beneficial trophic signaling in cardiac development, and that these α_1AR-mediated effects in the adult can counteract the negative effects of β_1AR overstimulation in HF [21]. The α_1AR-dependent protective role in failing myocardium has been associated with the induction of adaptive or physiological hypertrophy and also to prevention of cardiac myocyte death, thus augmenting contractile function [22–24]. Importantly, total α_1AR levels are not altered in vivo by HF [21, 25], and α_1AR inotropic effects are maintained or increased, in contrast to βARs, which are downregulated. Partial explanation for the differences in desensitization of α_1AR and βARs might reside in their expression and regulation by specific GRKs [21, 26–28].

2.3 Angiotensin II Receptors (AIIRs)

Angiotensin II (Ang II) is the key component of the renin–angiotensin–aldosterone system (RAAS) and plays an important role in cardiac physiology. Ang II can activate 2 primary receptors, Ang II type 1 and type 2 receptors (AT$_1$R and AT$_2$R, respectively). However, the AT$_1$R mediates most of the known cardiac physiological effects of Ang II, such as positive chronotropy and inotropy, NE release from cardiac sympathetic nerve terminals, coronary vessel vasoconstriction, aldosterone release, cardiac hypertrophy, and interstitial fibrosis [29, 30]. It has been recently proposed that AT_2R is also involved in some important activities of Ang II [31, 32]. However, whereas the AT_1R has been identified in the heart and in most vascular tissues of adults, AT_2R expression is limited mainly to fetal organs including the heart [33]. For this reason, most cardiac pharmacology is focused on drugs capable of inhibiting only the AT_1R. Consistently, experimental and clinical studies have demonstrated that AT_1R antagonism attenuates most of the deleterious effects of Ang II in the heart [34].

The AT_1R is a classic $G_{q/11}$-coupled receptor and activates a similar signaling pathway as seen for α_1ARs (see above). In addition, it signals via β-arrestins independently of G proteins [35]. Analogous to other G_q-coupled receptors, the AT_1R is believed to play an important role in the pathogenesis of HF. In fact, hallmarks of HF like contractile dysfunction, myocyte hypertrophy, increased cardiac cell death and fibrosis [36], can be worsened by activation of G_q-coupled receptors [37].

2.4 Sphingosine-1 Phosphate (S1P) Receptors (S1PRs)

The lysophospholipid, S1P, is a circulating bioactive lipid metabolite that can act through a GPCR. In the heart there are currently three GPCRs for which S1P is a high-affinity ligand and thereby activate different G-protein signaling pathways. In particular, cardiomyocytes express $S1PR_1$, $S1PR_2$, and $S1PR_3$ receptors. The $S1PR_1$ receptor couples exclusively to the G_i protein [38–40]. In contrast, the $S1PR_2$ and $S1PR_3$ receptors couple to G_i and G_q proteins [41]. In the heart, all of these receptors have been linked to cardioprotective signaling with effects that include the induction of adaptative hypertrophy, inhibition of contractility, and activation of anti-apoptotic molecules [42]. The $S1PR_1$ is the predominant subtype in cardiomyocytes and has been shown to be regulated by both GRK2 and PKC through phosphorylation [43].

Interestingly, it has been recently shown that $S1PR_1$, through its coupling to the G_i protein, has a signaling that opposes β_1AR-mediated AC activation [44]. Moreover, $S1PR_1$ is able to antagonize the effects mediated by isoproterenol (ISO) and other βAR agonists [44, 45]. Recently, our group has reported in cardiomyocytes a direct cross-talk between β_1AR and $S1PR_1$ that is orchestrated by GRK2 [46]. In fact, we and others demonstrated that catecholamines can exert a hypertrophic response in cardiomyocytes by influencing the $S1PR_1$ signaling pathway [45, 46]. This mechanism seems to be strongly reduced during HF where adrenergic overstimulation increases the levels of GRK2, which then induces the downregulation of both $S1PR_1$ and β_1AR with a consistent negative effect on cardiac function [46].

3   GRKs in Cardiac Physiology and Pathology

As discussed above, heart function is primarily regulated by βARs that are activated by circulating catecholamines. High levels of these hormones released following any kind of injury or stress on the heart can induce a persistent activation of βARs that could be detrimental in the absence of a kinase able to uncouple these receptors from their downstream signaling machinery [47]. Under most circumstances, βAR hyperstimulation is acutely regulated by GRKs. However, continuous stimulation of βARs results in their profound desensitization and loss of responsiveness to catecholamine, which appears to contribute to HF development [48]. Almost two decades ago, it was found that this marked desensitization of βARs in the failing myocardium is accompanied by robust GRK2 upregulation [49, 50]. These increased levels exacerbate the unresponsiveness of βARs and induce their chronic downregulation. Indeed, overexpression of GRK2 in the heart results in decreased isoproterenol (βARs agonist)-stimulated contractility and reduced cAMP production [51], impaired cardiac function [52], and increased apoptosis [53]. GRK2 is not the only GRK isoform expressed in the heart. In fact, of the seven mammalian GRKs, GRK2, GRK3, and GRK5 are expressed in the heart [8]. However, studies have shown GRK2 and GRK5 to be the most involved in cardiac physiology and pathophysiology [54].

Regarding their structure, all GRKs are serine/threonine kinases with similar structural architecture as they all have a highly conserved N-terminal domain, unique to the GRK family, a catalytic region containing the kinase domain [55] and a carboxyl-terminal (CT) domain that contains specific regulatory sites [8]. The N-terminal domain harbors several regulatory motifs including a regulator of G-protein signaling (RGS) homology domain, whereas the CT domain mediates interactions with lipids and membrane proteins that control the subcellular localization of GRKs [8]. Importantly, the CT domain of GRK2 (and the related GRK3) contains a pleckstrin homology domain (PH), which interacts with phosphatidylinositol 4,5-biphosphate (PIP_2) and free Gβγ subunits [56]. Following these interactions, GRK2 translocates from the cytoplasm to the plasma membrane enhancing activated GPCR phosphorylation. GRK5 does not have this domain and does not use Gβγ to target the plasma membrane, but its membrane localization is facilitated by the CT-lipid-binding domain [57, 58].

GRK targeting to activated GPCRs generally requires N-terminus-mediated allosteric activation by the agonist-bound GPCR [59], a feature distinguishing them from other serine–threonine protein kinases [60]. Subsequently, GRK-mediated GPCR phosphorylation, in combination with recruitment of β-arrestin to the receptor, leads to functional repression of G protein-mediated signaling. GRK-mediated phosphorylation of diverse serine and threonine GPCR residues creates a specific pattern (or "barcode") that controls differential activation of downstream signaling—a feature recently termed "biased signaling" [61]. This occurs via modulating β-arrestin scaffolding with divergent interacting partners [62]. For example, phosphorylation of the angiotensin II receptor by GRK2 and 3 mediated receptor internalization, whereas phosphorylation by GRK5 promoted activation of the extracellular signal-related kinase (ERK) [62].

In animal studies, it has been shown that overexpression of GRK3 did not influence the activity of βARs [63]; whereas inhibition of GRK3 in the heart improved the sensitivity to stimulation of α1ARs and caused increased systolic blood pressure due to augmented cardiac output [64]. In contrast, cardiac-specific overexpression of GRK5 diminished the βARs response to isoproterenol [27] and compromised cardiac function [65], suggesting that this kinase GRK5 can have a role in HF development. Interestingly, high mRNA and protein levels of GRK5 have been reported in experimental models of HF [66, 67] and also in humans [68].

Over the last two decades, GRK2 inhibition has been shown to be beneficial in the failing heart [8]. This has primarily been done through the transgene expression of a peptide designed from the CT domain of GRK2, called the βARKct, which competes with endogenous GRK2 for Gβγ binding and targeting to agonist bound GPCRs [51, 56]. Expression of the βARKct in cardiomyocytes, including failing human cardiomyocytes, reverses βAR desensitization and improves cardiac contractile function [51].

Transgene βARKct expression has prevented in mice [27] and reversed in preclinical studies in pig [69] the development of HF. The importance of GRK2 in the regulation of cardiac function and HF pathology has been confirmed in GRK2 knockout (KO) mice including global KOs [70] and cardiac-specific GRK2 KO mice [71, 72].

Other strategies have been recently developed in order to inhibit GRK2 in the failing heart. The discovery that an FDA-approved drug, paroxetine, has significant GRK2 inhibitory properties both in vitro and in vivo has opened a new scenario in cardiac pharmacology and drug design [73, 74]. Paroxetine binds in the active site of GRK2 and stabilizes the kinase domain in a novel conformation in which a unique regulatory loop forms part of the ligand binding site [73]. Interestingly, pretreatment of mice with this drug significantly increases left ventricular inotropic reserve with no significant effect on heart rate following isoproterenol stimulation [73]. Of note, in a mouse model of HF it has been recently shown that chronic paroxetine treatment significantly reversed cardiac dysfunction and induced beneficial effects on remodeling including a complete restoration of βAR system, which was shown to be due to GRK2 inhibition [74]. Consistently, as previously shown [75], the observed effects with pharmacological GRK2 inhibition were more beneficial than those with βAR blockade [74].

Recently, GRKs have been found to phosphorylate a variety of non-GPCR proteins, including transcription factors and tyrosine kinases, further broadening their functional roles in cardiac physiology. These noncanonical roles for GRKs may result from their innate basal activity or, perhaps, through phosphorylation of proteins following GPCR activation [8, 76–80].

In this context, recent data support GRK2 being a key negative modulator of myocyte energy substrate use, especially following myocardial infarction. In fact, GRK2 can regulate the insulin receptor substrate-1 (IRS-1) or the non-GPCR adiponectin receptor 1 (Adipo R1) through direct phosphorylation, thus impairing glucose uptake [76, 77].

GRK5 has an interesting noncanonical activity that appears to be constitutively involved in pathological cardiomyopathy. In this regard, it has been recently demonstrated that GRK5 has an active nuclear localization signal (NLS), and this is functional in cardiomyocytes [81]. In particular, our group has found that GRK5 in cardiac myocytes, following G_q-dependent signaling, translocates to the nucleus [78]. Nuclear GRK5 is able to regulate the hypertrophic response through direct interaction and phosphorylation of histone deacetylase 5 (HDAC5) leading to activation of the myocytes enhance factor-2 (MEF-2) transcription. Importantly, the nuclear activity of GRK5 exclusively related to an increased maladaptive cardiac hypertrophic response as recently demonstrated in animal models of pressure overload [82, 83]. Indeed, GRK5 appears to function as a physiological HDAC kinase, as GRK5 KO mice display less hypertrophy after left-ventricular pressure overload with lower amount of HDAC5 in the cytoplasm [83]. Moreover, our group has also found that nuclear GRK5 mediates pathological cardiac hypertrophy through its kinase-independent ability to bind the DNA, thus enhancing the activation of both nuclear factor of activated T cells (NFATc3) and nuclear factor-κB (NF-κB) [79, 80]. Thus, the nuclear noncanonical activity of GRK5 represents a novel target for maladaptive hypertrophy and HF.

4   Conclusions

Over the past 3 decades, characterization of GPCR-related structures and signaling, especially obtained thanks to Robert Lefkowitz and Brian Kobilka, for which they recently received a Nobel prize in chemistry [1], has provided key clinical and pharmacological information that has advanced our understanding of cardiac

278   Alessandro Cannavo et al.

physiology and how to go about counteracting the development and progression of cardiac diseases like HF. In this regard, molecules capable of directly interacting with GPCRs or that can target specific proteins involved in cardiac GPCR signaling, such as GRKs and β-arrestins, represent the most exciting area for cardiac pharmacology. For example, GRK2 blockade, which can provide both a positive inotropic and sympatholytic therapy at the same time [2], has been widely demonstrated to be one of the strongest potential therapies that could be used in synergy with conventional therapies used to fight chronic HF [8]. The noncanonical actions of GRKs, independent of their canonical GPCR regulation, also represent novel targets for future HF intervention.

References

1. Lin HH (2013) G-protein-coupled receptors and their (Bio) chemical significance win 2012 Nobel Prize in chemistry. Biomed J 36(3):118–124
2. Lymperopoulos A, Rengo G, Koch WJ (2013) Adrenergic nervous system in heart failure: pathophysiology and therapy. Circ Res 113:739–753
3. Lymperopoulos A, Bathgate A (2013) Arrestins in the cardiovascular system. Prog Mol Biol Transl Sci 118:297–334
4. Benovic JL, Strasser RH, Caron MG et al (1986) Beta-adrenergic receptor kinase: identification of a novel protein kinase that phosphorylates the agonist-occupied form of the receptor. Proc Natl Acad Sci U S A 83:2797–2801
5. Benovic JL, Mayor F Jr, Staniszewski C et al (1987) Purification and characterization of the beta-adrenergic receptor kinase. J Biol Chem 262:9026–9032
6. Lohse MJ, Benovic JL, Codina J et al (1990) Beta-arrestin: a protein that regulates beta-adrenergic receptor function. Science 248:1547
7. O'Connell TD, Jensen BC, Baker AJ et al (2013) Cardiac alpha1-adrenergic receptors: novel aspects of expression, signaling mechanisms, physiologic function, and clinical importance. Pharmacol Rev 66(1):308–333
8. Cannavo A, Liccardo D, Koch WJ (2013) Targeting cardiac β-adrenergic signaling via GRK2 inhibition for heart failure therapy. Front Physiol 4:264
9. Siryk-Bathgate A, Dabul S, Lymperopoulos A (2013) Current and future G protein-coupled receptor signaling targets for heart failure therapy. Drug Des Devel Ther 7:1209–1222
10. Bristow MR, Hershberger RE, Port JD et al (1990) Beta-adrenergic pathways in nonfailing and failing human ventricular myocardium. Circulation 82(Suppl 2):I12–I25
11. Huang ZM, Gold JI, Koch WJ (2011) G protein-coupled receptor kinases in normal and failing myocardium. Front Biosci (Landmark Ed) 16:3047–3060
12. Xiao RP (2001) Beta-adrenergic signaling in the heart: dual coupling of the beta2-adrenergic receptor to G(s) and G(i) proteins. Sci STKE 2001(104):re15
13. Zhu WZ, Zheng M, Koch WJ et al (2001) Dual modulation of cell survival and cell death by β2-adrenergic signaling in adult mouse cardiac myocytes. Proc Natl Acad Sci U S A 98:1607–1612
14. Dessy C, Balligand JL (2010) Beta3-adrenergic receptors in cardiac and vascular tissues emerging concepts and therapeutic perspectives. Adv Pharmacol 59:135–163
15. Cheng HJ, Zhang ZS, Onishi K, Ukai T, Sane DC, Cheng CP (2001) Upregulation of functional beta(3)-adrenergic receptor in the failing canine myocardium. Circ Res 89:599–606
16. Moniotte S, Kobzik L, Feron O et al (2001) Upregulation of beta(3)-adrenoceptors and altered contractile response to inotropic amines in human failing myocardium. Circulation 103:1649–1655
17. Sharma V, Parsons H, Allard MF et al (2008) Metoprolol increases the expression of beta(3)-adrenoceptors in the diabetic heart: effects on nitric oxide signaling and forkhead transcription factor-3. Eur J Pharmacol 595:44–51
18. Zhao Q, Wu TG, Jiang ZF et al (2007) Effect of beta-blockers on beta3-adrenoceptor expression in chronic heart failure. Cardiovasc Drugs Ther 21:85–90
19. Trappanese DM, Liu Y, McCormick RC et al (2015) Chronic β1-adrenergic blockade

enhances myocardial β3-adrenergic coupling with nitric oxide-cGMP signaling in a canine model of chronic volume overload: new insight into mechanisms of cardiac benefit with selective β1-blocker therapy. Basic Res Cardiol 110(1):456

20. Montó F, Oliver E, Vicente D et al (2012) Different expression of adrenoceptors and GRKs in the human myocardium depends on heart failure etiology and correlates to clinical variables. Am J Physiol Heart Circ Physiol 303(3):H368–H376

21. Sjaastad I, Schiander I, Sjetnan A et al (2003) Increased contribution of alpha 1- vs. beta-adrenoceptor-mediated inotropic response in rats with congestive heart failure. Acta Physiol Scand 177(4):449–458

22. Knowlton KU, Michel MC, Itani M et al (1993) The alpha 1 A-adrenergic receptor subtype mediates biochemical, molecular, and morphologic features of cultured myocardial cell hypertrophy. J Biol Chem 268(21): 15374–15380

23. Du XJ, Gao XM, Kiriazis H et al (2006) Transgenic alpha1 A-adrenergic activation limits post-infarct ventricular remodeling and dysfunction and improves survival. Cardiovasc Res 71(4):735–743

24. Huang Y, Wright CD, Merkwan CL et al (2007) An alpha1A-adrenergic extracellular signal-regulated kinase survival signaling pathway in cardiac myocytes. Circulation 115(6):763–772

25. Rokosh DG, Stewart AF, Chang KC et al (1996) Alpha1-adrenergic receptor subtype mRNAs are differentially regulated by alpha1-adrenergic and other hypertrophic stimuli in cardiac myocytes in culture and in vivo. Repression of alpha1B and alpha1D but induction of alpha1C. J Biol Chem 271(10): 5839–5843

26. Vinge LE, Øie E, Andersson Y et al (2001) Myocardial distribution and regulation of GRK and beta-arrestin isoforms in congestive heart failure in rats. Am J Physiol Heart Circ Physiol 281(6):H2490–H2499

27. Rockman HA, Choi DJ, Rahman NU et al (1996) Receptor-specific in vivo desensitization by the G protein-coupled receptor kinase-5 in transgenic mice. Proc Natl Acad Sci U S A 93:9954–9959

28. Eckhart AD, Duncan SJ, Penn RB et al (2000) Hybrid transgenic mice reveal in vivo specificity of G protein-coupled receptor kinases in the heart. Circ Res 86:43–50

29. Reaves PY, Gelband CH, Wang H et al (1999) Permanent cardiovascular protection from hypertension by the AT1 receptor antisense gene therapy in hypertensive rat offspring. Circ Res 85:E44–E50

30. Kawano H, Do YS, Kawano Y et al (2000) Angiotensin II has multiple profibrotic effects in human cardiac fibroblasts. Circulation 101:1130–1137

31. Hein L, Barsh GS, Pratt RE et al (1995) Behavioural and cardiovascular effects of disrupting the angiotensin II type-2 receptor in mice. Nature 377:744–747

32. Yang Z, Bove CM, French BA et al (2002) Angiotensin II type 2 receptor overexpression preserves left ventricular function after myocardial infarction. Circulation 106:106–111

33. Zhu YC, Zhu YZ, Lu N et al (2003) Role of angiotensin AT1 and AT2 receptors in cardiac hypertrophy and cardiac remodelling. Clin Exp Pharmacol Physiol 30(12):911–918

34. Cerbai E, Crucitti A, Sartiani L et al (2000) Long-term treatment of spontaneously hypertensive rats with losartan and electrophysiological remodeling of cardiac myocytes. Cardiovasc Res 45:388–396

35. Wei H, Ahn S, Shenoy SK et al (2003) Independent beta-arrestin 2 and G protein-mediated pathways for angiotensin II activation of extracellular signal-regulated kinases 1 and 2. Proc Natl Acad Sci U S A 100(19): 10782–10787

36. Anand IS, Florea VG (2003) Alterations in ventricular structure: role of left ventricular remodeling. In: Mann DL (ed) Heart failure: a companion to Braunwald's Heart Disease. WB Saunders Co, Philadelphia, pp 229–245

37. Salazar NC, Chen J, Rockman HA (2007) Cardiac GPCRs: GPCR signaling in healthy and failing hearts. Biochim Biophys Acta 1768:1006–1018

38. Lee MJ, Evans M, Hla T (1996) The inducible G protein-coupled receptor edg-1 signals via the G(i)/mitogen-activated protein kinase pathway. J Biol Chem 271:11272–11279

39. Lee MJ, Van Brocklyn JR, Thangada S, Liu CH, Hand AR, Menzeleev R et al (1998) Sphingosine-1-phosphate as a ligand for the G protein-coupled receptor EDG-1. Science 279:1552–1555

40. Zondag GC, Postma FR, Etten IV et al (1998) Sphingosine 1-phosphate signalling through the G-protein-coupled receptor Edg-1. Biochem J 330:605–609

41. Windh RT, Lee M-J, Hla T et al (1999) Differential coupling of the sphingosine 1-phosphate receptors Edg-1, Edg-3, and h218/Edg-5 to the Gi, Gq, and G12 families

of heterotrimeric G proteins. J Biol Chem 274:27351–27358

42. Means CK, Brown JH (2009) Sphingosine-1-phosphate receptor signalling in the heart. Cardiovasc Res 82(2):193–200

43. Watterson KR, Johnston E, Chalmers C et al (2002) Dual regulation of EDG1/S1P(1) receptor phosphorylation and internalization by protein kinase C and G-protein-coupled receptor kinase 2. J Biol Chem 277(8):5767–5777

44. Means CK, Miyamoto S, Chun J et al (2008) S1PR1 receptor localization confers selectivity for Gi-mediated cAMP and contractile responses. J Biol Chem 283:11954–11963

45. Errami M, Galindo CL, Tassa AT et al (2008) Doxycycline attenuates isoproterenol- and transverse aortic banding-induced cardiac hypertrophy in mice. J Pharmacol Exp Ther 324:1196–1203

46. Cannavo A, Rengo G, Liccardo D et al (2013) β1-adrenergic receptor and sphingosine-1-phosphate receptor 1 (S1PR1) reciprocal downregulation influences cardiac hypertrophic response and progression to heart failure: protective role of S1PR1 cardiac gene therapy. Circulation 128(15):1612–1622

47. Matkovich SJ, Diwan A, Klanke JL et al (2006) Cardiac-specific ablation of G-protein receptor kinase 2 redefines its roles in heart development and beta-adrenergic signaling. Circ Res 99(9):996–1003

48. Eschenhagen T (2008) Beta-adrenergic signaling in heart failure-adapt or die. Nat Med 14(5):485–487

49. Ungerer M, Böhm M, Elce JS et al (1993) Altered expression of beta-adrenergic receptor kinase and beta 1-adrenergic receptors in the failing human heart. Circulation 87:454–463

50. Ungerer M, Parruti G, Böhm M et al (1994) Expression of beta-arrestins and beta-adrenergic receptor kinases in the failing human heart. Circ Res 74:206–213

51. Koch WJ, Rockman HA, Samama P et al (1995) Cardiac function in mice overexpressing the beta-adrenergic receptor kinase or a beta ARK inhibitor. Science 268:1350–1353

52. Chen EP, Bittner HB, Akhter SA et al (1998) Myocardial recovery after ischemia and reperfusion injury is significantly impaired in hearts with transgenic overexpression of beta-adrenergic receptor kinase. Circulation 98(19 Suppl):I1249–I1253

53. Brinks H, Boucher M, Gao E et al (2010) Level of G protein-coupled receptor kinase-2 determines myocardial ischemia/reperfusion injury via pro- and anti-apoptotic mechanisms. Circ Res 107:1140–1149

54. Belmonte SL, Blaxall BC (2011) G protein coupled receptor kinases as therapeutic targets in cardiovascular disease. Circ Res 109:309–319

55. Siderovski DP, Hessel A, Chung S et al (1996) A new family of regulators of G-protein-coupled receptors? Curr Biol 6:211–212

56. Koch WJ, Inglese J, Stone WC et al (1993) The binding site for the beta gamma subunits of heterotrimeric G proteins on the beta-adrenergic receptor kinase. J Biol Chem 268(11):8256–8260

57. Pitcher JA, Inglese J, Higgins JB et al (1992) Role of beta gamma subunits of G proteins in targeting the beta-adrenergic receptor kinase to membrane-bound receptors. Science 257:1264–1267

58. Stoffel RH, Randall RR, Premont RT et al (1994) Palmitoylation of G protein-coupled receptor kinase, GRK6. Lipid modification diversity in the GRK family. J Biol Chem 269:27791–27794

59. Huang CC, Tesmer JJ (2011) Recognition in the face of diversity: Interactions of heterotrimeric G proteins and G protein-coupled receptor (GPCR) kinases with activated GPCRs. J Biol Chem 286:7715–7721

60. Lodowski DT, Tesmer VM, Benovic JL et al (2006) The structure of G protein-coupled receptor kinase (GRK)-6 defines a second lineage of GRKs. J Biol Chem 281:16785–16793

61. Patel CB, Noor N, Rockman HA (2010) Functional selectivity in adrenergic and angiotensin signaling systems. Mol Pharmacol 78:983–992

62. Kim J, Ahn S, Ren XR et al (2005) Functional antagonism of different G protein-coupled receptor kinases for beta-arrestin-mediated angiotensin II receptor signaling. Proc Natl Acad Sci U S A 102:1442–1447

63. Iaccarino G, Rockman HA, Shotwell KF et al (1998) Myocardial overexpression of GRK3 in transgenic mice: evidence for in vivo selectivity of GRKs. Am J Physiol 275(4 Pt 2):H1298–H1306

64. Vinge LE, von Lueder TG, Aasum E et al (2008) Cardiac-restricted expression of the carboxyl-terminal fragment of GRK3 uncovers distinct functions of GRK3 in regulation of cardiac contractility and growth: GRK3 controls cardiac alpha1-adrenergic receptor responsiveness. J Biol Chem 283(16):10601–10610

65. Chen EP, Bittner HB, Akhter SA et al (2001) Myocardial function in hearts with transgenic overexpression of the G protein-coupled receptor kinase 5. Ann Thorac Surg 71:1320–1324

66. Takagi C, Urasawa K, Yoshida I et al (1999) Enhanced GRK5 expression in the hearts of cardiomyopathic hamsters, J2N-k. Biochem Biophys Res Commun 262:206–210

67. Ping P, Anzai T, Gao M, Hammond HK (1997) Adenylyl cyclase and G protein receptor kinase expression during development of heart failure. Am J Physiol 273(2 Pt 2): H707–H717

68. Dzimiri N, Muiya P, Andres E et al (2004) Differential functional expression of human myocardial G protein receptor kinases in left ventricular cardiac diseases. Eur J Pharmacol 489(3):167–177

69. Raake PW, Schlegel P, Ksienzyk J et al (2013) AAV6.βARKct cardiac gene therapy ameliorates cardiac function and normalizes the catecholaminergic axis in a clinically relevant large animal heart failure model. Eur Heart J 34(19):1437–1447

70. Rockman HA, Choi DJ, Akhter SA et al (1998) Control of myocardial contractile function by the level of beta-adrenergic receptor kinase 1 in gene-targeted mice. J Biol Chem 273(29): 18180–18184

71. Raake PW, Vinge LE, Gao E et al (2008) G protein-coupled receptor kinase 2 ablation in cardiac myocytes before or after myocardial infarction prevents heart failure. Circ Res 103(4):413–422

72. Fan Q, Chen M, Zuo L et al (2013) Myocardial ablation of G protein-coupled receptor kinase 2 (GRK2) decreases ischemia/reperfusion injury through an anti-intrinsic apoptotic pathway. PLoS One 8(6):e66234

73. Thal DM, Homan KT, Chen J et al (2012) Paroxetine is a direct inhibitor of g protein-coupled receptor kinase 2 and increases myocardial contractility. ACS Chem Biol 7(11): 1830–1839

74. Fan Q, Chen M, Zuo L et al (2013) Myocardial ablation of G protein-coupled receptor kinase 2 (GRK2) decreases ischemia/reperfusion injury through an anti-intrinsic apoptotic pathway. PLoS One 8(6):277ra31

75. Rengo G, Lymperopoulos A, Zincarelli C et al (2009) Myocardial adeno-associated virus serotype 6-betaARKct gene therapy improves cardiac function and normalizes the neurohormonal axis in chronic heart failure. Circulation 119(1):89–98

76. Woodall MC, Ciccarelli M, Woodall BP et al (2014) G protein-coupled receptor kinase 2: a link between myocardial contractile function and cardiac metabolism. Circ Res 114(10): 1661–1670

77. Wang Y, Gao E, Lau WB et al (2015) GRK2-mediated desensitization of AdipoR1 in failing heart. Circulation 131(16):1392–1404.

78. Martini JS, Raake P, Vinge LE et al (2008) Uncovering G protein-coupled receptor kinase-5 as a histone deacetylase kinase in the nucleus of cardiomyocytes. Proc Natl Acad Sci U S A 105(34):12457–12462

79. Hullmann JE, Grisanti LA, Makarewich CA et al (2014) GRK5-mediated exacerbation of pathological cardiac hypertrophy involves facilitation of nuclear NFAT activity. Circ Res 115(12):976–985

80. Islam KN, Bae JW, Gao E et al (2013) Regulation of nuclear factor κB (NF-κB) in the nucleus of cardiomyocytes by G protein–coupled receptor kinase 5 (GRK5). J Biol Chem 288:35683–35689

81. Johnson LR, Robinson JD, Lester KN et al (2013) Distinct structural features of G protein-coupled receptor kinase 5 (GRK5) regulate its nuclear localization and DNA-binding ability. PLoS One 8(5):e62508

82. Gold JI, Martini JS, Hullmann J et al (2013) Nuclear translocation of cardiac G protein-coupled receptor kinase 5 downstream of select Gq-activating hypertrophic ligands is a calmodulin-dependent process. PLoS One 8(3):e57324

83. Gold JI, Gao E, Shang X et al (2012) Determining the absolute requirement of G protein-coupled receptor kinase 5 for pathological cardiac hypertrophy: short communication. Circ Res 111(8):1048–1053

Chapter 13

GRK Roles in *C. elegans*

Jordan F. Wood and Denise M. Ferkey

Abstract

G-protein-coupled receptor kinases (GRKs) are serine/threonine kinases that specifically phosphorylate activated (agonist bound) GPCRs to terminate signaling. Proteins of the arrestin family then bind to the phosphorylated receptor, blocking both receptor and G-protein reactivation. Thus, GRKs are critical regulators of GPCR signaling that function to protect cells against receptor overstimulation, maintain sensitivity to changing environmental signals and allow signal integration. When considering the extent to which *C. elegans* rely upon GPCR-mediated chemosensation to navigate their native environments, the involvement of GRKs in the regulation of *C. elegans* chemosensation is logical. While *C. elegans grk-1* plays a minor modulatory role in dopamine signaling, *C. elegans grk-2* is involved in numerous aspects of chemosensation, from regulation of specialized sensory structures to circadian control over chemosensory sensitivity. In this chapter, we discuss the functions of both in detail and, to avoid confusion with the mammalian gene names, we refer to the *C. elegans* genes as *Ce-grk-1* and *Ce-grk-2*, respectively.

Key words *C. elegans*, Nematode, Chemosensation, Olfaction, Taste, GPCR, Cilia, Circadian

1 Introduction

1.1 The Nematode *C. elegans*

Although widely recognized as one of the principal contributors to the history of molecular biology, Sydney Brenner is perhaps best known for his introduction of *C. elegans* as a research model organism [1, 2]. Continually drawn to solving large biological problems, in the 1960s Brenner became keenly interested in applying newly established regulatory tenets of molecular genetics toward understanding organismal development and physiological function, with a specific focus on the nervous system. Bridging this intellectual gulf required an organism with a sufficiently simple nervous system that could also be easily cultivated and experimentally manipulated. Brenner settled on the nematode *C. elegans* as best fitting these criteria [1]. In doing so, he established the worm as the model organism of choice now utilized by over 1100 laboratories worldwide.

C. elegans are small, free-living nematodes that are believed to naturally inhabit composting soil environments in temperate climates around the globe. In 1998, *C. elegans* became the first

Vsevolod V. Gurevich et al. (eds.), *G Protein-Coupled Receptor Kinases*, Methods in Pharmacology and Toxicology, DOI 10.1007/978-1-4939-3798-1_13, © Springer Science+Business Media New York 2016

multicellular organism to have its full genome sequenced [3], finally pairing specific genetic sequence to decades of functional mutant analysis. Subsequent comparative genomic analyses have revealed extensive genetic orthology from *C. elegans* to humans, allowing the simple nematode to facilitate insights into widely conserved genes and pathways across species.

Isogenic populations of *C. elegans* are easily maintained, as the animals exist primarily as self-fertilizing hermaphrodites. Owing to the fact that *C. elegans* are only ~1 mm in length and transparent, cellular and subcellular structures and events are easily visualized via microscopy. This allowed for developmental fate mapping of every single somatic cell in the animal (959 in the adult hermaphrodite and 1031 in the adult male) [4, 5]. In addition, serial electron microscopy was used to compile complete maps of nervous system connectivity [6, 7]. These attributes, combined with ease of transgenesis and rapid generational time, make *C. elegans* a powerful model for understanding the genetics and mechanisms of organismal development, physiology, and nervous system function.

1.2 G-Protein-Coupled Signaling in C. elegans

Many of the genes that play critical roles in chemosensation in diverse species are conserved in *C. elegans* [8, 9]. Chemosensation is generally mediated by G-protein-coupled receptor signaling and the *C. elegans* genome encodes numerous GPCRs, G-protein subunits, downstream effectors, and regulatory factors [9–13]. Moreover, there are well-established physiological roles for non-chemosensory GPCR signaling in the regulation of egg laying, pharyngeal pumping, and the innate immune system [14, 15].

Coupled to this functionally diverse array of GPCRs are 21 $G\alpha$ subunits, among which are single orthologs of the mammalian $G\alpha$ families G_s (GSA-1), $G_{q/11}$ (EGL-30), $G_{i/o}$ (GOA-1), and G_{12} (GPA-12) [11]. Interestingly, fourteen of the remaining seventeen *C. elegans* $G\alpha$ subunits are most similar to $G_{i/o}$ and are expressed almost exclusively in a subset of sensory neurons [16–20]. The *C. elegans* genome also encodes 2 $G\beta$ (GPB-1 and GPB-2) and 2 $G\gamma$ (GPC-1 and GPC-2) subunits. GPB-1 is ubiquitously expressed and is broadly required for heterotrimeric G-protein signaling, including sensory signaling [21, 22]. GPB-2 is similar to the vertebrate $G\beta_5$ subunit and may regulate GOA-1 ($G\alpha_o$) and EGL-30 ($G\alpha_{q/11}$) signaling [11, 23–25]. GPC-1 is expressed in a subset of sensory neurons and is required for response and adaptation to a variety of chemosensory cues [26, 27]. The broadly expressed GPC-2 is required for proper spindle orientation during *C. elegans* embryogenesis and has no reported sensory function [28]. To regulate these various G-protein-coupled signaling pathways, the *C. elegans* genome encodes numerous regulatory factors, including two GRKs (*G*-protein-coupled *r*eceptor *k*inases), thirteen RGS (*r*egulator of *G*-protein *s*ignaling) proteins, and one arrestin [29–34].

1.3 Chemosensation in C. elegans

As mammals, most of us have the benefit of five senses to gather the information about our surroundings that ultimately influences our behaviors. However, since *C. elegans* have neither eyes nor ears, they depend largely upon the senses of taste and smell (chemosensation). *C. elegans* gather chemical information about their surrounding environment primarily through GPCRs located in the specialized sensory cilia of chemosensory neurons [10, 35–37]. Receptor activation initiates chemotaxis toward odorants that indicate a food source and movement away from odorants that indicate a harmful or toxic environment. In *C. elegans*, five pairs of chemosensory neurons (AWA, AWC, ASH, ADL, and AWB) have been shown to detect volatile chemicals [38]. The AWA and AWC chemosensory neurons detect attractive volatile odorants that animals chemotax toward. In contrast, the ASH, ADL, and AWB chemosensory neurons detect aversive stimuli, which animals avoid by rapidly initiating backward locomotion upon stimulus detection. The ASH sensory neurons are polymodal and, thus, respond to a broad range of aversive stimuli, including volatile and soluble chemicals, ions, high osmolarity, and touch to the nose [9, 39–46]. Appropriate behavioral responses are generated when signals are relayed from the sensory neurons to downstream interneurons and motor neurons [7]. These responses are determined by both the cellular expression patterns of individual GPCRs and the invariant *C. elegans* neural circuitry [7, 35].

Specifically functioning downstream of GPCRs in chemosensory signaling, AWC neurons utilize three stimulatory $G\alpha_{i/o}$-like proteins, ODR-3, GPA-3, and GPA-13, while the AWA and ASH sensory neurons signal primarily through ODR-3 and GPA-3 [16–19, 22, 41, 43]. AWC-mediated chemotaxis requires the guanylyl cyclase ODR-1 and the cyclic nucleotide gated channel composed of the TAX-2/TAX-4 subunits [47–49]. Conversely, both the AWA and ASH sensory neurons appear to use *poly*unsaturated *f*atty *a*cids (PUFAs) as second messengers that act upstream of or directly on the OSM-9/OCR-2 TRPV-related channel [50–52]. Calcium influx is likely a unifying downstream consequence of signaling in all of these neurons, required for efficient synaptic release of neurotransmitters and proper signal communication within the sensory circuit.

Taken together, *C. elegans* provides a genetically tractable in vivo model that is manipulated in ways not easily accomplished in mammalian systems. Given its sophisticated repertoire of reproducible chemosensory behaviors mediated by well-characterized neuronal circuits, *C. elegans* is an ideal system in which to identify and functionally characterize the molecules and molecular mechanisms that underlie GPCR signal transduction and regulation [8–10].

2   *C. elegans* GRK-1 (Ce-GRK-1)

Ce-GRK-1 is the single worm ortholog of the mammalian GRK4/5/6 family, sharing 56% identity with human GRK5 [29]. To date, the only function ascribed to Ce-GRK-1 is the regulation of dopamine-induced locomotor abnormalities [53], possibly functioning as a negative regulator of both D1-like (DOP-1) and D2-like (DOP-3) dopamine GPCR signaling.

2.1   Ce-GRK-1 Modulates Dopamine-Mediated Swimming-Induced Paralysis

The *C. elegans* dopamine transporter DAT-1 clears dopamine from synaptic clefts, and *dat-1* loss-of-function (lof) results in accumulation of synaptic dopamine and subsequent elevated signaling through the inhibitory D2-like DOP-3 dopamine receptor in motor neurons [53–55]. This increased DOP-3-mediated signaling manifests generally as reduced locomotion and eventual paralysis, including swimming-induced paralysis (SWIP) [54–56]. While wild-type *C. elegans* swim continuously for more than 30 min when placed in water, *dat-1(lof)* animals develop paralysis within just 6–10 min [53].

Loss of Ce-GRK-1 function also results in increased SWIP [53]. Although the basis of this phenotype is unknown, one possibility is that in conditions of normal synaptic dopamine levels, loss of Ce-GRK-1-mediated downregulation of DOP-3 signaling may bias antagonistic D1-like/D2-like receptor signaling toward inhibitory signaling through the D2-like receptors. Such a shift in the balance of signaling strength between the opposing pathways could subsequently lead to increased SWIP, as was observed in the *Ce-grk-1(lof)* animals.

Surprisingly, although loss of either DAT-1 or Ce-GRK-1 function leads to increased SWIP, *Ce-grk-1(lof)* partially suppresses the *dat-1(lof)*-mediated heightened SWIP phenotype [53, 56]. While the nature of this genetic interaction is not immediately clear, it could be explained in the following way. As the highly penetrant SWIP phenotype observed in the *dat-1(lof)* animals results from elevated synaptic dopamine and subsequent increased DOP-3 signaling [54], under such conditions loss of Ce-GRK-1-mediated downregulation of DOP-3 may not be able to further enhance signaling through the DOP-3 pathway. Thus, the partial suppression of the *dat-1(lof)* SWIP phenotype may result from the loss of Ce-GRK-1-mediated negative regulation of DOP-1 (D1-like receptor) signaling. This loss of DOP-1 downregulation may then be sufficient to antagonize the paralytic effect of increased synaptic dopamine acting on the D2-like DOP-3 receptors. However, alternate models could also be consistent with this genetic interaction.

3   *C. elegans* GRK-2 (Ce-GRK-2)

Ce-GRK-2 is the single worm ortholog of the mammalian GRK2/3 family and displays 66% identity with human GRK3 and 65% with human GRK2 [29]. Ce-GRK-2 is expressed throughout the *C. elegans* nervous system, including chemosensory neurons [29]. Thus, analysis of *C. elegans* chemosensation provides an organismal paradigm in which to analyze the in vivo role(s) of this GRK family member in the regulation of neuronal signaling.

3.1   Loss of Ce-GRK-2 Function Broadly Disrupts Chemosensation

In most described instances, the absence of GRK-mediated desensitization results in prolonged responses to receptor-activating ligands [57–61]. However, there are descriptions of reduced signaling resulting from loss of GRK function. For example, although GRK6$^{-/-}$ mice are hypersensitive to stimulants including cocaine, T cells from these mice fail to chemotax toward the stimulatory chemokine CXCL12 [59, 62]. Moreover, loss of GRK3 function in mouse olfactory epithelia results in significant reduction in the odorant-induced generation of secondary messengers, in addition to the lack of agonist-induced receptor desensitization following odorant exposure [63–65].

Worms lacking Ce-GRK-2 function are not hypersensitive to chemosensory stimuli due to increased sensory signaling, as would be expected for loss of a negative regulator of GPCR signaling. Instead, loss of Ce-GRK-2 function in adult sensory neurons broadly disrupts chemosensation [29]. Loss of Ce-GRK-2 eliminates two different sets of G-protein-coupled behaviors: (1) chemotaxis toward attractive odorants detected by the AWA and AWC olfactory sensory neurons (including diacetyl, isoamyl alchohol, and benzaldehyde) and (2) avoidance of the ASH-detected aversive chemicals 1-octanol (odorant) and quinine (bitter tastant) [29, 66]. Although some chemosensory neurons also mediate other sensory behaviors, *Ce-grk-2(lof)* animals respond normally to mechanosensory stimuli, SDS, and Cu^{2+} [29, 66]. This indicates that loss of Ce-GRK-2 function affects GPCR-mediated chemosensation, without broadly disrupting neuronal signaling or animal locomotion.

3.1.1   Loss of Ce-GRK-2 Function Leads to Reduced G-Protein-Coupled Signaling

Ce-grk-2(lof) animals show reduced stimulus-evoked calcium signaling in sensory neurons [29]. Accordingly, increasing sensory signaling via overexpression of the chemosensory Gα ODR-3 (Gα$_{i/o}$) significantly restored the response of *Ce-grk-2(lof)* animals to the ASH-detected odorant 1-octanol [29]. Similarly, increasing sensory signaling through the removal of the negative regulatory protein EAT-16 (an RGS GTPase activating protein) was sufficient to restore *Ce-grk-2(lof)* chemotaxis to the attractive AWA-detected odorant diacetyl [29]. Importantly, heat shock rescue of Ce-GRK-2 in adult animals was sufficient to restore ASH-mediated response to 1-octanol, indicating that Ce-GRK-2 function in adult stages is sufficient for normal chemosensory response [29]. Taken together, loss of Ce-GRK-2 function was shown to lead to decreased signaling in *C. elegans* sensory neurons, reminiscent of the loss of mammalian GRK3 function in olfactory epithelia [29, 65]. Moreover, these results suggested that compensatory inhibitory mechanisms function to downregulate G-protein-coupled signaling and dampen sensory signaling in the absence of Ce-GRK-2 function [29]. These compensatory pathways may serve to protect the sensory neurons from overstimulation in the absence of Ce-GRK-2.

3.2   *C. elegans* TRPV Channels Regulate Aberrant Sensory Signaling

To identify mechanisms responsible for regulating chemosensory GPCR signaling in the absence of Ce-GRK-2 function, a genetic screen was performed to identify genetic suppressors of the *Ce-grk-2(lof)* chemosensory defects [66]. Second-site mutations in the genes encoding the transient receptor potential vanilloid (TRPV) channels OSM-9 and OCR-2 were identified in *Ce-grk-2(lof)* animals that displayed restored chemosensory sensitivity [66]. Interestingly, loss of TRPV function specifically restored *Ce-grk-2(lof)* sensory sensitivity to ASH-detected bitter tastants, including quinine, primaquine, and amodiaquine, but not to other ASH-detected stimuli. Moreover, loss of TRPV signaling failed to restore *Ce-grk-2(lof)* chemotaxis to the AWA-detected odorants diacetyl and pyrazine [66], even though, like ASH, AWA also utilizes the OSM-9/OCR-2 channel in primary sensory signaling [51, 52]. The selective restoration of chemosensory behaviors that occurs upon loss of OSM-9/OCR-2 function in *Ce-grk-2(lof)* mutants indicates that these channels function in both a cell-specific and modality-specific manner to modulate sensory signaling in the absence of Ce-GRK-2 function [66]; signaling components specific to bitter taste may be selectively regulated by OSM-9/OCR-2 in the ASH sensory neurons.

Downstream of their roles in primary signal transduction, the OSM-9/OCR-2 TRPV channels affect transcriptional levels of sensory genes [67, 68]. Suppression of the *Ce-grk-2(lof)* defect in avoidance of bitter tastants by a TRPV channel null mutant does not distinguish between these two functional roles [66]. Two well-characterized alleles for the *ocr-2* gene are available that allow for separation of the channel's role in primary signal transduction versus regulation of activity-dependent gene expression. *ocr-2(ak47)* is a predicted null that fails to form functional channels and disrupts AWA-mediated chemosensory behaviors [52]. In contrast, *ocr-2(yz5)* contains a single amino acid substitution (G36E) in the cytoplasmic amino-terminal tail that disrupts the expression of the serotonin biosynthetic enzyme gene *tph-1* in the ADF sensory neurons, but does not disrupt channel localization or AWA-mediated signaling [67, 68]. Moreover, expression of the OCR-2 amino-terminal tail in a chimeric channel is sufficient to increase *tph-1* expression, supporting the role of this domain in regulating transcription [68].

Similar to the *ocr-2(ak47)* null allele, disruption of OCR-2 amino-terminal tail-mediated regulation of gene expression using the *yz5* allele also selectively restored *Ce-grk-2(lof)* animals' behavioral sensitivity to bitter tastants [66]. This suggests that restoration of behavioral sensitivity does not arise from reduced primary signaling through loss of the OCR-2 TRPV channel [66]. Instead, it suggests that loss of a downstream function or pathway coupled to the amino-terminal motif of OCR-2 underlies the restoration of bitter taste responses in *Ce-grk-2(lof)* animals. For example, the G36E change in OCR-2 may disrupt interactions with adaptor signaling proteins required for TRPV-mediated changes in gene expression [68].

3.3 Ce-GRK-2 Regulates Sensory Neuron Structure

Nonmotile primary cilia are sensory organelles often found on sensory neurons, consisting of a microtubule-based axoneme surrounded by a membrane that houses GPCR signaling components utilized in sensory detection and signaling [69, 70]. The *C. elegans* nervous system contains 60 ciliated neurons, 12 pairs of which are located in the amphid chemosensory organ in the head [6, 71, 72]. Eight pairs of sensory neurons utilize single, channel-shaped sensory cilia to detect aqueous chemical cues [6, 70, 71, 73]. To detect volatile odorants, three pairs of chemosensory neurons (including the AWB nociceptive neurons) utilize specialized, structurally elaborate wing-shaped cilia [6, 38, 71]. In both types of *C. elegans* amphid sensory cilia, the molecular motors kinesin-II and dynein transport molecules essential for ciliary assembly and function in a highly conserved process referred to as intraflagellar transport (IFT) [72, 74–76]. Moreover, both channel and wing cilia contain transmembrane proteins required for sensory signaling and a portion of these signaling components depend on IFT for proper localization [77].

To understand the molecules and pathways required to generate and modulate ciliary structures on specific sensory neurons, the characteristic slender, Y-shaped wing sensory cilia of the AWB neurons were examined in worms carrying mutations for genes expressed in and required for AWB sensory signaling [36]. Included among the loss-of-function signaling mutants that displayed dramatic and highly penetrant ciliary structural defects was *Ce-grk-2(lof)* [36]. Whereas wild-type AWB sensory cilia display a slender Y-shaped architecture, loss of Ce-GRK-2 function results in fan-like membraneous expansions that significantly increase the surface area of the AWB ciliary fork [36]. GPCRs that are present normally throughout the AWB cilia were observed in the ectopic ciliary fan observed in *Ce-grk-2(lof)* animals and this ciliary expansion requires IFT; a loss-of-function mutation in the kinesin-II subunit gene *klp-11* suppressed the ectopic expansions of the AWB sensory cilia in *Ce-grk-2(lof)* animals [36].

Similar ectopic ciliary structures were observed in *C. elegans* lacking cGMP signaling proteins that function in AWB, suggesting that the fan-like membraneous expansions on the ends of the Y-shaped AWB sensory cilia reflect a compensatory mechanism resulting from reduced sensory signaling [36]. In addition, consistent with the ability of $G\alpha_{i/o}$ subunit ODR-3 overexpression to rescue ASH chemosensory sensitivity in the absence of Ce-GRK-2 function [29], increased calcium signaling mediated by a gain-of-function mutation in the L-type voltage-gated calcium channel gene *egl-19* suppressed the AWB ciliary defects of *Ce-grk-2(lof)* animals [36]. Collectively, these data suggest that the AWB neurons actively monitor sensory signaling levels to responsively regulate ciliary structure and function, and lend further support to the model that loss of Ce-GRK-2 function ultimately results in reduced chemosensory signaling.

3.4 Regulation of Gustatory Plasticity by Ce-GRK-2

An animal's ability to detect and properly respond to environmental salt is critical for the maintenance of water and ion homeostasis. Accordingly, *C. elegans* display three distinct behavioral responses to NaCl: (1) chemoattraction to low (0.1–200 mM) NaCl, (2) avoidance of high (>250 mM) concentrations of NaCl, and (3) avoidance of attractive NaCl concentrations following NaCl pre-exposure, referred to as gustatory plasticity [46, 78–80].

Gustatory behaviors may ultimately result from the competing output of sensory neurons or modulatory interactions [80]. For example, chemoattraction to low NaCl is primarily mediated by the ASE gustatory neurons [73], relying upon cGMP generation by several guanylyl cyclases and activity of the TAX-2/TAX-4 cyclic nucleotide-gated channel for sensory signaling [48–50]. In contrast, avoidance of high concentrations of NaCl is mediated by the nociceptive ASH sensory neurons [46]. In the ASHs, high NaCl activates TMC-1 channels, which then signal through the OSM-9/OCR-2 TRPV channels to activate ASH and drive avoidance behavior [46].

Supporting the model that signals from multiple sensory neurons are integrated to generate appropriate context-dependent gustatory behaviors, Ce-GRK-2 function is required in the ASH nociceptors for ASE-mediated attraction to 25–100 mM NaCl, and *Ce-grk-2(lof)* animals display defective NaCl chemotaxis behaviors that are indistinguishable from those of animals lacking ASE function [80]. However, Ce-GRK-2 function is not required in the ASHs for avoidance of 1 M NaCl [80]. *Ce-grk-2(lof)* mutants also develop gustatory plasticity more rapidly than wild-type animals [80]. In contrast, gustatory plasticity is disrupted in animals lacking ASE sensory function [80]. These data suggest that, upon prolonged exposure to attractive NaCl concentrations, the ASEs signal to and activate the nociceptive ASHs, resulting in the avoidance of NaCl concentrations that would normally be attractive [80]. It is unlikely, however, that the ASE–ASH interaction modulating gustatory plasticity results in increased ASH sensitivity to low NaCl concentrations, as the only known ASH-expressed salt detector, TMC-1, is activated by NaCl concentrations above 250 mM [46]. Rather, the ASE-derived signal that functions to stimulate ASH activity following prolonged exposure to low NaCl concentrations likely acts through GPCR-mediated signaling, a point emphasized by both the requirement of the $G\alpha_{i/o}$ subunit ODR-3 in gustatory plasticity and the important role that Ce-GRK-2 plays in regulating NaCl chemotaxis and gustatory plasticity [80].

3.5 Circadian Regulation of Ce-GRK-2 and Aversive Olfaction in C. elegans

In response to the highly predictable nature of daily cycles of light and dark, organisms have evolved to use light as a reference point for time. Environmental cues such as temperature also can be sufficiently oscillatory to reflect the 24-h daily light cycle [81, 82]. The biological systems that sense and maintain a distinct orientation in time are referred to as circadian clocks. These biological clocks regulate processes ranging from gene expression to behavior within cells, organisms, and populations [83–85]. Analysis of *C. elegans* following cultivation in a 24-h temperature cycle (13–16 °C) for 5 days revealed phasic regulation of the highly conserved circadian protein target PRDX-2, validating this approach to study circadian clocks in the nematode [86–88].

Circadian regulation of olfaction has been observed in flies and mice [89, 90]. Interestingly, *C. elegans* response to the aversive odorant 1-octanol was shown to undergo circadian modulation as well [86]. Worms displayed reduced chemosensory sensitivity to 1-octanol in the subjective night (13 °C) and increased sensitivity during the subjective day (16 °C) [86]. Likely underlying these aversive behavioral dynamics, Ce-GRK-2 protein abundance fluctuated rhythmically, being elevated in the subjective night and decreased during the subjective day [86]. This anti-phase correlation between Ce-GRK-2 protein levels and 1-octanol sensitivity is what would be expected if Ce-GRK-2 acts as a negative regulator of chemosensory GPCRs and, thus, behavioral sensitivity to sensory stimuli. Although Ce-GRK-2 protein levels fluctuated, *Ce-grk-2* transcript levels did not display circadian control following temperature entrainment [86]. Thus, a yet undetermined mode of translational or posttranslational regulation of Ce-GRK-2 functions to regulate circadian cycles of sensory sensitivity [86].

3.6 In Vivo Structure–Function Analysis of Ce-GRK-2

The mammalian GRK2/3 family of receptor kinases has been extensively characterized, both structurally and biochemically, revealing the following in vitro functional contributions from structural domains. The amphipathic amino-terminal α-helix (αN) stabilizes interaction with ligand-bound GPCRs, the regulator of G-protein signaling homology (RH) domain binds activated $G\alpha_{q/11}$, and the pleckstrin homology (PH) domain mediates membrane localization via $G\beta\gamma$ and phospholipid interactions [91–97].

However, despite extensive in vitro characterization, little is known about the in vivo contribution of these described GRK structural domains and interactions to proper GRK function in signal regulation in mammalian systems.

Each of the key functional domains of mammalian GRK2/3 is conserved in Ce-GRK-2. Thus, the disrupted chemosensory behavior characteristic of *Ce-grk-2(lof)* mutants [29] provided a unique opportunity to determine which biochemically defined GRK2/3 interactions are required for function and cell signaling in vivo. Specifically, selective mutation of biochemically defined Ce-GRK-2 residues, and subsequent expression and chemosensory behavioral analysis in worms lacking endogenous Ce-GRK-2 function, were used to delineate the domains and associated interactions critical for Ce-GRK-2 function in vivo [98].

3.6.1 Ce-GRK-2 Likely Regulates Chemosensory Signaling via Direct Phosphorylation of Chemosensory GPCRs

While GRKs have been classically characterized to downregulate G-protein-coupled signaling pathways by directly phosphorylating activated GPCRs, mammalian GRKs have also been shown to interact with and/or phosphorylate additional proteins, including signaling molecules [92, 99]. However, three lines of evidence support the model that the primary in vivo function of Ce-GRK-2 in the regulation of chemosensory signaling is the phosphorylation of agonist-bound chemosensory GPCRs. First, the importance of catalytic activity was demonstrated when expression of the putative kinase-dead Ce-GRK-2(K220R) failed to restore chemosensory responses in *Ce-grk-2(lof)* animals [98, 100]. However, this result does not distinguish between a role for Ce-GRK-2 in receptor phosphorylation versus phosphorylation of other potential substrates [98]. Second, the extreme amino-terminal residues of mammalian GRKs, including GRK2, form an amphipathic α-helix required specifically for GPCR phosphorylation, but not GRK–receptor interaction or kinase activity [91, 92, 97, 101]. This structure is highly conserved, including in Ce-GRK-2, and mutation of any of the constituent amino acid residues (Asp3, Leu4, Val7/Leu8, or Asp10) abrogated Ce-GRK-2 chemosensory function in vivo [98]. Lastly, an exposed arginine residue on the small kinase lobe (Arg190 in bGRK6) forms both hydrogen bonds and apolar contacts with the amino-terminal α-helix, stabilizing GRKs in their active GPCR- and ATP-bound conformation [92]. This arginine is conserved among all GRKs and mutation in bGRK1 (Arg191) and bGRK2 (Arg195) severely compromised phosphorylation of rhodopsin in vitro, β_2AR phosphorylation in cell culture and, importantly, phosphorylation of off-target substrates [91]. Thus, this conserved arginine residue is critical for mediating conformational changes required for overall GRK catalytic function [91, 97]. *Ce-grk-2(lof)* animals expressing Ce-GRK-2(R195A) remained defective in chemosensory behaviors [98]. Thus, kinase activity, GPCR interaction and predicted intramolecular stabilizing interactions, all required for effective receptor phosphorylation by mammalian GRKs, are also required for Ce-GRK-2 chemosensory function [91, 92, 96–98, 101, 102].

3.6.2 Ce-GRK-2 Function Supports a Universal Model for GRK Activation

A variety of approaches have shown that contact between the GRK amino-terminal α-helix and the small kinase lobe likely forms a receptor docking site that is crucial for both GRK recognition of activated GPCRs and GRK catalytic function [91, 97, 102]. Furthermore, interaction between an activated GPCR and the putative receptor docking site likely mediates both catalytic structure stabilization and proper GPCR phospho-acceptor site positioning in the active ATP-bound GRK catalytic cleft [91, 92, 102]. As GRKs specifically regulate agonist-bound GPCRs, an activation mechanism that selectively requires GRK association with activated receptors would provide intrinsic substrate specificity among the diversity of membrane-bound and associated proteins within the cell. Such a mechanism of activation would also explain why alteration of any of the conserved residues involved in these interactions disrupts effective chemosensory function of Ce-GRK-2 in vivo, and effective receptor phosphorylation among all mammalian GRKs tested (GRK1, 2, 5, and 6) in vitro [91, 92, 97, 101, 102]. These required residues and structures, therefore, comprise highly conserved structural features that couple enzymatic activation with GPCR interaction, and the structure–function experiments in *C. elegans* provide in vivo support for a universal mechanism of GRK activation.

3.6.3 Gα, Gβγ, and Phospholipid Interactions Differentially Contribute to Ce-GRK-2 Chemosensory Function

In addition to primarily phosphorylating activated GPCRs, mammalian GRK2/3 also interact with $G\alpha_{q/11}$, Gβγ, and phospholipids to regulate signaling [93–95, 103–105]. These interactions are mediated by the RH and PH domains [93–95, 103, 104].

Biochemical and structural evidence suggest that the RH domain of mammalian GRK2 interacts with both GPCRs and the $G\alpha_{q/11}$ subunit, physically separating the receptor and $G\alpha_{q/11}$, thereby blocking subsequent rounds of G-protein activation and interfering with $G\alpha_{q/11}$-mediated activation of downstream effectors [93–95, 103, 104]. However, mutations predicted to disrupt Ce-GRK-2 binding to $G\alpha_{q/11}$ (R106A, Y109I, and D110A) had no effect on Ce-GRK-2's ability to restore chemosensory behavioral responses in *Ce-grk-2(lof)* animals [98]. This is likely explained by the fact that the predominant chemosensory signaling Gα subunits in ASH (ODR-3 and GPA-3) are $G\alpha_{i/o}$-like and do not contain GRK-2 RH domain-binding sites [17, 19, 41, 98]. Thus, $G\alpha_{q/11}$ binding or sequestration are not likely a significant aspect of Ce-GRK-2 function in chemosensory signaling. However, as the RH domain-binding residues of $bG\alpha_{q/11}$ are completely conserved in the *C. elegans* $G\alpha_{q/11}$ ortholog EGL-30, a more significant regulatory role for the Ce-GRK-2 RH domain is possible in different cells or physiological processes where EGL-30 is the primary signaling Gα protein, such as acetylcholine release at neuromuscular junctions, locomotion, or egg laying [11].

PH domain interactions with membrane phospholipids and Gβγ subunits mediate mammalian GRK2/3 translocation to the cell membrane and activated GPCRs located therein, and thus are critical for effective receptor phosphorylation [64, 94, 106–108]. Specific mammalian GRK2 PH domain residues contribute to these interactions: K567 mediates phospholipid binding while R587 is required for effective Gβγ interaction [94]. Disruption of either of these interactions dramatically reduces effective receptor phosphorylation [94]. Expression of Ce-GRK-2(K567E) significantly restored chemosensory avoidance, indicating that changing this residue alone is not sufficient to disrupt Ce-GRK-2 function [98]. In contrast, introducing the R587Q amino acid substitution significantly reduced the ability of Ce-GRK-2 to restore chemosensory responses in *Ce-grk-2(lof)* animals, suggesting that Gβγ interaction contributes to Ce-GRK-2 regulation of chemosensory signaling [98]. Compounding the effects of disrupted membrane localization that likely result from the R587Q change, the mammalian GRK2 kinase domain rotates 10–15° away from the membrane upon binding Gβγ, positioning GRK2 for efficient GPCR binding, and potentially enhancing receptor phosphorylation [109]. Thus, it is likely that loss of both membrane recruitment and optimal kinase domain positioning contributes to the pronounced reduction in Ce-GRK-2(R587Q) function. While Ce-GRK-2(R587Q) did retain low-level activity, introducing the K567E and R587Q changes in combination to disrupt both phospholipid and Gβγ binding showed an enhanced effect, suggesting that the PH domain of Ce-GRK-2 utilizes both interactions to mediate the regulation of chemosensory signaling in vivo [98].

4 Concluding Remarks

The regulatory functions and mechanisms reviewed in this chapter reflect, as sagely envisioned by Sydney Brenner decades ago, the utility of leveraging the simplicity of *C. elegans* to enhance our understanding of primary signaling and regulatory mechanisms controlling animal development, physiology, and behavior. Although the scope of this chapter is generally limited to the realm of GRK roles in sensory function, the experimental potential for investigation in other physiological contexts reflects the true scientific value of *C. elegans*. Considering the extensive evolutionary conservation of signaling cascades across species, *C. elegans* is poised to continue providing valuable insights into the varied roles these receptor kinases play in vivo, as well as the cellular and physiological responses to loss of appropriate signal regulation.

References

1. Brenner S (1974) The genetics of *Caenorhabditis elegans*. Genetics 77(1):71–94

2. Hoffenberg R (2003) Brenner, the worm and the prize. Clin Med 3(3):285–286

3. Consortium CeS (1998) Genome sequence of the nematode *C. elegans*: a platform for investigating biology. Science 282(5396):2012–2018

4. Sulston JE, Horvitz HR (1977) Post-embryonic cell lineages of the nematode, *Caenorhabditis elegans*. Dev Biol 56(1):110–156

5. Kimble J, Hirsh D (1979) The postembryonic cell lineages of the hermaphrodite and male gonads in *Caenorhabditis elegans*. Dev Biol 70(2):396–417

6. Ward S, Thomson N, White JG, Brenner S (1975) Electron microscopical reconstruction of the anterior sensory anatomy of the nematode *Caenorhabditis elegans*. J Comp Neurol 160(3):313–337

7. White JG, Southgate E, Thomson JN, Brenner S (1986) The structure of the nervous system of the nematode *Caenorhabditis elegans*. Philos Trans R Soc Lond B Biol Sci 314(1165):1–340

8. Prasad BC, Reed RR (1999) Chemosensation: molecular mechanisms in worms and mammals. Trends Genet 15(4):150–153

9. Troemel ER (1999) Chemosensory signaling in *C. elegans*. Bioessays 21(12):1011–1020

10. Bargmann CI (2006, October 25) Chemosensation in C. elegans. In: WormBook (ed) The C. elegans Research Community, WormBook. doi:10.1895/wormbook.1.123.1. http://www.wormbook.org

11. Bastiani C, Mendel J (2006, October 13) Heterotrimeric G proteins in C. elegans. In: WormBook, (ed) The C. elegans Research Community, WormBook. doi:10.1895/wormbook.1.75.1. http://www.wormbook.org

12. Robertson HM, Thomas JH (2006, January 06) The putative chemoreceptor families of C. elegans. In: WormBook (ed) The C. elegans Research Community, WormBook. doi:10.1895/wormbook.1.66.1, http://www.wormbook.org

13. Bargmann CI (2006) Comparative chemosensation from receptors to ecology. Nature 444(7117):295–301

14. Hobson RJ, Hapiak VM, Xiao H, Buehrer KL, Komuniecki PR, Komuniecki RW (2006) SER-7, a *Caenorhabditis elegans* 5-HT7-like receptor, is essential for the 5-HT stimulation of pharyngeal pumping and egg laying. Genetics 172(1):159–169

15. Sun J, Singh V, Kajino-Sakamoto R, Aballay A (2011) Neuronal GPCR controls innate immunity by regulating noncanonical unfolded protein response genes. Science 332(6030):729–732

16. Zwaal RR, Mendel JE, Sternberg PW, Plasterk RH (1997) Two neuronal G proteins are involved in chemosensation of the *Caenorhabditis elegans* Dauer-inducing pheromone. Genetics 145(3):715–727

17. Roayaie K, Crump JG, Sagasti A, Bargmann CI (1998) The Gα protein ODR-3 mediates olfactory and nociceptive function and controls cilium morphogenesis in *C. elegans* olfactory neurons. Neuron 20(1):55–67

18. Lans H, Rademakers S, Jansen G (2004) A network of stimulatory and inhibitory Gα-subunits regulates olfaction in *Caenorhabditis elegans*. Genetics 167(4):1677–1687

19. Jansen G, Thijssen KL, Werner P, van der Horst M, Hazendonk E, Plasterk RH (1999) The complete family of genes encoding G proteins of *Caenorhabditis elegans*. Nat Genet 21(4):414–419

20. Cuppen E, van der Linden AM, Jansen G, Plasterk RH (2003) Proteins interacting with *Caenorhabditis elegans* Gα subunits. Comp Funct Genom 4(5):479–491

21. van der Voorn L, Gebbink M, Plasterk RH, Ploegh HL (1990) Characterization of a G-protein β-subunit gene from the nematode *Caenorhabditis elegans*. J Mol Biol 213(1):17–26

22. Zwaal RR, Ahringer J, van Luenen HG, Rushforth A, Anderson P, Plasterk RH (1996) G proteins are required for spatial orientation of early cell cleavages in *C. elegans* embryos. Cell 86(4):619–629

23. Chase DL, Patikoglou GA, Koelle MR (2001) Two RGS proteins that inhibit Gα$_o$ and Gα$_q$ signaling in *C. elegans* neurons require a Gβ$_5$-like subunit for function. Curr Biol 11(4):222–231

24. Robatzek M, Niacaris T, Steger K, Avery L, Thomas JH (2001) *eat-11* encodes GPB-2, a Gβ$_5$ ortholog that interacts with G$_o$α and G$_q$α to regulate *C. elegans* behavior. Curr Biol 11(4):288–293

25. van der Linden AM, Simmer F, Cuppen E, Plasterk RH (2001) The G-protein β-subunit GPB-2 in *Caenorhabditis elegans* regulates the G$_o$α-G$_q$α signaling network through interactions with the regulator of G-protein signaling proteins EGL-10 and EAT-16. Genetics 158(1):221–235

26. Jansen G, Weinkove D, Plasterk RH (2002) The G-protein γ subunit *gpc-1* of the nematode *C. elegans* is involved in taste adaptation. EMBO J 21(5):986–994

27. Yamada K, Hirotsu T, Matsuki M, Kunitomo H, Iino Y (2009) GPC-1, a G protein γ-subunit, regulates olfactory adaptation in *Caenorhabditis elegans*. Genetics 181(4): 1347–1357

28. Gotta M, Ahringer J (2001) Distinct roles for Gα and Gβγ in regulating spindle position and orientation in *Caenorhabditis elegans* embryos. Nat Cell Biol 3(3):297–300

29. Fukuto HS, Ferkey DM, Apicella AJ, Lans H, Sharmeen T, Chen W, Lefkowitz RJ, Jansen G, Schafer WR, Hart AC (2004) G protein-coupled receptor kinase function is essential for chemosensation in *C. elegans*. Neuron 42(4):581–593

30. Dong MQ, Chase D, Patikoglou GA, Koelle MR (2000) Multiple RGS proteins alter neural G protein signaling to allow *C. elegans* to rapidly change behavior when fed. Genes Dev 14(16):2003–2014

31. Palmitessa A, Hess HA, Bany IA, Kim YM, Koelle MR, Benovic JL (2005) *Caenorhabditus elegans* arrestin regulates neural G protein signaling and olfactory adaptation and recovery. J Biol Chem 280(26):24649–24662

32. Ahola TM, Manninen T, Alkio N, Ylikomi T (2002) G protein-coupled receptor 30 is critical for a progestin-induced growth inhibition in MCF-7 breast cancer cells. Endocrinology 143(9):3376–3384

33. Bargmann CI (1998) Neurobiology of the *Caenorhabditis elegans* genome. Science 282(5396):2028–2033

34. Hess HA, Roper JC, Grill SW, Koelle MR (2004) RGS-7 completes a receptor-independent heterotrimeric G protein cycle to asymmetrically regulate mitotic spindle positioning in *C. elegans*. Cell 119(2):209–218

35. Sengupta P, Chou JH, Bargmann CI (1996) *odr-10* encodes a seven transmembrane domain olfactory receptor required for responses to the odorant diacetyl. Cell 84(6):899–909

36. Mukhopadhyay S, Lu Y, Shaham S, Sengupta P (2008) Sensory signaling-dependent remodeling of olfactory cilia architecture in *C. elegans*. Dev Cell 14(5):762–774

37. Troemel ER, Chou JH, Dwyer ND, Colbert HA, Bargmann CI (1995) Divergent seven transmembrane receptors are candidate chemosensory receptors in *C. elegans*. Cell 83(2):207–218

38. Bargmann CI, Hartwieg E, Horvitz HR (1993) Odorant-selective genes and neurons mediate olfaction in *C. elegans*. Cell 74(3): 515–527

39. Kaplan JM, Horvitz HR (1993) A dual mechanosensory and chemosensory neuron in *Caenorhabditis elegans*. Proc Natl Acad Sci U S A 90(6):2227–2231

40. Bargmann CI, Thomas JH, Horvitz HR (1990) Chemosensory cell function in the behavior and development of *Caenorhabditis elegans*. Cold Spring Harb Symp Quant Biol 55:529–538

41. Hilliard MA, Bergamasco C, Arbucci S, Plasterk RH, Bazzicalupo P (2004) Worms taste bitter: ASH neurons, QUI-1, GPA-3 and ODR-3 mediate quinine avoidance in *Caenorhabditis elegans*. EMBO J 23(5): 1101–1111

42. Hilliard MA, Bargmann CI, Bazzicalupo P (2002) *C. elegans* responds to chemical repellents by integrating sensory inputs from the head and the tail. Curr Biol 12(9):730–734

43. Hilliard MA, Apicella AJ, Kerr R, Suzuki H, Bazzicalupo P, Schafer WR (2005) In vivo imaging of *C. elegans* ASH neurons: cellular response and adaptation to chemical repellents. EMBO J 24(1):63–72

44. Sambongi Y, Nagae T, Liu Y, Yoshimizu T, Takeda K, Wada Y, Futai M (1999) Sensing of cadmium and copper ions by externally exposed ADL, ASE, and ASH neurons elicits avoidance response in *Caenorhabditis elegans*. Neuroreport 10(4):753–757

45. Hart AC, Kass J, Shapiro JE, Kaplan JM (1999) Distinct signaling pathways mediate touch and osmosensory responses in a polymodal sensory neuron. J Neurosci 19(6): 1952–1958

46. Chatzigeorgiou M, Bang S, Hwang SW, Schafer WR (2013) *tmc-1* encodes a sodium-sensitive channel required for salt chemosensation in *C. elegans*. Nature 494(7435):95–99

47. L'Etoile ND, Bargmann CI (2000) Olfaction and odor discrimination are mediated by the *C. elegans* guanylyl cyclase ODR-1. Neuron 25(3):575–586

48. Komatsu H, Mori I, Rhee JS, Akaike N, Ohshima Y (1996) Mutations in a cyclic nucleotide-gated channel lead to abnormal thermosensation and chemosensation in *C. elegans*. Neuron 17(4):707–718

49. Coburn CM, Bargmann CI (1996) A putative cyclic nucleotide-gated channel is required for sensory development and function in *C. elegans*. Neuron 17(4):695–706

50. Kahn-Kirby AH, Dantzker JL, Apicella AJ, Schafer WR, Browse J, Bargmann CI, Watts JL (2004) Specific polyunsaturated fatty acids drive TRPV-dependent sensory signaling in vivo. Cell 119(6):889–900

51. Colbert HA, Smith TL, Bargmann CI (1997) OSM-9, a novel protein with structural similarity to channels, is required for olfaction,

mechanosensation, and olfactory adaptation in *Caenorhabditis elegans*. J Neurosci 17(21):8259–8269

52. Tobin D, Madsen D, Kahn-Kirby A, Peckol E, Moulder G, Barstead R, Maricq A, Bargmann C (2002) Combinatorial expression of TRPV channel proteins defines their sensory functions and subcellular localization in *C. elegans* neurons. Neuron 35(2):307–318

53. Wani KA, Catanese M, Normantowicz R, Herd M, Maher KN, Chase DL (2012) D1 dopamine receptor signaling is modulated by the R7 RGS protein EAT-16 and the R7 binding protein RSBP-1 in *Caenoerhabditis elegans* motor neurons. PLoS One 7(5):e37831

54. McDonald PW, Hardie SL, Jessen TN, Carvelli L, Matthies DS, Blakely RD (2007) Vigorous motor activity in *Caenorhabditis elegans* requires efficient clearance of dopamine mediated by synaptic localization of the dopamine transporter DAT-1. J Neurosci 27(51):14216–14227

55. Chase DL, Pepper JS, Koelle MR (2004) Mechanism of extrasynaptic dopamine signaling in *Caenorhabditis elegans*. Nat Neurosci 7(10):1096–1103

56. Allen AT, Maher KN, Wani KA, Betts KE, Chase DL (2011) Coexpressed D1- and D2-like dopamine receptors antagonistically modulate acetylcholine release in *Caenorhabditis elegans*. Genetics 188(3):579–590

57. Jaber M, Koch WJ, Rockman H, Smith B, Bond RA, Sulik KK, Ross J Jr, Lefkowitz RJ, Caron MG, Giros B (1996) Essential role of β-adrenergic receptor kinase 1 in cardiac development and function. Proc Natl Acad Sci U S A 93(23):12974–12979

58. Rockman HA, Choi DJ, Akhter SA, Jaber M, Giros B, Lefkowitz RJ, Caron MG, Koch WJ (1998) Control of myocardial contractile function by the level of β-adrenergic receptor kinase 1 in gene-targeted mice. J Biol Chem 273(29):18180–18184

59. Gainetdinov RR, Bohn LM, Sotnikova TD, Cyr M, Laakso A, Macrae AD, Torres GE, Kim KM, Lefkowitz RJ, Caron MG, Premont RT (2003) Dopaminergic supersensitivity in G protein-coupled receptor kinase 6-deficient mice. Neuron 38(2):291–303

60. Gainetdinov RR, Bohn LM, Walker JK, Laporte SA, Macrae AD, Caron MG, Lefkowitz RJ, Premont RT (1999) Muscarinic supersensitivity and impaired receptor desensitization in G protein-coupled receptor kinase 5-deficient mice. Neuron 24(4):1029–1036

61. Premont RT, Gainetdinov RR (2007) Physiological roles of G protein-coupled receptor kinases and arrestins. Annu Rev Physiol 69:511–534

62. Fong AM, Premont RT, Richardson RM, Yu YR, Lefkowitz RJ, Patel DD (2002) Defective lymphocyte chemotaxis in β-arrestin2- and GRK6-deficient mice. Proc Natl Acad Sci U S A 99(11):7478–7483

63. Schleicher S, Boekhoff I, Arriza J, Lefkowitz RJ, Breer H (1993) A β-adrenergic receptor kinase-like enzyme is involved in olfactory signal termination. Proc Natl Acad Sci U S A 90(4):1420–1424

64. Boekhoff I, Inglese J, Schleicher S, Koch WJ, Lefkowitz RJ, Breer H (1994) Olfactory desensitization requires membrane targeting of receptor kinase mediated by βγ subunits of heterotrimeric G proteins. J Biol Chem 269(1):37–40

65. Peppel K, Boekhoff I, McDonald P, Breer H, Caron MG, Lefkowitz RJ (1997) G protein-coupled receptor kinase 3 (GRK3) gene disruption leads to loss of odorant receptor desensitization. J Biol Chem 272(41):25425–25428

66. Ezak MJ, Hong E, Chaparro-Garcia A, Ferkey DM (2010) *Caenorhabditis elegans* TRPV channels function in a modality-specific pathway to regulate response to aberrant sensory signaling. Genetics 185(1):233–244

67. Zhang S, Sokolchik I, Blanco G, Sze JY (2004) *Caenorhabditis elegans* TRPV ion channel regulates 5HT biosynthesis in chemosensory neurons. Development 131(7):1629–1638

68. Sokolchik I, Tanabe T, Baldi PF, Sze JY (2005) Polymodal sensory function of the *Caenorhabditis elegans* OCR-2 channel arises from distinct intrinsic determinants within the protein and is selectively conserved in mammalian TRPV proteins. J Neurosci 25(4):1015–1023

69. Scholey JM, Anderson KV (2006) Intraflagellar transport and cilium-based signaling. Cell 125(3):439–442

70. Singla V, Reiter JF (2006) The primary cilium as the cell's antenna: signaling at a sensory organelle. Science 313(5787):629–633

71. Perkins LA, Hedgecock EM, Thomson JN, Culotti JG (1986) Mutant sensory cilia in the nematode *Caenorhabditis elegans*. Dev Biol 117(2):456–487

72. Inglis PN, Ou G, Leroux MR, Scholey JM (2006, November 27) The sensory cilia of Caenorhabditis elegans. In: WormBook (ed) The C. elegans Research Community, WormBook. doi:10.1895/wormbook.1.126.1, http://www.wormbook.org

73. Bargmann CI, Horvitz HR (1991) Chemosensory neurons with overlapping functions direct chemotaxis to multiple chemicals in *C. elegans*. Neuron 7(5):729–742

74. Cole DG, Diener DR, Himelblau AL, Beech PL, Fuster JC, Rosenbaum JL (1998) *Chlamydomonas* kinesin-II-dependent intraflagellar transport (IFT): IFT particles contain proteins required for ciliary assembly in *Caenorhabditis elegans* sensory neurons. J Cell Biol 141(4):993–1008

75. Rosenbaum JL, Witman GB (2002) Intraflagellar transport. Nat Rev Mol Cell Biol 3(11):813–825

76. Scholey JM (2003) Intraflagellar transport. Annu Rev Cell Dev Biol 19:423–443

77. Qin H, Burnette DT, Bae YK, Forscher P, Barr MM, Rosenbaum JL (2005) Intraflagellar transport is required for the vectorial movement of TRPV channels in the ciliary membrane. Curr Biol 15(18):1695–1699

78. Ward S (1973) Chemotaxis by the nematode *Caenorhabditis elegans*: identification of attractants and analysis of the response by use of mutants. Proc Natl Acad Sci U S A 70(3):817–821

79. Dusenbery DB, Sheridan RE, Russell RL (1975) Chemotaxis-defective mutants of the nematode *Caenorhabditis elegans*. Genetics 80(2):297–309

80. Hukema RK, Rademakers S, Dekkers MP, Burghoorn J, Jansen G (2006) Antagonistic sensory cues generate gustatory plasticity in *Caenorhabditis elegans*. EMBO J 25(2): 312–322

81. Brown SA, Zumbrunn G, Fleury-Olela F, Preitner N, Schibler U (2002) Rhythms of mammalian body temperature can sustain peripheral circadian clocks. Curr Biol 12(18):1574–1583

82. Merrow M, Brunner M, Roenneberg T (1999) Assignment of circadian function for the *Neurospora* clock gene frequency. Nature 399(6736):584–586

83. McWatters HG, Devlin PF (2011) Timing in plants—a rhythmic arrangement. FEBS Lett 585(10):1474–1484

84. Ripperger JA, Jud C, Albrecht U (2011) The daily rhythm of mice. FEBS Lett 585(10):1384–1392

85. Merrow M, Spoelstra K, Roenneberg T (2005) The circadian cycle: daily rhythms from behaviour to genes. EMBO Rep 6(10):930–935

86. Olmedo M, O'Neill JS, Edgar RS, Valekunja UK, Reddy AB, Merrow M (2012) Circadian regulation of olfaction and an evolutionarily conserved, nontranscriptional marker in *Caenorhabditis elegans*. Proc Natl Acad Sci U S A 109(50):20479–20484

87. Edgar RS, Green EW, Zhao Y, van Ooijen G, Olmedo M, Qin X, Xu Y, Pan M, Valekunja UK, Feeney KA, Maywood ES, Hastings MH, Baliga NS, Merrow M, Millar AJ, Johnson CH, Kyriacou CP, O'Neill JS, Reddy AB (2012) Peroxiredoxins are conserved markers of circadian rhythms. Nature 485(7399):459–464

88. O'Neill JS, Reddy AB (2011) Circadian clocks in human red blood cells. Nature 469(7331):498–503

89. Tanoue S, Krishnan P, Chatterjee A, Hardin PE (2008) G protein-coupled receptor kinase 2 is required for rhythmic olfactory responses in *Drosophila*. Curr Biol 18(11):787–794

90. Granados-Fuentes D, Tseng A, Herzog ED (2006) A circadian clock in the olfactory bulb controls olfactory responsivity. J Neurosci 26(47):12219–12225

91. Huang CC, Yoshino-Koh K, Tesmer JJ (2009) A surface of the kinase domain critical for the allosteric activation of G protein-coupled receptor kinases. J Biol Chem 284(25):17206–17215

92. Boguth CA, Singh P, Huang CC, Tesmer JJ (2010) Molecular basis for activation of G protein-coupled receptor kinases. EMBO J 29(19):3249–3259

93. Sterne-Marr R, Tesmer JJ, Day PW, Stracquatanio RP, Cilente JA, O'Connor KE, Pronin AN, Benovic JL, Wedegaertner PB (2003) G protein-coupled receptor Kinase 2/Gα(q/11) interaction. A novel surface on a regulator of G protein signaling homology domain for binding Gα subunits. J Biol Chem 278(8):6050–6058

94. Carman CV, Barak LS, Chen C, Liu-Chen LY, Onorato JJ, Kennedy SP, Caron MG, Benovic JL (2000) Mutational analysis of Gβγ and phospholipid interaction with G protein-coupled receptor kinase 2. J Biol Chem 275(14):10443–10452

95. Carman CV, Parent JL, Day PW, Pronin AN, Sternweis PM, Wedegaertner PB, Gilman AG, Benovic JL, Kozasa T (1999) Selective regulation of Gα$_{(q/11)}$ by an RGS domain in the G protein-coupled receptor kinase, GRK2. J Biol Chem 274(48):34483–34492

96. Noble B, Kallal LA, Pausch MH, Benovic JL (2003) Development of a yeast bioassay to characterize G protein-coupled receptor kinases. Identification of an NH2-terminal region essential for receptor phosphorylation. J Biol Chem 278(48):47466–47476

97. Pao CS, Barker BL, Benovic JL (2009) Role of the amino terminus of G protein-coupled receptor kinase 2 in receptor phosphorylation. Biochemistry 48(30):7325–7333

98. Wood JF, Wang J, Benovic JL, Ferkey DM (2012) Structural domains required for *Caenorhabditis elegans* G protein-coupled receptor kinase 2 (GRK-2) function in vivo. J Biol Chem 287(16):12634–12644

99. Ribas C, Penela P, Murga C, Salcedo A, Garcia-Hoz C, Jurado-Pueyo M, Aymerich I, Mayor F Jr (2007) The G protein-coupled receptor kinase (GRK) interactome: role of GRKs in GPCR regulation and signaling. Biochim Biophys Acta 1768(4):913–922

100. Kong G, Penn R, Benovic JL (1994) A β-adrenergic receptor kinase dominant negative mutant attenuates desensitization of the β2-adrenergic receptor. J Biol Chem 269(18):13084–13087

101. Huang CC, Tesmer JJ (2011) Recognition in the face of diversity: interactions of heterotrimeric G proteins and G protein-coupled receptor (GPCR) kinases with activated GPCRs. J Biol Chem 286(10):7715–7721

102. Beautrait A, Michalski KR, Lopez TS, Mannix KM, McDonald DJ, Cutter AR, Medina CB, Hebert AM, Francis CJ, Bouvier M, Tesmer JJ, Sterne-Marr R (2014) Mapping the putative G protein-coupled receptor (GPCR) docking site on GPCR kinase 2: insights from intact cell phosphorylation and recruitment assays. J Biol Chem 289(36):25262–25275

103. Tesmer VM, Kawano T, Shankaranarayanan A, Kozasa T, Tesmer JJ (2005) Snapshot of activated G proteins at the membrane: the Gα(q)-GRK2-Gβγ complex. Science 310(5754):1686–1690

104. Lodowski DT, Tesmer VM, Benovic JL, Tesmer JJ (2006) The structure of G protein-coupled receptor kinase (GRK)-6 defines a second lineage of GRKs. J Biol Chem 281(24):16785–16793

105. Dhami GK, Dale LB, Anborgh PH, O'Connor-Halligan KE, Sterne-Marr R, Ferguson SS (2004) G Protein-coupled receptor kinase 2 regulator of G protein signaling homology domain binds to both metabotropic glutamate receptor 1a and $G\alpha_q$ to attenuate signaling. J Biol Chem 279(16):16614–16620

106. Touhara K, Koch WJ, Hawes BE, Lefkowitz RJ (1995) Mutational analysis of the pleckstrin homology domain of the β-adrenergic receptor kinase. Differential effects on Gβγ and phosphatidylinositol 4,5-bisphosphate binding. J Biol Chem 270(28):17000–17005

107. Koch WJ, Inglese J, Stone WC, Lefkowitz RJ (1993) The binding site for the βγ subunits of heterotrimeric G proteins on the β-adrenergic receptor kinase. J Biol Chem 268(11):8256–8260

108. Pitcher JA, Inglese J, Higgins JB, Arriza JL, Casey PJ, Kim C, Benovic JL, Kwatra MM, Caron MG, Lefkowitz RJ (1992) Role of βγ subunits of G proteins in targeting the β-adrenergic receptor kinase to membrane-bound receptors. Science 257(5074):1264–1267

109. Boughton AP, Yang P, Tesmer VM, Ding B, Tesmer JJ, Chen Z (2011) Heterotrimeric G protein β1γ2 subunits change orientation upon complex formation with G protein-coupled receptor kinase 2 (GRK2) on a model membrane. Proc Natl Acad Sci U S A 108(37):E667–E673

Chapter 14

Evolutionarily Conserved Role of G-Protein-Coupled Receptor Kinases in the Hedgehog Signaling Pathway

Dominic Maier and David R. Hipfner

Abstract

Hedgehog (Hh) signaling plays a crucial role in the formation and maintenance of tissues in most animals. The key activator of cytoplasmic Hh signaling is an atypical G-protein-coupled receptor (GPCR) family protein called Smoothened (Smo). In response to binding of Hh ligands to their receptor Patched, Smo is conformationally activated by extensive phosphorylation of its cytoplasmic C-terminus and engages downstream pathway components to promote Hh target gene expression. GPCR kinases (GRKs) positively regulate Hh signaling, a function that has been conserved in both invertebrates and vertebrates. Direct phosphorylation of highly conserved clusters of Ser/Thr residues in the proximal Smo C-terminus by GRKs is important in controlling Smo trafficking and activating signaling. GRKs also indirectly affect Hh pathway activity by influencing cellular cAMP levels and thus the activity of protein kinase A, a key regulator of the Cubitus interruptus/GLI family transcription factors that mediate Hh transcriptional responses. This indirect role hints at a broader interconnectivity between GRKs, GPCR signaling, and Hh pathway function, an idea supported by the recent identification of several GPCRs that are capable of modulating Hh target gene expression.

Key words G-protein-coupled receptor kinase, Hedgehog signaling, Smoothened, G-protein-coupled receptor, Cubitus interruptus/GLI, protein kinase A, phosphorylation

1 Introduction

Secreted Hedgehog (Hh) family proteins control a signaling cascade crucial not only for embryonic development in most animals but also for adult tissue homeostasis [1, 2]. The Hh pathway is highly conserved throughout evolution and its misregulation is associated with severe human pathologies including congenital defects and many types of cancer, most prominently medulloblastoma and basal cell carcinoma [3, 4]. Identifying suitable therapeutic targets within the Hh pathway is imperative; however, this requires a complete understanding of its molecular biology. Work in the 1980s and 1990s identified the core proteins and the general architecture of the signaling cascade whereas the last 15 years of Hh research has uncovered proteins that modulate the Hh response by regulating the core components [5].

Vsevolod V. Gurevich et al. (eds.), *G Protein-Coupled Receptor Kinases*, Methods in Pharmacology and Toxicology,
DOI 10.1007/978-1-4939-3798-1_14, © Springer Science+Business Media New York 2016

G-protein-coupled receptor kinases (GRKs) are modulators of Hh signaling in species as diverse as fruit flies, fish, and mice [6–9]. The link between GRKs and the Hh pathway was not obvious as GRKs are a subgroup of Ser/Thr kinases most closely associated with classical G-protein-coupled receptor (GPCR) signaling [10]. Studies in *Drosophila* and mammals have demonstrated that GRKs directly regulate Smoothened (Smo), the central signal transducer of the pathway and distant member of the GPCR superfamily, through an evolutionarily conserved mechanism [11, 12]. Work in *Drosophila* further suggests that GRKs can affect Hh signaling indirectly by helping maintain conditions permissive for signaling in Hh-responsive cells [13]. In this chapter, we first outline some physiological functions and basic mechanisms of Hh signal transduction leading to target gene expression, and then summarize our current understanding of the dual role of GRKs in this pathway.

2   Role of Hh in Tissue Patterning

2.1 Hh Patterns Embryonic Tissues in a Concentration-Dependent Manner

Secreted Hh proteins contribute to the process of embryonic patterning of numerous tissues by specifying cell fates in a concentration-dependent manner. This morphogen function of Hh is well-described in several processes including patterning of the anterior–posterior axis of the developing *Drosophila* wing, digit formation in the vertebrate limb, and specification of neural cell-type identity in the developing vertebrate neural tube [4, 14]. In each system, Hh ligands form a concentration gradient extending away from their source of secretion and regulate transcription of different sets of target genes at different thresholds in surrounding cells [14].

2.2 Hh Patterns the Drosophila Wing Imaginal Disk

The wing imaginal disk is the embryonic precursor to the adult fly wing, and is divided into separate anterior (A) and posterior (P) populations of cells, or compartments [15]. The Hh protein is produced solely in the P compartment of the wing disk (Fig. 1a) [16]. However, P cells are not responsive to Hh because they do not express the gene encoding Cubitus interruptus (Ci), the key transcription factor of the pathway (see below) [17]. Instead, Hh diffuses into the A compartment and forms a concentration gradient spanning ~15–20 cell diameters, with cells close to the A/P boundary exposed to the highest concentration of Hh [16, 18]. Hh-responsive genes are roughly divided into high, medium, and low threshold Hh targets. Low amounts of Hh are sufficient to induce transcription of so-called low threshold Hh target genes; consequently, these genes are expressed essentially throughout the entire region of Hh diffusion. The most notable low threshold target gene is *decapentaplegic* (*dpp*), whose transcription is induced in a wide stripe of A cells [19]. Expression of high threshold Hh target genes requires high concentrations of Hh and they are

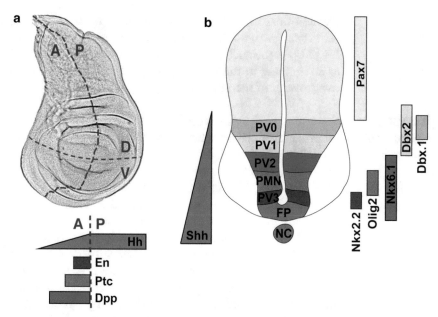

Fig. 1 Hh proteins act as morphogens in embryonic tissue patterning. (**a**) Hh patterns the anterior (A)–posterior (P) axis of the *Drosophila* wing imaginal disk. Hh is produced by P cells (representation of protein levels in *orange*). Because they do not express Ci, P cells do not activate Hh target genes. Hh diffuses and forms a concentration gradient in the A compartment. Hh target genes are activated in a concentration-dependent manner in a central stripe of A cells adjacent to the A/P boundary. High-threshold targets (like *en*) are activated in only a few rows of A cells, where Hh levels are highest. Activation of medium-threshold targets (like *ptc*) requires less Hh, so these genes are expressed in a broader stripe of cells. Low-threshold targets (like *dpp*) require little Hh for activation, and are thus expressed throughout most of the region where Hh diffuses. The combination of the various Hh target genes patterns the portion of the wing disk that will give rise to the central region of the adult wing. (**b**) Shh directs neural cell type identity in the developing vertebrate neural tube. Shh secreted by cells of the notochord, which underlies the neural tube, induces expression of Shh in the floor plate. Shh diffuses away from the floorplate throughout the ventral half of the neural tube, forming a ventral-to-dorsal concentration gradient. High-threshold target genes like the transcription factor Nkx2.2 are expressed only in cells adjacent to the floorplate, where Shh levels are highest. Others, like Olig2 and Nkx6.1, are expressed at increasing distances from the floorplate and represent medium-threshold target genes. Pax7 is an example of a low-threshold target gene whose expression is repressed throughout much of the region spanning the Shh gradient. Dbx1 and 2 are activated in response to low levels of Shh. The identities of neural progenitor cells (FP, PV0-3, PMN) in the ventral neural tube are dictated by the different combinations of these and other transcription factors along the dorsal–ventral axis

therefore only induced in a few rows of cells in the A compartment, adjacent to the A/P boundary. Examples include *collier* (*col*) and *engrailed* (*en*), with the latter representing the highest known Hh threshold target and expressed in only a very narrow stripe of A cells. Finally, medium threshold target genes like *patched* (*ptc*) are activated by intermediate levels of Hh. The *ptc* expression domain is narrower than that of *dpp* but substantially wider than that of *col* or *en* [20]. Hh signaling defects in the wing disk lead to defects in the size and venation of the adult fly wing. Complete loss of Hh signaling in the wing disk results in the absence of the wing, while partial impairment leads to a smaller wing, more specifically to a reduction in the central space between longitudinal veins L3 and L4 [21]. Conversely, inappropriate pathway activity manifests itself as an increase in the vein L3-L4 space and in more severe cases in overgrowth of the entire A wing compartment [16].

2.3   In Vertebrates Sonic Hedgehog (Shh) Directs Neural Cell Type Identity in the Vertebrate Neural Tube

Patterning of the embryonic neural tube defines the identity of neural progenitor cell populations that will later give rise to neurons of the adult spinal cord. In the ventral half of the neural tube, a Shh gradient specifies the progenitor cells PV3, PMN, PV2, PV1, and PV0 (Fig. 1b) [22]. Shh is secreted by cells of the notochord, which underlies the neural tube. Shh induces its own expression in the floor plate generating a Shh diffusion gradient throughout the ventral half of the neural tube. Analogous to the situation in the wing disk, Shh triggers expression of different subsets of genes at different concentrations. For instance, the transcription factor Nk2 homeobox 2 (Nkx2.2) is expressed only in cells adjacent to the floorplate, and is thus classified as a high threshold target gene, whereas oligodendrocyte transcription factor 2 (Olig2) and Nkx6.1 are expressed at increasing distances from the floorplate and represent medium threshold target genes. Low levels of Shh are sufficient to repress Pax7 expression, so this transcription factor is absent from most cells throughout the Shh gradient. The spatially differentiated combinations of these and other transcription factors determines the cell identity of progenitor cells in the ventral neural tube [22].

3   Molecular Biology of the Pathway

The proteins involved in the Hh pathway trace back at least as far as the origins of eumetazoans and consequently Hh signaling cascades have been described for many different bilaterian species. In all examples known to date, the key components and the general architecture of the Hh pathway are well conserved [23]. The essential components of the pathway include the secreted Hh ligands, two transmembrane proteins (Patched (Ptc) and Smo), a cytosolic complex of proteins called the Hh signaling complex (HSC), and the transcription factor(s) of the pathway (Ci in *Drosophila* and Glioma-associated oncogenes (Gli) -1, -2, and -3 in vertebrates) (Fig. 2). Ptc is the Hh receptor and a key negative regulator of Smo, which is itself the central signal transducer of the pathway. In brief, Hh activates Smo indirectly by inhibiting Ptc. In turn, activated Smo induces transcription of Hh target genes by controlling the activity of the Ci/Gli transcription factors via the HSC.

3.1   Regulation of Ci/Gli

The Hh concentration gradient is ultimately translated into an activity gradient of the bifunctional Ci/Gli transcription factors [24]. In the absence of Hh, the full-length Ci/Gli proteins are proteolytically processed into truncated versions (Ci^{75}/Gli^R) capable of binding DNA via their zinc finger domains and acting as transcriptional repressors for some Hh target genes. Upon exposure to Hh, the equilibrium shifts in favor of the full-length transcriptional activator forms (Ci^{155}/Gli^A) because proteolytic processing of Ci/Gli proteins is blocked [25–27]. The nature of the transcriptional response, that is, whether low or high threshold target genes are expressed, depends on the state of the Ci/Gli transcription factors. High- threshold Hh target genes require strong Ci/Gli activation. Low-threshold target gene expression in flies can be achieved simply by relieving the transcriptional inhibition of Ci^{75} (i.e. by blocking Ci processing), although transcription is further enhanced by Ci^{155} activation [26]. How Hh controls this balance between activator and repressor forms of Ci/Gli is best illustrated by examining the Hh pathway in its "on" and "off" state. We focus first on Hh signaling in the fruit fly where the pathway is still best understood. The similarities and differences between Ci regulation in *Drosophila* and Gli regulation in vertebrates are discussed below.

3.2 Drosophila Hh Pathway in the "Off" State

In the absence of Hh, Smo activity is constitutively blocked by Ptc through a poorly defined mechanism. Ptc keeps Smo protein levels low and traps Smo in internal endocytic vesicles [28]. In this condition, Smo seems to reside in an inactive state and is targeted for proteasomal degradation through ubiquitination (Fig. 2a) [29, 30]. Ptc is a twelve-pass membrane protein with structural homology to bacterial transporters and it has long been speculated that Ptc controls the availability of a naturally occurring Smo ligand, possibly a sterol-like compound [31, 32]. This model is compelling, because Smo is a member of the GPCR superfamily of seven-pass transmembrane receptors, whose conformation and activity are often modulated by natural ligands acting either as agonists or antagonists. Ptc might deliver an antagonist to Smo or limit the availability of a Smo agonist. The result in both cases is the same—Smo remains in an inactive conformation and is subsequently ubiquitinated and degraded. Ptc also seems to play another role in Smo degradation. Ptc mediates the recruitment of internalized lipoproteins, called lipophorins in flies, to Smo-rich endosomes. Lipids delivered by the lipophorins get incorporated in the membranes of the Smo-containing vesicles and this process might be required for lysosomal Smo degradation [33, 34].

Inhibition of Smo by Ptc has consequences for Ci processing. Ci^{155} associates with the HSC, composed of Costal2 (Cos2), an atypical kinesin acting as molecular scaffold, the Ser/Thr kinase Fused (Fu), and Suppressor of Fused (SuFu), a small protein whose function is to retain Ci^{155} in the cytoplasm [35–40]. Cos2 recruits several kinases (protein kinase A (PKA), casein kinase 1 (Ck1), glycogen synthase kinase-3β (Gsk3β)), which extensively phosphorylate Ci [41–45]. PKA acts as the master kinase for this step, as Ck1- and

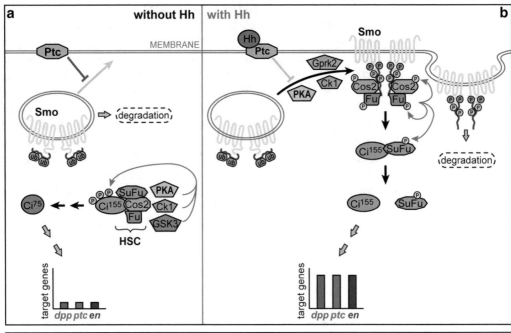

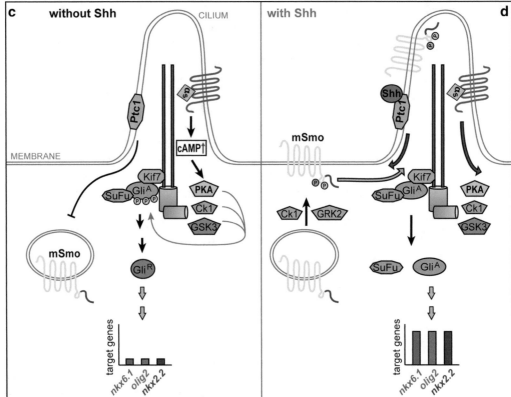

Fig. 2 Transduction of the Hh signal. (**a**) In *Drosophila melanogaster*, in the absence of Hh Ptc at the plasma membrane prevents Smo from becoming activated and accumulating at the cell surface. Smo is instead subject to ubiquitin-dependent degradation. In this condition, Cos2 acts as a scaffold, assembling a microtubule-associated Hedgehog signaling complex (HSC) that includes Fu, SuFu, and the full-length form of Ci (Ci155).

Gsk3β-dependent phosphorylation requires priming at adjacent PKA sites. Phosphorylated Ci[155] is targeted for partial proteolysis by the proteasome and processed into the transcriptional repressor Ci[75].

3.3 The "On" State of the Drosophila Hh Pathway

Upon binding of Hh by Ptc, its inhibition of Smo is released and hyper-phosphorylated Smo homodimers accumulate at the plasma membrane (Fig. 2b) [28, 46]. All known Smo phosphorylation sites are situated in the cytoplasmic C-terminal tail of the protein, and several Smo kinases have been identified. Similar to the situation with Ci, PKA is the master regulator of *Drosophila* Smo. PKA phosphorylates Smo at three consensus sites located in the "Smo autoinhibitory domain" (SAID), triggering additional phosphorylation by Ck1 at adjacent Ser residues [47–49]. Interspersed between these three clusters of phosphorylation sites are stretches of positively charged Arg/Lys residues, which serve two functions in Smo autoinhibition. First, they help maintain Smo in an inactive conformation, perhaps by interacting with negatively charged residues in the distal Smo C-terminus [46]. Second, several Lys residues in this region are ubiquitinated to promote endocytosis and degradation of Smo, helping to keep the pathway off [29, 30]. Collectively, PKA/Ck1 phosphorylation at the three Ser/Thr clusters in the SAID prevents Smo ubiquitination, leading to its accumulation at the cell surface [29, 30]. It also neutralizes the local positive charge of the SAID, thereby inducing a conformational change within the Smo C-terminus, which can be detected by intramolecular fluorescence resonance energy transfer (FRET) analysis of tagged Smo proteins,

---

Fig. 2 (continued) Cos2 also recruits three kinases (PKA, Ck1, and Gsk3β), which sequentially phosphorylate Ci[155]. Phosphorylation promotes limited proteolysis of Ci[155] to the cleaved repressor form (Ci[75]). This has two effects: Ci[75] directly represses expression of certain target genes (e.g. *dpp*), and the processing of Ci[155] reduces the levels of this transcriptional activator, preventing expression of many Hh target genes. (**b**) Binding of Hh inactivates Ptc, relieving its repression of Smo. Smo becomes phosphorylated in its C-terminus, first by PKA and Ck1 (causing it to translocate to the cell surface) and then by Gprk2. Phosphorylation promotes Smo dimerization and recruitment of the HSC to its cytoplasmic tail. Recruited Fu autophosphorylates and activates itself. Fu then phosphorylates Cos2, inactivating it and causing dissociation and accumulation of Ci[155]. Fu also phosphorylates SuFu, which may prevent it from tethering Ci[155] in the cytoplasm. Ci[155] enters the nucleus, and activates target gene expression. Phosphorylation of Smo by Gprk2 also promotes internalization and degradation of activated Smo, perhaps in a manner resembling homologous desensitization, helping to terminate signaling. (**c**) In the absence of Shh, mammalian Ptc localizes to and prevents Smo trafficking to the cilium. Gpr161 also localizes to the cilium, where it activates $G_{\alpha s}$ to increase cAMP production and PKA activity. PKA, Ck1, and Gsk3β phosphorylate Gli2/3, a reaction likely scaffolded by Kif7, to promote their limited proteolysis. This reduces the levels of the activator forms (Gli[A]) and increases levels of the repressor forms (Gli[R]) of these transcription factors to keep target gene expression "off." (**d**) Binding of Shh triggers Ptc removal from the cilium. Gpr161 also exits the cilium, terminating its signaling. Smo becomes phosphorylated in its cytoplasmic tail by GRK2 and Ck1, and traffics into the cilium in a GRK2/β-arrestin-dependent manner. Although the precise molecular details remain unclear, Gli2/3 processing ceases and the Gli[A] proteins are released from Sufu, exit the cilium, and move to the nucleus to activate target gene expression

resulting in a more open conformation and dimerization of Smo C-tails [46]. This is thought to expose HSC binding sites within the distal Smo C-terminus and leads to the recruitment of HSC proteins to Smo [50–53]. This interaction between Smo and the HSC interferes with the recruitment of PKA, Ck1, and Gsk3β to the HSC and triggers the release of full-length Ci^{155}, such that processing of Ci^{155} into Ci^{75} ceases [50, 53]. Ci^{155} accumulates and can now enter the nucleus to activate expression of Hh target genes.

Interestingly, the degree of Smo conformational shift and dimerization of its C-terminal tail detected by FRET correlates with endogenous Hh concentrations in the wing disk and with the extent of PKA/Ck1-dependent Smo phosphorylation [46]. This could be because the conformational change of Smo is gradual rather than all-or-none, with activity correlating with the extent of conformational change. Alternatively, Smo might have only one active conformation, with more extensive phosphorylation increasing the likelihood of Smo adopting and remaining in this active conformation. In either case, the outcome is that the Hh ligand concentration gradient gets translated into a Smo phosphorylation gradient, leading in turn to a gradient of Smo activity and ultimately of Ci activation.

3.4 Differences Between Hh Signaling in Drosophila and Mammals

Generally, Hh pathway components are well conserved, but gene duplication events in mammals have increased the complexity for some pathway components. For instance, mammals have three functional Hh genes: Indian (Ihh), Desert (Dhh), and Shh, the latter being the most widely expressed paralog [54]. The Hh-responsive transcription factor in mammals also exists as three gene variants, Gli1, 2, and 3 [55]. Analogous to the *Drosophila* Ci protein, Gli2 and 3 are bifunctional transcriptional repressors and activators and are also regulated by PKA, Ck1, and Gsk3β. Gli1, however, plays only a minor role as a transcriptional activator and transcriptional target of the pathway [55].

Hh signaling in mammals follows the same general architecture as described for *Drosophila*. However, there are several important distinctions between mammals and flies. For instance, proper functioning of the Hh pathway in mammals requires the primary cilium [56], a microtubule-based membrane protrusion, present in most mammalian cells but largely absent in flies. Key Hh pathway components such as Ptc, Smo, and the Gli transcription factors are dynamically trafficked in and out of the cilium in the response to Shh making this organelle a Hh signaling hub (Fig. 2c, d). Consequently, disruption of ciliogenesis or ciliary trafficking also results in Hh signaling defects in mammals [56]. It should be noted that in the few cell types that are ciliated in the fly, the cilium may also be implicated in Hh signaling [57].

Signaling downstream of Smo, both in terms of the role and composition of the HSC, also differs somewhat between *Drosophila* and mammals. In flies, the HSC (Cos2, Fu, SuFu) is recruited to active, hyper-phosphorylated and dimerized Smo C-terminal tails in the presence of Hh, facilitating Fu autoactivation, which in turn phosphorylates Cos2 and SuFu (Fig. 2b) [51, 53, 58]. These phosphorylation events are thought to trigger the release of Ci[155] from Cos2 and inhibit SuFu, allowing Ci[155] to enter the nucleus [37, 44, 51, 53, 59, 60]. Signaling downstream of mammalian Smo is less well understood, but it is clear that it differs (Fig. 2d). The ortholog of Fu, STK36, has no function in the mammalian pathway [61, 62]. Kif7, the ortholog of Cos2, seems to perform similar functions as Cos2, but the molecular details are still not well characterized [63–65]. Lastly, SuFu, which has only a minor inhibitory role in the fly Hh pathway, is a major negative regulator in the mammalian pathway although it remains unknown how SuFu is itself controlled [66, 67].

Some of these differences are explainable at the level of the primary sequence of Smo. Most vertebrate genomes including those of mammals encode one Smo ortholog. Vertebrate and invertebrate Smo orthologs show a fair degree of conservation throughout large parts of the proteins including the N-terminal and transmembrane domains. However, only the ~100 most membrane-proximal amino acids of the cytoplasmic C-terminus are broadly conserved (Fig. 3) [12]. The rest of the tail diverges substantially in different clades. This distal, non-conserved part of the Smo C-terminus comprises roughly an additional 100 amino acids in most species. However, arthropod Smo proteins possess a much longer tail of approximately 350 amino acids. Interestingly, the SAID containing the PKA/Ck1 phosphorylation clusters crucial for the conformational regulation of Smo as well as most binding sites for *Drosophila* HSC proteins fall into this non-conserved region (Fig. 3a) [24]. This suggests that the mechanism of Smo activation and the means by which it engages the downstream signaling machinery has diverged. In fact, vertebrate Smo orthologs do not contain PKA phosphorylation sites and there is no evidence that they are regulated by PKA. It was a long-standing puzzle in the field as to whether or not there is a vertebrate Smo kinase that serves a function analogous to PKA in *Drosophila*. The answer emerged over the last decade through the collective efforts of several laboratories. As further elaborated below, GRK2 in conjunction with Ck1α fills the role of the activating vertebrate Smo kinase.

4   Role of GRKs

4.1   GRKs Participate in Hh Signaling in Vertebrates and Invertebrates

The first connection between GRKs and the Hh pathway was established in mammalian cell culture experiments. The fact that Smo is a distant member of the GPCR superfamily suggested that proteins involved in GPCR regulation such as GRKs and β-arrestins

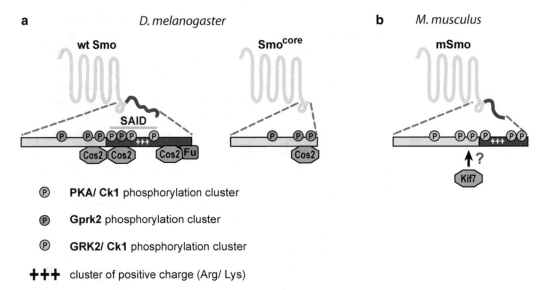

a   *D. melanogaster*   **b**   *M. musculus*

Fig. 3 Conservation and divergence of functional elements in the *Drosophila* and mammalian Smo C-terminus. The Smo N-terminus, 7-transmembrane domain region, and the first ~100 amino acids of the cytoplasmic tail are well conserved in bilaterians (yellow). However, the C-terminal regions are highly divergent in different clades. (**a**) In *Drosophila* Smo (left panel), the divergent C-terminus (*blue*) includes the Smo autoinhibitory domain (SAID) containing three clusters of PKA/Ck1 phosphorylation sites and a highly positively charged stretch that plays an important negative role in controlling Smo levels and activity. Several binding sites for the downstream HSC components Cos2 and Fu have also been mapped to this divergent region. Three of four Gprk2 phosphorylation clusters (including the functionally most important first two) are situated in the more membrane-proximal conserved region of the cytoplasmic tail. Phosphorylation at these sites regulates interaction with Cos2 at a proximal binding site. Smo^core (*right*), a truncated form of *Drosophila* Smo, lacks the non-conserved cytoplasmic tail but retains most of the Gprk2 sites and the proximal Cos2 interaction domain. Smo^core can activate signaling, suggesting that the non-conserved elements are not essential. (**b**) The divergent tail of mouse Smo (*purple*) lacks PKA phosphorylation sites, although it too has a (non-conserved) stretch of positively charged residues. Rather than PKA, mSmo is activated by GRK2 and Ck1 phosphorylation at six clusters of residues, three of which (including the functionally most important first two) are highly conserved. By analogy with *Drosophila* Smo, mSmo may interact with Kif7 through a conserved binding site

might also affect Smo and, by extension, Hh pathway activity. Metabolic labeling revealed that GRK2 does indeed promote Smo phosphorylation in HEK293 cells, and both β-arrestin and GRK2 are recruited to active Smo localized at the plasma membrane [68]. The functional relevance of these findings was confirmed in a subsequent study demonstrating that GRK2 phosphorylation and β-arrestin recruitment are required for the expression of Hh-responsive reporter genes in C3H10T1/2 cells [69].

These results led to a careful evaluation of GRK loss-of-function phenotypes in vivo. Depletion of zGRK2/3 in zebrafish causes several phenotypes associated with mild Hh loss-of-function, including somite malformation and abnormal neural tube patterning, as well as lower transcription of Hh target genes [9]. GRK2 knockout mice die embryonically due to abnormalities in the development of the heart that are independent of the Hh pathway. However, at embryonic day (E)11.5, GRK2 knockout mouse embryos display defects in limb development and neural tube patterning, consistent with an impairment of Hh signaling [9]. The phenotypes in both model organisms clearly confirmed that GRK2 is required for vertebrate Hh signaling.

The discovery of Hh signaling defects in *Drosophila* GRK mutants demonstrated that the role of GRKs in Hh signaling is more broadly conserved. In contrast to mammals, which have genes encoding seven distinct GRKs, the fly genome encodes only two, Gprk1 and 2 [70]. Gprk1 shows homology to the mammalian GRK2 group consisting of GRKs 2 and 3. Gprk2 corresponds to the mammalian GRK5 group encompassing GRK4, 5, and 6. Several independent studies, based on either depletion of the protein by RNAi or classic loss-of-function genetic analysis, reported a moderate Hh loss-of-function phenotype in response to the loss of Gprk2 [6–8]. Wings of *gprk2* mutant flies displayed a marked reduction in the area between longitudinal veins L3 and L4 caused by an earlier impairment of Hh target gene expression in the developing wing disk. Specifically, expression of high (*en*, *col*) and medium (*ptc*) threshold Hh target genes was either lost or strongly decreased, respectively. However, expression of the low threshold target gene *dpp* was unaffected. These analyses indicated that Gprk2 function is specifically required for cells to mount a strong Hh response. Interestingly, in addition to being ubiquitously expressed at basal levels, *gprk2* is a Hh target gene and both mRNA and protein levels are strongly induced in Hh-responding cells [7, 8]. This suggests that Gprk2 acts as part of a positive feedback mechanism to enhance Hh signaling.

Mechanistically, Gprk2 acts in the Hh pathway at the level of Smo, consistent with the typical function of GRKs in regulating GPCRs and with the observations in mammalian cells [68]. In the absence of Gprk2, Smo regulation is clearly impaired. In normal wing disks, Smo protein levels are low in most A Hh-responding cells (although it is actively signaling). In *gprk2* mutant disks, however, Smo accumulates to high levels in Hh-responding cells [7, 8]. This accumulated Smo protein is less extensively phosphorylated than normal [7]. Similarly, depletion of Gprk2 in *Drosophila* S2 cells in the presence of Hh causes the accumulation of hypophosphorylated Smo at the plasma membrane [7]. This suggests that Gprk2 normally promotes the internalization and degradation of Smo in cells where it is activated, perhaps through a mechanism resembling homologous desensitization.

4.2   Mapping of GRK Phosphorylation Sites in Smo

The fact that loss of GRK function in vivo results in Hh loss-of-function phenotypes in both vertebrate and invertebrate species suggests they play a conserved and positive role in Hh signaling. The most straightforward model is that GRK-dependent Smo phosphorylation, and possibly β-arrestin recruitment, is required for Smo activation and Hh target gene expression. The aforementioned experiments in mammalian cells supported this view. However, formal proof of this hypothesis required that GRK phosphorylation sites in Smo be mapped and functionally characterized.

The first attempt employed in vitro kinase assays using mammalian GRK5 and fragments of the *Drosophila* Smo C-terminus as substrates to map phosphorylation sites. Chen and colleagues identified four Ser/Thr residues located at two different clusters (GPS1 and GPS2) within the cytoplasmic tail of Smo, neither of which is conserved [6]. Of the two clusters only GPS1 (Ser[741] and Ser[742]) seemed of some functional relevance. However, mutation of these sites to Asp to mimic the negative charge of the phosphate groups was not sufficient to rescue the *gprk2* loss-of-function phenotype as expected. To explain this, the authors proposed that Gprk2 also has a kinase activity-independent function. According to their model, in addition to regulating Smo activity by phosphorylating it, the dimerization of Gprk2 bound to the Smo cytoplasmic tail stabilizes the open conformation of the Smo C-terminus and facilitates Smo dimerization, both of which are required for efficient Hh signaling [6].

Several lines of evidence call this model into question, including the observation that mutation of GPS1 and GPS2 sites to Ala does not impair Smo activity [12]. By employing complementary cell-based approaches including direct monitoring of Smo phosphopeptides in control and Gprk2-depleted cells using a label-free semi-quantitative liquid chromatography/tandem mass spectrometry (LC-MS/MS) method, we identified four clusters of Gprk2-responsive Ser/Thr residues in the membrane-proximal region of the Smo cytoplasmic tail (Fig. 3a). These four clusters harbor a total of 18 phosphorylated Ser/Thr residues [12]. Mutation of all 18 sites to Ala recapitulates the specific effect that loss of Gprk2 has on Smo accumulation in Hh-responding cells in vivo, confirming that these are the functionally important phosphorylation sites. The phosphoproteomic analysis also detected phosphorylation at the two GPS1 residues. However, the observed decrease in phosphopeptide abundance in control versus Gprk2-depleted cells was relatively small, indicating that Gprk2 is not the major kinase responsible for phosphorylating the GPS1 sites under physiological conditions [12].

Functional characterization of the four clusters of Gprk2 phosphorylation sites strongly supports a strictly catalytic activity-dependent function for Gprk2 in regulating Smo. Mutation of the phosphorylation sites to Ala decreased but did not abolish Smo activity (measured using a dual luciferase-based Hh target gene transcriptional reporter assay), consistent with the in vivo phenotypes. Mutation of individual clusters or individual residues within a cluster had partial effects, suggesting that increasing levels of Gprk2 phosphorylation have a graded effect on Smo activity.

Gprk2-dependent phosphorylation affects Smo signaling in at least two ways. First, bioluminescence resonance energy transfer (BRET) experiments demonstrated that phosphorylation enhances dimerization of the Smo C-terminus. Second, phosphorylation is required for recruitment of Cos2 to a novel binding site located between residues 625 and 651 in the Smo cytoplasmic tail. Both functions require Gprk2 kinase activity and can be rescued in the absence of the kinase itself by mutating the Gprk2 sites in Smo to Asp. Interestingly, not all four clusters are equally important—Ala substitution of the first two clusters (c1/2) but not the last two clusters strongly impairs Smo activity, and mimicking phosphorylation at c1/2 is sufficient to circumvent the loss of Gprk2 [12]. In contrast to the PKA phosphomimetic form of Smo [48], mimicking Gprk2 phosphorylation is not sufficient to constitutively activate Smo, suggesting Gprk2 acts downstream of PKA in Smo activation.

Mapping studies using mouse Smo (mSmo) uncovered conserved regulatory phosphorylation sites in vertebrate Smo orthologs. A total of 12 Ser/Thr residues grouped in six clusters (PS0-5) in mSmo are phosphorylated by GRK2 and Ck1α in response to Shh stimulation (Fig. 3b) [11]. Phosphorylation at these sites appears to be graded in response to various Shh dosages and it is necessary and sufficient to promote Smo activation, dimerization of the cytoplasmic tail, β-arrestin recruitment, and translocation of Smo into the cilium in NIH 3T3 cells and mouse embryonic fibroblasts. Transgenic expression of a series of Smo constructs carrying different combinations of Ala or Asp substitutions at the GRK2/Ck1α phosphorylation sites in the chick neural tube confirmed the crucial activating role of these two kinases in vivo. Most importantly, phosphomimetic substitutions of the GRK2/Ck1α sites caused ectopic expression of Shh target genes such as Nkx2.2, Nkx6.1, and Olig2 and reduced expression of the dorsal marker Pax7. Of note, not all sites are equally important, as the first two clusters (PS0/1 with four and three Ser/Thr residues, respectively) account for the majority of the activating effect. The authors proposed a model similar to that of Smo activation by PKA in flies: the Shh gradient gets translated into graded mSmo phosphorylation and activation. GRK2/Ck1α phosphorylation causes a conformational change within the mSmo protein and leads to dimerization of C-termini, the extent of which correlates with the number of phosphorylated residues [11]. Only maximally phosphorylated mSmo is capable of inducing expression of high-threshold Shh target gene such as Nkx2.2 in the neural tube. Phosphorylation at the GRK2/Ck1α sites is also required for ciliary localization, most likely through the recruitment of β-arrestins [11]. This is in line with earlier work establishing that translocation of Smo into the cilium depends on β-arrestin recruitment [68]. However, the precise mechanism by which GRK2/Ck1α-dependent Smo activation and ciliary accumulation of Smo are coordinated is still unclear.

At first glance, GRK2/Ck1α regulation of mSmo and PKA/Ck1 regulation of *Drosophila* Smo appear quite similar. In both systems, the Hh gradient is translated into distinct Smo phosphorylation and activation states correlating with the extent of the Smo conformational change and C-terminal dimerization. It is important to note, however, that the principal kinase and the sites that are phosphorylated in each species are different. While this would appear to suggest that a similar regulatory mechanism arose independently in different lineages, this is not the case. In fact, the precise mechanism of GRK regulation appears to be operative in all bilaterian lineages. In multiple sequence alignments of the conserved first 98 amino acids of the cytoplasmic tail of Smo orthologs from all three branches of Bilateria (corresponding to residues 554–651 in *Drosophila* Smo), there is a striking near-perfect alignment of the first two phosphorylation clusters in the mouse and fly proteins (c1/2 in *Drosophila* Smo and PS0/1 in mSmo), and these are highly conserved in all Smo orthologs [12]. Notably, these are the sites that are most important for activation of both the mouse and fly proteins by GRKs. Thus phosphorylation by GRKs appears to be an evolutionarily ancient mechanism for regulating Smo activity that has been retained in all species in which it is found [12].

A compelling argument in support of this idea came from the analysis of a C-terminally truncated form of *Drosophila* Smo consisting of just the evolutionarily conserved portion (Smo^{core}). Smo^{core} is capable of activating cytoplasmic Hh signaling in both tissue culture cells and in vivo, although to a lesser extent than full-length Smo [12]. Smo^{core} lacks the PKA phosphorylation sites and most of the mapped binding sites of HSC proteins (Fig. 3a), suggesting that these arthropod-specific additions to Smo are not essential for its activity. Retained in Smo^{core}, however, are the first three conserved Gprk2 phosphorylation clusters and a newly identified membrane-proximal Cos2 binding site. Rather than being regulated by PKA, Smo^{core} signaling is exclusively and absolutely dependent on GRK phosphorylation, making its regulation more similar to mSmo. GRK phosphorylation is required for the interaction of Smo^{core} with Cos2 [12]. It will be interesting to see whether GRK2 phosphorylation promotes the recruitment of the mammalian Cos2 ortholog Kif7 to the comparable conserved region of mSmo to promote signaling.

It seems, then, that the GRK-driven mechanism of Smo regulation employed by mammalian Smo proteins is used in flies as well. However, whereas GRK2 is functionally equivalent to PKA in the fly, in that it turns on mSmo, Gprk2 seems to play more of a fine-tuning role by increasing the signaling strength of *Drosophila* Smo. The most straightforward explanation is that, while the functional GRK-regulated core has been retained, additional regulatory elements were acquired early during the evolution of arthropods. These rendered Smo activity subject to control principally by PKA, and added additional HSC binding sites that enabled PKA-dependent engagement of the downstream signaling machinery. This PKA-dependent mechanism may be how Smo signals when initially activated in response to low levels of Hh (Fig. 4). As Hh levels increase, so too does the extent of PKA/Ck1 phosphorylation of Smo [71], leading to increased signaling and target gene expression. As *gprk2* is itself a medium/high threshold Hh target gene [7, 8], signaling above a certain threshold will activate its transcription, initiating a positive feedback mechanism. Increased Gprk2 phosphorylation of Smo will then enhance Smo dimerization and Cos2 binding via the proximal binding site. Maximal Smo signaling activity is thus the combined output of separate PKA- and GRK-regulated mechanisms.

The shift from a GRK-regulated to a primarily PKA-regulated signaling mechanism could explain the mismatching roles of

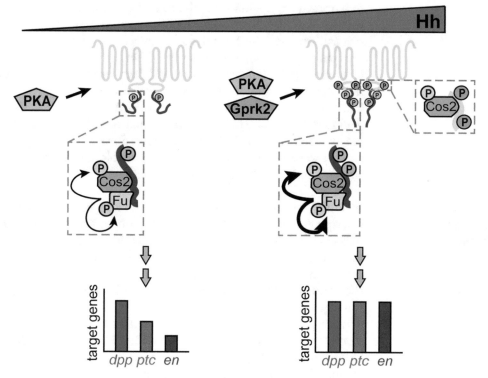

Fig. 4 Model for increasing *Drosophila* Smo activity in response to a gradient of Hh ligand. In response to low levels of Hh, Smo becomes partially phosphorylated by PKA (and Ck1—not shown) at sites in the SAID. This leads to partial conformational activation and dimerization of Smo and subsequent engagement of the HSC components Cos2 and Fu via the non-conserved, distal C-terminus. Fu engagement leads to its autoactivation and phosphorylation of Cos2 (and Sufu—not shown), releasing some Ci[155] to partially activate transcription of target genes, particularly low/intermediate threshold targets. In response to higher levels of Hh, Smo is more heavily phosphorylated by PKA. At a certain point, Smo activity is sufficient to activate *gprk2* transcription, triggering a positive feedback loop. As Gprk2 levels increase, it increasingly phosphorylates Smo, leading to additional engagement of Cos2 through the conserved proximal binding site to enhance downstream signaling. The combined actions of PKA/Ck1 and Gprk2 on Smo are required for maximal signaling activity

β-arrestins seen in the *Drosophila* and mammalian Hh pathways. In the vertebrate Hh pathway, GRK2/Ck1α-dependent Smo phosphorylation triggers β-arrestin recruitment and this is required for Smo activation and trafficking to the cilium [68, 69]. The positive role of β-arrestin in the Hh pathway was confirmed in vivo, as zebrafish morphants depleted for β-arrestin2 show similar Hh defects as zGRK2/3 morphants [9, 72]. In flies, the role of β-arrestins is less clear. The interaction between Smo and Kurtz (Krz), the only typical β-arrestin in flies, can be visualized biochemically through co-immunoprecipitation in tissue culture cells, when both proteins are overexpressed. In vivo, expression of Krz causes downregulation of Smo and a reduction in Hh target gene expression [7, 73]. However, loss of Krz fails to produce any misregulation of Smo or Hh signaling, raising questions about the physiological importance of this interaction [73]. It is possible that other fly arrestins, such as the two visual arrestins (Arr1 and Arr2), functionally compensate for the loss of Krz. Alternatively, regulation of Smo by Krz might represent an evolutionarily ancient mechanism that has been largely replaced by a PKA-dependent mechanism. Indeed, protein levels of *Drosophila* Smo are thought to be regulated by ubiquitination and proteasome-dependent degradation. The ubiquitination sites are in close proximity to the PKA sites and phosphorylation at the PKA clusters prevents Smo degradation [29, 30]. This suggests that Smo turnover in flies is mainly controlled by PKA and ubiquitination rather than by Gprk2 and β-arrestin recruitment. It is also possible that both pathways coexist and have overlapping effects [29].

4.4 Indirect Role of GRKs in the Hh Pathway

In addition to their conserved role as Smo kinases, GRKs can affect Hh signaling indirectly by controlling cellular levels of the second messenger cAMP. Both in Gprk2-depleted S2 cells and in *gprk2* mutant flies, cAMP levels are abnormally low, by approximately 60% at the level of entire ovaries or whole animals [13, 74]. In fact, the abnormally low cAMP levels seem to be a major cause of the Hh signaling impairment in *gprk2* mutant animals because target gene expression can be largely, though not completely, rescued simply by stimulating cAMP production or activating PKA [13]. Consistent with this, Ala substitution of the four Gprk2 phosphorylation clusters in Smo did not recapitulate the full severity of the *gprk2* mutant phenotype in terms of target gene expression in vivo, as it led to a loss of high-threshold target genes but had little effect on the intermediate-threshold target *ptc* [12]. Thus in parallel to directly activating Smo, Gprk2 also influences Hh signaling indirectly, by keeping cAMP levels and PKA activity at levels permissive for Hh signaling. The fact that signaling in *gprk2* mutants could also be largely restored by expressing a PKA phosphomimetic form of Smo suggests that Smo is the target of this indirect effect—i.e. that PKA-dependent Smo activation is impaired in *gprk2* mutants.

4.5 Global Misregulation of GPCR/ Heterotrimeric G-Protein Signaling in gprk2 Mutants?

What could be the connection between a GRK and cellular cAMP levels? One plausible answer is GPCR/heterotrimeric G-protein signaling. In canonical GPCR signaling, ligand-occupied, active GPCRs act as GEFs for the G_α subunits of the heterotrimeric G-protein complex, triggering G-protein signaling. GRKs negatively regulate GPCR/heterotrimeric G-protein signaling by phosphorylating active GPCRs, generating high-affinity binding sites for β-arrestins. β-Arrestins in turn block the GEF activity of the GPCR by shielding the G-protein binding site and by triggering clathrin-dependent receptor endocytosis. Not surprisingly, loss of GRK activity can have severe consequences on GPCR function, often characterized by prolonged and exaggerated heterotrimeric G-protein signaling responses. For example, loss of GRK2 results in elevated cAMP levels in response to V2 Vasopressin stimulation [75]. Similarly, activation of the angiotensin II type 1A receptor causes an excessive accumulation of the lipid-derived second messenger diacyglycerol in GRK2-depleted cells [76]. The same phenomenon can be observed in vivo under certain circumstances. For instance, loss of GRK5 renders mice supersensitive to muscarinic, but not dopaminergic, stimulation [77]. However, it should be noted that germline knockouts of most GRK isoforms display surprisingly mild defects, possibly due to functional redundancies between GRKs [78]. More pronounced and severe impairment of GPCR signaling might be expected in double or triple knockouts.

Dysregulation of GPCR desensitization and signaling could explain the abnormally low cAMP levels in *gprk2* mutants (Fig. 5). One candidate for misregulation is Smo itself. Although Smo is a rather distant member of the GPCR superfamily, mounting evidence suggests that Smo is a functional GPCR that directly couples to and signals through $G_{\alpha i}$ to inhibit cAMP production. Activation of endogenous Smo both in *Drosophila* and in cultured mammalian cells lowered cAMP levels [79, 80]. Direct coupling of mouse Smo exclusively to members of the $G_{\alpha i}$ family of G proteins was observed in several cell lines when at least one of the interacting partners was overexpressed [80, 81]. Coupling of mammalian Smo to $G_{\alpha i}$ seems to be a physiologically relevant process, because the efficacy of Smo toward $G_{\alpha i}$ is similar to that measured for the 5-hydroxytryptamine 1A (5-HT1A) receptor, a well-defined $G_{\alpha i}$-coupled receptor. This fits with the observation that activation of endogenously expressed Smo decreases cellular cAMP levels to about the same extent as stimulation of the 5-HT1A receptor does [80]. Based on this it seems plausible that, in the absence of Gprk2, Smo-$G_{\alpha i}$ signaling is hyperactivated due to the lack of receptor desensitization. However, simultaneous elimination of Smo and Gprk2 in cells failed to rescue cAMP levels back to normal, indicating that the changes in cAMP levels upon removal of Gprk2 are not (only) Smo-dependent. Given that the fly genome encodes about 100 GPCRs but only two GRKs [82], each GRK must be capable of regulating many different GPCRs. It follows that the *gprk2* mutant phenotype might be complex, resulting from misregulation of several GPCRs. At least in *Drosophila*, the net outcome of this global GPCR misregulation is abnormally low cellular cAMP concentrations that are limiting for Smo activation and consequently for Hh target gene expression (Fig. 5).

5   Cross-Talk Between GPCR Signaling and the Hh Pathway

One implication of the indirect model of Smo regulation by GRKs is that the Hh pathway may normally be influenced by cross-talk with GPCR signaling. Consistent with this, several recent studies have described modulatory effects of GPCR signaling on Shh pathway responses in mammals. With respect to the role of PKA, the vertebrate pathway has a simpler setup than its *Drosophila* counterpart. In mammals, PKA has only one function in the Hh pathway, promoting degradation of Gli2/3 transcription factors [5]. Consequently, increasing cAMP levels or activating PKA blocks Hh target gene expression, whereas reducing cAMP levels promotes it. Several recent examples demonstrate that this regulatory mechanism is utilized in vivo. Gpr161, a $G_{\alpha s}$-coupled GPCR localized to the primary cilium of mice, plays an inhibitory role in Shh-dependent neural tube patterning. According to the proposed model, Gpr161 ensures Gli2/3 degradation in the absence of Shh by keeping cAMP concentration/ PKA activity at levels high enough to restrict accumulation of full-length $Gli2^A/3^A$. Therefore, Gpr161 functions in parallel to Ptc to keep the pathway off in the absence of Shh (Fig. 2c). Shh deactivates both Ptc and Gpr161 by triggering removal of the two proteins from the ciliary membrane, permitting $Gli2^A/3^A$ accumulation and activity (Fig. 2d) [83]. Another example is the GPCR PAC_1, which couples to $G_{\alpha s}$ and activates adenylyl cyclase in response to its ligand, the PACAP peptide. PAC_1 activation inhibits the formation of medulloblastomas in *ptc1* mutant mice. As medulloblastoma in these mice is caused by uncontrolled Shh pathway activation driving proliferation of cerebellar granular cells, this indicates that the PAC_1-dependent increase in cAMP levels inhibits Shh signaling [84, 85]. Interestingly, a positive influence of $G_{\alpha i}$-coupled GPCRs on Shh target gene expression and proliferation of cerebellar granular cells in mice has also been demonstrated. The GPCR CXCR4 signals through $G_{\alpha i}$, promotes

Fig. 5 (continued) Too much PKA activity forces Ci^{155} processing and diminishes target gene expression. Between these two extremes, increasing PKA activity promotes Smo activation in the presence of Hh, stimulating target gene expression. By controlling homologous desensitization of GPCRs, GRKs influence cAMP levels and so may impinge upon this normal regulation of Hh pathway activity. (**b**) In *Drosophila* cells lacking Gprk2, cAMP levels are abnormally low, perhaps due to GPCR misregulation. Under these conditions, PKA-dependent activation of Smo is diminished and Hh target gene expression is impaired

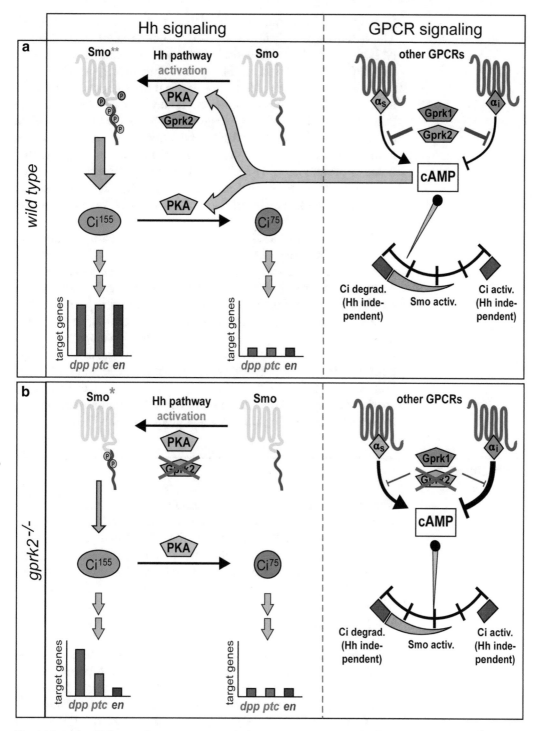

Fig. 5 Model for GRK regulation of Hh pathway–GPCR crosstalk via cAMP in *Drosophila*. (**a**) PKA plays two roles in the *Drosophila* Hh pathway. In the absence of Hh, PKA phosphorylation of Ci[155] promotes its processing to the Ci[75] repressor to prevent target gene expression. In the presence of Hh, PKA phosphorylation is required for Smo activation and expression of target genes. PKA activity (and by extension, cAMP levels) can set thresholds for pathway activity. Too little PKA activity leads to Ci[155] stabilization and Hh-independent target gene expression.

Shh signaling, and induces Shh-dependent cell proliferation [86]. These examples nicely illustrate that the Shh signaling outcomes can be both positively and negatively influenced, depending on whether the GPCR couples to an inhibitory or stimulatory G_α protein.

It should be pointed out, however, that the role of GPCR signaling in the Hh pathway is controversial and conflicting evidence has been reported. For instance, a large-scale RNAi screen in a *Drosophila* cell culture model, aimed at discovering novel components of the Hh pathway, failed to identify any GPCR or member of the heterotrimeric G-protein family [87]. In addition, the positive role of $G_{\alpha i}$ signaling in vertebrates was challenged by the finding that overexpression of $G_{\alpha i}$ in the chick neural tube had no obvious effect on its patterning [88]. Rather than being necessary and instructive, it may be more useful to view cAMP levels as being permissive for pathway function, by setting thresholds for activity. In cells where cAMP levels fall within a permissive range (for Smo activation in *Drosophila*, or Gli regulation in mammals), heterotrimeric G proteins may not be required for proper pathway function. This would fit well with the long-standing observation that a constitutively active, cAMP-insensitive form of PKA is capable of supporting Hh signaling in flies [89, 90]. However, the accumulating evidence in mammals clearly suggests that in some cell types, cross-talk with GPCRs does influence Shh pathway activity. Given that some 30–50% of medicinal drugs are directed against GPCRs [91], this could be an interesting avenue to pursue in developing therapeutic inhibitors of Shh signaling.

6 Conclusions

The combination of work in *Drosophila* and vertebrate models has led to substantial progress in our understanding of the role of GRKs in Hh signaling. GRKs activate Smo through an evolutionarily conserved mechanism involving phosphorylation of residues within the cytoplasmic tail. In mammals, this phosphorylation promotes dimerization, β-arrestin recruitment, and translocation of Smo into the cilium where it signals. In *Drosophila*, it promotes recruitment of Cos2 to a region in the conserved portion of the Smo cytoplasmic tail to enhance downstream signaling. In addition to this direct function, GRKs may act indirectly by controlling global GPCR/heterotrimeric G-protein signaling, thus maintaining cAMP at levels permissive for Hh pathway function. Research in mammalian systems has so far focused only on the direct role of GRK2 in Smo activation. The identification of additional GPCRs, including Gpr161, PAC_1, and CXCR4 that are capable of cross-talking with the Shh pathway via cAMP regulation greatly expands the potential complexity of the role of GRKs in Shh signaling. Future studies will have to take into consideration the potential indirect effects of manipulating GRKs and β-arrestins on these and other GPCRs when examining Shh-dependent signaling outputs.

References

1. Beachy PA, Karhadkar SS, Berman DM (2004) Tissue repair and stem cell renewal in carcinogenesis. Nature 432(7015):324–331

2. Varjosalo M, Taipale J (2008) Hedgehog: functions and mechanisms. Genes Dev 22(18):2454–2472

3. Jiang J, Hui CC (2008) Hedgehog signaling in development and cancer. Dev Cell 15(6):801–812

4. McMahon AP, Ingham PW, Tabin CJ (2003) Developmental roles and clinical significance of hedgehog signaling. Curr Top Dev Biol 53:1–114

5. Briscoe J, Therond PP (2013) The mechanisms of hedgehog signalling and its roles in development and disease. Nat Rev Mol Cell Biol 14(7):416–429

6. Chen Y, Li S, Tong C, Zhao Y, Wang B, Liu Y, Jia J, Jiang J (2010) G protein-coupled receptor kinase 2 promotes high-level hedgehog signaling by regulating the active state of Smo through kinase-dependent and kinase-independent mechanisms in Drosophila. Genes Dev 24(18):2054–2067

7. Cheng S, Maier D, Neubueser D, Hipfner DR (2010) Regulation of smoothened by Drosophila G-protein-coupled receptor kinases. Dev Biol 337(1):99–109

8. Molnar C, Holguin H, Mayor FJ, Ruiz-Gomez A, de Celis JF (2007) The G protein-coupled receptor regulatory kinase GPRK2 participates in hedgehog signaling in Drosophila. Proc Natl Acad Sci U S A 104:7963–7968

9. Philipp M, Fralish GB, Meloni AR, Chen W, MacInnes AW, Barak LS, Caron MG (2008) Smoothened signaling in vertebrates is facilitated by a G protein-coupled receptor kinase. Mol Cel Biol 19(12):5478–5489

10. Moore CA, Milano SK, Benovic JL (2007) Regulation of receptor trafficking by GRKs and arrestins. Annu Rev Physiol 69:451–482

11. Chen Y, Sasai N, Ma G, Yue T, Jia J, Briscoe J, Jiang J (2011) Sonic hedgehog dependent phosphorylation by CK1alpha and GRK2 is required for ciliary accumulation and activation of smoothened. PLoS Biol 9(6):e1001083

12. Maier D, Cheng S, Faubert D, Hipfner DR (2014) A broadly conserved g-protein-coupled receptor kinase phosphorylation mechanism controls Drosophila smoothened activity. PLoS Genet 10(7):e1004399

13. Cheng S, Maier D, Hipfner DR (2012) Drosophila G-protein-coupled receptor kinase 2 regulates cAMP-dependent hedgehog signaling. Development 139(1):85–94

14. Hooper JE, Scott VP (2005) Communicating with hedgehogs. Nat Rev Mol Cell Biol 6(4):306–317

15. Blair SS (1995) Compartments and appendage development in Drosophila. Bioessays 17(4):299–309

16. Tabata T, Kornberg TB (1994) Hedgehog is a signaling protein with a key role in patterning Drosophila imaginal discs. Cell 76(1):89–102

17. Eaton S, Kornberg TB (1990) Repression of ci-D in posterior compartments of Drosophila by engrailed. Genes Dev 4(6):1068–1077

18. Strigini M, Cohen SM (1997) A hedgehog activity gradient contributes to AP axial patterning of the Drosophila wing. Development 124(22):4697–4705

19. Capdevila J, Guerrero I (1994) Targeted expression of the signaling molecule decapentaplegic induces pattern duplications and growth alterations in Drosophila wings. EMBO J 13(19):4459–4468

20. Phillips RG, Roberts IJ, Ingham PW, Whittle JR (1990) The Drosophila segment polarity gene patched is involved in a position-signalling mechanism in imaginal discs. Development 110(1):105–114

21. Bier E (2005) Drosophila, the golden bug, emerges as a tool for human genetics. Nat Rev Genet 6(1):9–23

22. Ribes V, Briscoe J (2009) Establishing and interpreting graded sonic hedgehog signaling during vertebrate neural tube patterning: the role of negative feedback. Cold Spring Harb Perspect Biol 1(2):a002014

23. Ingham PW, Nakano Y, Seger C (2011) Mechanisms and functions of hedgehog signalling across the metazoa. Nat Rev Genet 12(6):393–406

24. Chen Y, Jiang J (2013) Decoding the phosphorylation code in hedgehog signal transduction. Cell Res 23(2):186–200

25. Aza-Blanc P, Ramírez-Weber FA, Laget MP, Schwartz C, Kornberg TB (1997) Proteolysis that is inhibited by hedgehog targets Cubitus interruptus protein to the nucleus and converts it to a repressor. Cell 89(7):1043–1053

26. Methot N, Basler K (1999) Hedgehog controls limb development by regulating the activities of distinct transcriptional activator and repressor forms of Cubitus interruptus. Cell 96(6):819–831

27. Wang B, Fallon JF, Beachy PA (2000) Hedgehog-regulated processing of Gli3 produces an anterior/posterior repressor gradient in the developing vertebrate limb. Cell 100(4):423–434

28. Denef N, Neubüser D, Perez L, Cohen SM (2000) Hedgehog induces opposite changes in turnover and subcellular localization of patched and smoothened. Cell 102(4):521–531

29. Li S, Chen Y, Shi Q, Yue T, Wang B, Jiang J (2012) Hedgehog-regulated ubiquitination controls smoothened trafficking and cell surface expression in Drosophila. PLoS Biol 10(1):e1001239

30. Xia R, Jia H, Fan J, Liu Y, Jia J (2012) USP8 promotes smoothened signaling by preventing its ubiquitination and changing its subcellular localization. PLoS Biol 10(1):e1001238

31. Nachtergaele S, Mydock LK, Krishnan K, Rammohan J, Schlesinger PH, Covey DF, Rohatgi R (2012) Oxysterols are allosteric activators of the oncoprotein smoothened. Nat Chem Biol 8(2):211–220

32. Taipale J, Chen JK, Cooper MK, Wang B, Mann RK, Milenkovic L, Scott MP, Beachy PA (2000) Effects of oncogenic mutations in smoothened and patched can be reversed by cyclopamine. Nature 406(6799):1005–1009

33. Callejo A, Culi J, Guerrero I (2008) Patched, the receptor of hedgehog, is a lipoprotein receptor. Proc Natl Acad Sci U S A 105(3):912–917

34. Khaliullina H, Panáková D, Eugster C, Riedel F, Carvalho M, Eaton S (2009) Patched regulates smoothened trafficking using lipoprotein-derived lipids. Development 136(24):4111–4121

35. Methot N, Basler K (2000) Suppressor of fused opposes hedgehog signal transduction by impeding nuclear accumulation of the activator form of Cubitus interruptus. Development 127(18):4001–4010

36. Monnier V, Dussillol F, Alves G, Lamour-Isnard C, Plessis A (1998) Suppressor of fused links fused and Cubitus interruptus on the hedgehog signalling pathway. Curr Biol 8(10):583–586

37. Robbins DJ, Nybakken KE, Kobayashi R, Sisson JC, Bishop JM, Thérond PP (1997) Hedgehog elicits signal transduction by means of a large complex containing the kinesin-related protein costal2. Cell 90(2):225–234

38. Sisson JC, Ho KS, Suyama K, Scott MP (1997) Costal2, a novel kinesin-related protein in the hedgehog signaling pathway. Cell 90(2):235–245

39. Stegman MA, Vallance JE, Elangovan G, Sosinski J, Cheng Y, Robbins DJ (2000) Identification of a tetrameric hedgehog signaling complex. J Biol Chem 275(29):21809–21812

40. Wang G, Amanai K, Wang B, Jiang J (2000) Interactions with Costal2 and suppressor of fused regulate nuclear translocation and activity of cubitus interruptus. Genes Dev 14(22):2893–2905

41. Price MA, Kalderon D (1999) Proteolysis of cubitus interruptus in Drosophila requires phosphorylation by protein kinase A. Development 126(19):4331–4339

42. Price MA, Kalderon D (2002) Proteolysis of the hedgehog signaling effector Cubitus interruptus requires phosphorylation by Glycogen Synthase Kinase 3 and Casein Kinase 1. Cell 108(6):823–835

43. Wang G, Wang B, Jiang J (1999) Protein kinase A antagonizes hedgehog signaling by regulating both the activator and repressor forms of Cubitus interruptus. Genes Dev 13(21):2828–2837

44. Zhang W, Zhao Y, Tong C, Wang G, Wang B, Jia J, Jiang J (2005) Hedgehog-regulated Costal2-kinase complexes control phosphorylation and proteolytic processing of Cubitus interruptus. Dev Cell 8(2):267–278

45. Jia J, Amanai K, Wang G, Tang J, Wang B, Jiang J (2002) Shaggy/GSK3 antagonizes hedgehog signalling by regulating Cubitus interruptus. Nature 416(6880):548–552

46. Zhao Y, Tong C, Jiang J (2007) Hedgehog regulates smoothened activity by inducing a conformational switch. Nature 450(7167):252–258

47. Apionishev S, Katanayeva NM, Marks SA, Kalderon D, Tomlinson A (2005) Drosophila smoothened phosphorylation sites essential for hedgehog signal transduction. Nat Cell Biol 7(1):86–92

48. Jia J, Tong C, Wang B, Luo L, Jiang J (2004) Hedgehog signalling activity of smoothened requires phosphorylation by protein kinase A and casein kinase I. Nature 432(7020):1045–1050

49. Zhang C, Williams EH, Guo Y, Lum L, Beachy PA (2004) Extensive phosphorylation of smoothened in hedgehog pathway activation. Proc Natl Acad Sci U S A 101(52):17900–17907

50. Jia J, Tong C, Jiang J (2003) Smoothened transduces hedgehog signal by physically interacting with Costal2/Fused complex through its C-terminal tail. Genes Dev 17(21):2709–2720

51. Lum L, Zhang C, Oh S, Mann RK, von Kessler DP, Taipale J, Weis-Garcia F, Gong R, Wang B, Beachy PA (2003) Hedgehog signal transduction via smoothened association with a cytoplasmic complex scaffolded by the atypical kinesin, Costal-2. Mol Cell 12(5):1261–1274

52. Ogden SK, Ascano MJ, Stegman MA, Suber LM, Hooper JE, Robbins DJ (2003) Identification of a functional interaction between the transmembrane protein smooth-

ened and the kinesin-related protein Costal2. Curr Biol 13(22):1998–2003

53. Ruel L, Rodriguez R, Gallet A, Lavenant-Staccini L, Thérond PP (2003) Stability and association of smoothened, Costal2 and fused with Cubitus interruptus are regulated by hedgehog. Nat Cell Biol 5(10):907–913

54. Ingham PW, McMahon AP (2001) Hedgehog signaling in animal development: paradigms and principles. Genes Dev 15(23):3059–3087

55. Hui CC, Angers S (2011) Gli proteins in development and disease. Annu Rev Cell Dev Biol 27:513–537

56. Goetz SC, Anderson KV (2010) The primary cilium: a signalling centre during vertebrate development. Nat Rev Genet 11(5):331–344

57. Kuzhandaivel A, Schultz SW, Alkhori L, Alenius M (2014) Cilia-mediated hedgehog signaling in Drosophila. Cell Rep 7(3):672–680

58. Thérond PP, Knight JD, Kornberg TB, Bishop JM (1996) Phosphorylation of the fused protein kinase in response to signaling from hedgehog. Proc Natl Acad Sci U S A 93(9):4224–4228

59. Liu Y, Cao X, Jiang J, Jia J (2007) Fused-Costal2 protein complex regulates hedgehog-induced Smo phosphorylation and cell-surface accumulation. Genes Dev 21(15):1949–1963

60. Ruel L, Gallet A, Raisin S, Truchi A, Staccini-Lavenant L, Cervantes A, Thérond PP (2007) Phosphorylation of the atypical kinesin Costal2 by the kinase fused induces the partial disassembly of the Smoothened-Fused-Costal2-Cubitus interruptus complex in hedgehog signalling. Development 134(20):3677–3689

61. Chen MH, Gao N, Kawakami T, Chuang PT (2005) Mice deficient in the fused homolog do not exhibit phenotypes indicative of perturbed hedgehog signaling during embryonic development. Mol Cell Biol 25(16):7042–7053

62. Merchant M, Evangelista M, Luoh SM, Frantz GD, Chalasani S, Carano RA, van Hoy M, Ramirez J, Ogasawara AK, McFarland LM, Filvaroff EH, French DM, de Sauvage FJ (2005) Loss of the serine/threonine kinase fused results in postnatal growth defects and lethality due to progressive hydrocephalus. Mol Cell Biol 25(16):7054–7068

63. Cheung HO, Zhang X, Ribeiro A, Mo R, Makino S, Puviindran V, Law KK, Briscoe J, Hui CC (2009) The kinesin protein Kif7 is a critical regulator of Gli transcription factors in mammalian hedgehog signaling. Sci Signal 2(76):ra29

64. Endoh-Yamagami S, Evangelista M, Wilson D, Wen X, Theunissen JW, Phamluong K, Davis M, Scales SJ, Solloway MJ, de Sauvage FJ, Peterson AS (2009) The mammalian Cos2

homolog Kif7 plays an essential role in modulating Hh signal transduction during development. Curr Biol 19(15):1320–1326

65. Liem KFJ, He M, Ocbina PJ, Anderson KV (2009) Mouse Kif7/Costal2 is a cilia-associated protein that regulates sonic hedgehog signaling. Proc Natl Acad Sci U S A 106(32):13377–13382

66. Cooper AF, Yu KP, Brueckner M, Brailey LL, Johnson L, McGrath JM, Bale AE (2005) Cardiac and CNS defects in a mouse with targeted disruption of suppressor of fused. Development 132(19):4407–4417

67. Svärd J, Heby-Henricson K, Persson-Lek M, Rozell B, Lauth M, Bergström A, Ericson J, Toftgård R, Teglund S (2006) Genetic elimination of suppressor of fused reveals an essential repressor function in the mammalian hedgehog signaling pathway. Dev Cell 10(2):187–197

68. Chen W, Ren XR, Nelson CD, Barak LS, Chen JK, Beachy PA, de Sauvage F, Lefkowitz RJ (2004) Activity-dependent internalization of smoothened mediated by beta-arrestin 2 and GRK2. Science 306:2257–2260

69. Meloni AR, Fralish GB, Kelly P, Salahpour A, Chen JK, Wechsler-Reya RJ, Lefkowitz RJ, Caron MG (2006) Smoothened signal transduction is promoted by G protein-coupled receptor kinase 2. Mol Cell Biol 26(20):7550–7560

70. Cassill JA, Whitney M, Joazeiro CAP, Becker A, Zuker CS (1991) Isolation of Drosophila genes encoding G protein-coupled receptor kinases. Proc Natl Acad Sci U S A 88:11067–11070

71. Fan J, Liu Y, Jia J (2012) Hh-induced smoothened conformational switch is mediated by differential phosphorylation at its C-terminal tail in a dose- and position-dependent manner. Dev Biol 366(2):172–184

72. Wilbanks AM, Fralish GB, Kirby ML, Barak LS, Li YX, Caron MG (2004) Beta-arrestin 2 regulates zebrafish development through the hedgehog signaling pathway. Science 306:2264–2267

73. Molnar C, Ruiz-Gómez A, Martín M, Rojo-Berciano S, Mayor F, de Celis JF (2011) Role of the Drosophila non-visual ss-arrestin kurtz in hedgehog signalling. PLoS Genet 7(3):e1001335

74. Lannutti BJ, Schneider LE (2001) Gprk2 controls cAMP levels in Drosophila development. Dev Biol 233(1):174–185

75. Ren XR, Reiter E, Ahn S, Kim J, Chen W, Lefkowitz RJ (2005) Different G protein-coupled receptor kinases govern G protein and beta-arrestin-mediated signaling of V2 vasopressin receptor. Proc Natl Acad Sci U S A 102:1448–1453

76. Violin JD, Dewire SM, Barnes WG, Lefkowitz RJ (2006) G protein-coupled receptor kinase and beta-arrestin-mediated desensitization of the angiotensin II type 1A receptor elucidated by diacylglycerol dynamics. J Biol Chem 281(47):36411–36419

77. Gainetdinov RR, Bohn LM, Walker JK, Laporte SA, Macrae AD, Caron MG, Lefkowitz RJ, Premont RT (1999) Muscarinic supersensitivity and impaired receptor desensitization in G protein-coupled receptor kinase 5-deficient mice. Neuron 24(4):1029–1036

78. Premont RT, Gainetdinov RR (2007) Physiological roles of G protein-coupled receptor kinases and arrestins. Annu Rev Physiol 69:511–534

79. Ogden SK, Fei DL, Schilling NS, Ahmed YF, Hwa J, Robbins DJ (2008) G protein Galphai functions immediately downstream of smoothened in hedgehog signalling. Nature 456(7224):967–970

80. Shen F, Cheng L, Douglas AE, Riobo NA, Manning DR (2013) Smoothened is a fully competent activator of the heterotrimeric G protein G(i). Mol Pharmacol 83(3):691–697

81. Riobo NA, Saucy B, Dilizio C, Manning DR (2006) Activation of heterotrimeric G proteins by smoothened. Proc Natl Acad Sci U S A 103(33):12607–12612

82. Brody T, Cravchik A (2000) Drosophila melanogaster G protein-coupled receptors. J Cell Biol 150(2):F83–F88

83. Mukhopadhyay S, Wen X, Ratti N, Loktev A, Rangell L, Scales SJ, Jackson PK (2013) The ciliary G-protein-coupled receptor Gpr161 negatively regulates the sonic hedgehog pathway via cAMP signaling. Cell 152(1–2):210–223

84. Lelievre V, Seksenyan A, Nobuta H, Yong WH, Chhith S, Niewiadomski P, Cohen JR, Dong H, Flores A, Liau LM, Kornblum HI, Scott MP, Waschek JA (2008) Disruption of the PACAP gene promotes medulloblastoma in ptc1 mutant mice. Dev Biol 313(1):359–370

85. Nicot A, Lelièvre V, Tam J, Waschek JA, DiCicco-Bloom E (2002) Pituitary adenylate cyclase-activating polypeptide and sonic hedgehog interact to control cerebellar granule precursor cell proliferation. J Neurosci 22(21):9244–9254

86. Klein RS, Rubin JB, Gibson HD, DeHaan EN, Alvarez-Hernandez X, Segal RA, Luster AD (2001) SDF-1 alpha induces chemotaxis and enhances sonic hedgehog-induced proliferation of cerebellar granule cells. Development 128(11):1971–1981

87. Lum L, Yao S, Mozer B, Rovescalli A, Von Kessler D, Nirenberg M, Beachy PA (2003) Identification of hedgehog pathway components by RNAi in Drosophila cultured cells. Science 299(5615):2039–2045

88. Low WC, Wang C, Pan Y, Huang XY, Chen JK, Wang B (2008) The decoupling of smoothened from Galphai proteins has little effect on Gli3 protein processing and hedgehog-regulated chick neural tube patterning. Dev Biol 321(1):188–196

89. Jiang J, Struhl G (1995) Protein kinase A and hedgehog signaling in Drosophila limb development. Cell 80(4):563–572

90. Li W, Ohlmeyer JT, Lane ME, Kalderon D (1995) Function of protein kinase A in hedgehog signal transduction and Drosophila imaginal disc development. Cell 80(4):553–562

91. Salon JA, Lodowski DT, Palczewski K (2011) The significance of G protein-coupled receptor crystallography for drug discovery. Pharmacol Rev 63(4):901–937

INDEX

Vsevolod V. Gurevich et al. (eds.), *G Protein-Coupled Receptor Kinases*, Methods in Pharmacology and Toxicology,
DOI 10.1007/978-1-4939-3798-1, © Springer Science+Business Media New York 2016

Printed in the United States
By Bookmasters